Food and Nutrition Information Guide

Food and Nutrition Information Guide

PAULA SZILARD

LIBRARIES UNLIMITED, INC.
Littleton, Colorado
1987

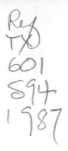
Copyright © 1987 Paula Szilard
All Rights Reserved
Printed in the United States of America

No part of this publication may be reproduced, stored in a retrieval
system, or transmitted, in any form or by any means, electronic,
mechanical, photocopying, recording, or otherwise, without the
prior written permission of the publisher.

LIBRARIES UNLIMITED, INC.
P.O. Box 263
Littleton, Colorado 80160-0263

Library of Congress Cataloging-in-Publication Data

Szilard, Paula.
    Food and nutrition information guide.

    Includes bibliographies and indexes.
    1. Nutrition--Bibliography. 2. Nutrition--
Information services. 3. Diet--Bibliography.
4. Diet--Information services. 5. Food--
Bibliography. 6. Food--Information services.
I. Title. [DNLM: 1. Food--abstracts. 2. Nu-
trition--abstracts. ZQU 145 S998f]
Z5776.N8S94   1987   [TX601]   016.6132   87-3852
ISBN 0-87287-457-5

Libraries Unlimited books are bound with Type II nonwoven material that meets
and exceeds National Association of State Textbook Administrators' Type II
nonwoven material specifications Class A through E.

This book is dedicated to my husband, Paul McCarthy, without whose constant love, support, encouragement, and help this book would have remained forever a good idea.

Contents

Part II
USING THE LITERATURE

Part III
NUTRITION

Part V
FOOD SCIENCE AND TECHNOLOGY

Part VI
RELATED AREAS

Preface

This book is devoted to reference materials on human nutrition, dietetics, food science and technology, and related subjects such as food service. It covers chiefly English-language materials published in the last ten years. Older materials have been included if they are currently useful. Material on animal nutrition is omitted except where it was considered useful for those interested in human nutrition.

Most of the citations in this book are annotated. Those which are presented without annotations are items for which bibliographic information was verified, but for which copies were difficult to locate. They were nonetheless considered potentially useful and were therefore included. Citations are arranged in one numerical sequence from the beginning to the end of the book. Under each heading the arrangement is alphabetical, except for a few instances where, because of their importance, outstanding reference works have been listed first.

Statements quoted in the annotations for which no sources are given are generally from prefatory material within the source described. Occasionally they are from a publisher's announcement, and, rarely, from abstracts found in the OCLC database.

Many materials, particularly in part IV, "Dietetics," were selected for inclusion on the basis of information obtained from questionnaires sent to state or local chapters of the American Dietetic Association with permanent mailing addresses. The decision was made to list all materials with useful information, even those of a more ephemeral nature. Addresses of organizations and prices of publications were included wherever possible for materials published outside the book trade and judged difficult to obtain. However, readers should be aware that these addresses may become dated.

In addition to materials from commercial publishers and organizations, all useful and substantial publications of the U.S. government, the Food and Agriculture Organization of the United Nations, and the World Health Organization have been listed.

Acknowledgments

A book like this is never simply the work of one person. It requires the harmonious efforts of many people. Although I take full responsibility for its contents, I am grateful for the assistance of the following people who contributed materially toward making it what it is: I want to thank my husband, Dr. Paul McCarthy, for his help on the chapter on how to get started on a term paper; Dr. Ira J. Lichton for his helpful suggestions on my original outline; Becky Clarke for her help in inputting the bibliographic citations; Virginia Richardson for helping proof the manuscript; Ginny Tangi for looking over the chapter on online searching; my sister, Selma Kristel (also a trained librarian) for annotating some of the titles which I did not have access to in Hawaii; Ellen Chapman for producing the illustrative material within the text; and Charlene Essling, R.D., MPH, for reading the edited manuscript. Finally, I would like to thank the colleagues who helped with Japanese, Chinese, and Korean references: Hisami Springer, Catherine Lee, Sam Hahn, and Susie Cheng.

How to Use This Book

This book is intended for students, professionals, researchers, and librarians who use the literature in human nutrition, dietetics, and food science and technology. Its purpose is twofold: first, to provide a background on the variety and types of publications available, the kinds of information they contain, and how they are organized in libraries; second, to serve as a type of "map" for locating specific information in nutrition, dietetics, and food science and technology.

Unfortunately, people who look for information in libraries often approach this task in a roundabout manner — for example, looking for specific information by browsing randomly through journals. A more structured approach is necessary. The library user who has a plan or mental map for locating the information is more apt to be successful.

This book provides the necessary structure and tools for developing such mental maps or plans. The word *structure* in this context means the different categories of information and the types of publications in which they appear. The word *tools* is defined as the electronic or printed reference sources used to retrieve information.

To discover what this structure is and to become acquainted with the tools necessary for retrieving information from it, the user should first read the general chapters in parts I and II. These provide an overview and orientation to the various types of materials being published and describe the major indexing/abstracting services (the keys to published research), how to make use of computer technologies to retrieve information, how to keep up with new research, how to use a research library, and how to get started on a research paper. Next, those chapters which deal with specific areas of interest will help the reader to become acquainted with the major sources of information in these fields, with particular emphasis on indexing/abstracting services. The chart in this section will help to determine the most suitable type of information source to use. The extensive subject index also provides access to the sources usually consulted for information on specific topics.

DOING A SEARCH

During the search, pay close attention to "road signs." They provide instant feedback about whether a search is on target. Occasionally it may be necessary to rethink the strategy or refer to the "map" again for a reorientation. Sometimes, it may even be necessary to stop at a reference desk more than once to ask for directions.

To illustrate this approach, let's assume the topic of interest is the relationship between dietary calcium and osteoporosis. After reading through parts I and II and relevant chapters in part III, "Nutrition," and reviewing the chart below, one approach might be to start out by looking for background information in a book on osteoporosis. Yet although the book may provide extensive information, including a discussion of the major studies on the subject, it will probably be dated. The next logical step would be to use information sources that identify more recent research on the subject, for instance, indexing/abstracting services which provide access to recent research published in nutrition and medical journals. To select the one best suited to a particular subject, consult the chart on pages 42-43.

On another occasion the topic may be as specific as the vitamin E content of sunflower seeds. Through reading chapter 11 and consulting the chart below, it should be clear that the answer is probably contained in a food composition table. Unfortunately, general tables of food composition frequently omit vitamin E values. Check the index to this book, or browse through chapter 11. There are several references to data on vitamin E and tocopherol values in publications readily available in many libraries.

One of the goals of this book is to convey a more structured, systematic approach to information seeking so that the less practiced library user can approach each problem with a plan for locating information, whether it is retrieved using an online search, a traditional indexing/abstracting service, handbooks, encyclopedias, tables, or other sources of information.

But in the beginning, the summary reference chart presented below is a good place to start any search.

CATEGORIZING INFORMATION NEEDS

For	Consult
Definitions of terms	Specialized dictionaries in all fields; books or textbooks for difficult to locate terms.
Addresses or information about people, organizations or products	Directories in specialized fields, for example on beverages or food science and technology.
Data, formulas, facts	Handbooks, manuals, tables, or reference texts, such as Goodhart and Shils's *Modern Nutrition in Health and Disease.*
Brief discussion of a topic	Specialized encyclopedias or reference texts.
Extensive or background information on a topic	Books or indexing/abstracting services to locate review articles.
Research on a topic particularly recently published research	Indexing/abstracting services to locate articles in periodicals.
Food composition data	Food composition tables, or use indexing/abstracting services to locate articles in periodicals for values not found in tables.
Nutrition and food consumption surveys	The Nationwide Food Consumption Surveys (NFCS) and the National Health and Nutrition Examination Surveys (NHANES or HANES), or an indexing/abstracting service for more specialized surveys.
Analytical methods	The major compilations containing standard methods of analysis published by major organizations found in chapter 20.
Food standards, regulations, and legislation	The *Code of Federal Regulations* and its indexes, the *Federal Register* and its indexes, or other sources described in chapter 21.

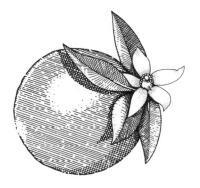

Part I

GENERAL INFORMATION

1
Present Scope of the Field

When it is unqualified, the term nutrition can refer to the science of nourishment as applied to animals or humans. Almost from the beginning, animal and human nutrition have been studied separately. Animal nutrition generally is studied in departments of animal science (formerly called animal husbandry) and human nutrition is studied as a biomedical science, though sometimes in tandem with food science and technology, and occasionally within a college of agriculture or home economics.

Dietetics is a specialized, applied academic program within nutrition curricula leading to a bachelor's degree and requiring a subsequent internship and professional registration. In addition, there are a number of ancillary applied fields: clinical nutrition, public health nutrition, nutrition education, community nutrition, home economics extension work, and food service administration. Each of these applies the principles of nutrition to a given setting.

Nutrition as a discipline can be defined broadly or narrowly. Generally, the younger a discipline, the more its practitioners or investigators find a need to set limits on what are proper subjects of investigation. The joint definition of the AMA Council on Food and Nutrition and the Nutrition Foundation encompasses both biological and behavioral aspects of nutrition:

> The science of food, the nutrients and other substances therein, their action, interaction, and balance in relation to health and disease, and the processes by which the organism ingests, digests, absorbs, transports, utilizes, and excretes food substances. In addition, nutrition must be concerned with certain social, economic, cultural and psychological implications of food and eating (American Medical Association, 1963).

This definition concentrates on the pure science, social, and cultural aspects of nutrition while neglecting the applied nutrition areas. The most conspicuously absent is dietetics, the only legally defined nutrition profession in the United States:

> A profession concerned with the science and art of human nutritional care, an essential component of the health sciences. It includes the extending and imparting of knowledge concerning foods which will provide nutrients sufficient for health and during disease throughout the life cycle and [includes] the management of group feeding for these purposes (American Dietetic Association, 1969).

In this book the broadest possible definition of nutrition is used, covering the study of human nourishment including all of the applied areas. The ADA definition of dietetics will be applied without amendment.

Although food science and technology both focus on food, there are differences between them. "Food technology is the application of science and engineering to the production, processing, storage, packaging, distribution, and utilization of foods" (Tape and Sabry, 1969). "Food science is distinct from food technology in that it involves the why of food processes.... Food science explains to the cheesemaker why acid develops in the vat and why cheese matures, and therefore, how he may produce a better flavor and texture to protect his product from spoilage" (Farrar, 1972).

Food scientists often know little about nutrition and nutritionists frequently know little about food science. Tape and Sabry (1969) provide an interesting argument for combining these academic disciplines, contending that without a knowledge of nutrition food technologists focus primarily on color, flavor, texture, appearance, and stability, and ignore nutritional parameters in developing new products. If nutritionists were informed about food science and technology the two disciplines could work more closely together to develop new, more nutritious products and help solve the world food problem. On the other hand, there are probably academics in both fields who are uneasy with this alliance, fearing perhaps that one or both of these curricula will receive short shrift if they are combined.

Nutrition information comes from a number of biomedical disciplines — nutritional biochemistry, physiology, genetics, microbiology, food chemistry, food science, dietetics, home economics, various branches of medicine including pediatrics and pathology, public health, and psychology and other behavioral sciences. Knowledge in food science and technology also comes from a variety of disciplines, such as chemistry, microbiology, biochemistry, biology, physics, and engineering.

Nutrition and food science and technology are at the same time basic, applied, and integrating and coordinating sciences, because they integrate knowledge from a variety of disciplines. They are multidisciplinary and diffuse, and the variety of their published literature reflects this diversity.

SELECTED REFERENCES

Akroyd, W. R. "What Do We Mean by Nutrition?" *Nutrition Today* 7 (November/December 1972): 30-31.

Barnes, R. H. "The Inseparability of Nutrition from the Social and Biological Sciences." *Nutritio et Dieta* 10 (1968): 1-8.

Day, Harry G. "The Science of Nutrition." *Journal of the NAL Associates* 5 (January-June 1980): 27-30.

Griffith, W. H. "The Scope of Nutrition." *Federation Proceedings* 26 (1967): 153-57.

Jowitt, Ronald. "The Scope of Food Engineering." *Journal of Food Engineering* 1 (1982): 3-16.

Leveitle, G. A. "Food Science and Human Nutrition." *Food Technology* 26 (August 1975): 77-78.

Mrak, Emil H. "Food Science and Technology: Past, Present, and Future." *Nutrition Reviews* 34 (1976): 193-200.

Olson, Robert E., and Alice A. Doisy. "Clinical Nutrition, an Interface between Human Ecology and Internal Medicine." *Nutrition Reviews* 36 (June 1978): 161-78.

NOTES

American Dietetic Association. Committee on Goals of Education for Dietetics. (1969). Goals of the lifetime education of the dietitian. *Journal of the American Dietetic Association, 54,* 91-93.

American Medical Association. Council on Foods and Nutrition. (1963). Report of the Council on Foods and Nutrition. *Journal of the American Medical Association, 193,* 955-57.

Farrar, K. T. H. (1972, January/February). The interaction of food science, technology, and nutrition. *Search, 3,* 31-37.

Tape, N. W. and Sabry, Z. I. (1969). The marriage of food technology and nutrition. *World Review of Nutrition and Dietetics, 10,* 1-12.

2
Historical Evolution
Nutrition and Food Science and Technology

NUTRITION

Nutrition is a relatively young science. Its beginnings date from 1783, the year of Antoine de Lavoisier's classic experiments in respiratory metabolism. Lavoisier was a chemist, but is commonly regarded as the father of modern nutrition because he proved that respiration is essentially a process of combustion, similar to what happens in the burning of a candle.

Scientists who first investigated phenomena in nutrition came from various fields such as chemistry, medicine, and physiology. Nutrition was not recognized as an independent discipline until the beginning of the twentieth century.

During the nineteenth century the scope of the field coincided closely with what today is the study of metabolism in physiology. Researchers of the period studied energy metabolism, caloric values of various foods, and basal metabolic rate. They identified the three major classes of organic nutrients: carbohydrates, fats, and proteins. By the end of this period some of the minerals, such as calcium and iron, were also known to be essential in human nutrition.

By the beginning of the twentieth century most of the amino acids had been identified. Although vitamin deficiency diseases had been known for centuries, the vitamins themselves were not discovered until after 1920. It strikes us as odd today that throughout the history of nutrition there was ample evidence linking scurvy with the absence of fresh fruits and vegetables, beri-beri with the consumption of polished rice, and pellagra with the widespread reliance on corn among the poor, but scientists of the time failed to see these relationships. This was especially true after the germ theory of disease gained a solid foothold. It was simply considered impossible for a disease to result from the absence of something and scientists went down many blind alleys looking for bacterial infections and toxins.

Knowledge and understanding of nutrition changed greatly with the advent of the vitamin theory advocated by Casimir Funk in 1911. Although he is not credited with the discovery of any particular vitamin, Funk proposed the existence of organic substances which, in minute quantities, were essential to life. He referred to these as "vitamines." The new era of vitamin discovery was ushered in by an American researcher, E. V. McCollum, who discovered vitamins A and D in the 1920s. Most vitamins were discovered between 1920 and 1940, although a few, like vitamin B-12, were not discovered until the 1950s.

The legacy of this era of discovery, however, was an overemphasis on nutritional deficiencies. The accent was on "getting enough." There was concern that the population was getting insufficient quantities of essential nutrients.

The period of concern over "getting enough" was followed by the era of "too much" as nutritionists became increasingly aware of the health problems related to an affluent Western diet. Many major killers such as coronary heart disease were found to have a strong nutritional component and it was usually a question of "too much" rather than "too little."

Currently there is a kind of equilibrium between these two orientations. Many researchers continue to focus on deficiency problems, particularly of the lesser known nutrients, such as the trace elements. Others focus on dietary patterns and disease relationships and on problems of affluence such as obesity and a variety of other concerns.

At the same time medicine has become more open to the investigation of nutritional factors in disease. Consequently, there is now a flood of nutrition-related medical literature where only a trickle existed 10 or 15 years ago.

FOOD SCIENCE AND TECHNOLOGY

A number of modern developments in food processing stand out as most important in the evolution of food science. One of the earliest of these was the invention of the digester by Denis Papin in 1679. This was the forerunner of the modern pressure cooker or autoclaver and Papin used it to make gelatin, which was then erroneously viewed as a possible meat substitute for the poor.

Canning, another important technological development, was invented in 1812 by Nicolas Appert, for a contest held by Napoleon Bonaparte in his search for a new and better method to preserve food for his armies. Introduced into the United States in 1821, this technology paved the way for later developments such as Gale Borden's invention of condensed milk in the 1850s.

A milestone in the history of food science and technology in the United States was the passage of the Food and Drug Act of 1906, the result of increased public awareness of food adulteration and poor sanitation in food plants. Upton Sinclair's *The Jungle*, a grisly account of abuses in Chicago's meat packing plants, is credited with shocking the public into action. Another major development was the process of quick freezing, developed in the late 1920s by Clarence Birdseye. This method became extremely popular because it allowed foods to retain more of their natural texture and flavor than did previously existing methods of preservation.

In the 1950s and 1960s food science and technology came of age as an academic discipline with defined curricula based on a combined fund of knowledge from chemistry, biochemistry, microbiology, engineering, and other disciplines.

CONVERGENCE

Although throughout most of their history nutrition and food science and technology have gone their separate ways, their paths began to converge in the late 1930s, when nutritionists concerned about widespread deficiencies resulting from the consumption of refined foods lobbied for enrichment of basic foods such as flour. Today greater sophistication and knowledge of nutrition among consumers is forcing the food industry to pay closer attention to nutrition in developing and marketing new products.

SOURCES FOR THE STUDY OF THE HISTORY OF NUTRITION AND FOOD SCIENCE

1. Beatty, William K. "The History of Nutrition: A Tour of the Literature." **Federation Proceedings** 37 (1977): 2511-13.
    A brief guide to important reference sources on the history of nutrition.

2. **Bibliography of the History of Medicine**. Vol. 1- (1964-). Washington, D.C.: Government Printing Office, 1965- . annual. ISSN 0067-7280. HE20.3615: .
    This annual bibliography has five-year cumulations and is an excellent source of books and articles on the history of nutrition. Coverage is from 1964 to date. Search under "Nutrition and Diet" or "Foods and Food Supply." To some extent this bibliography duplicates materials in *Index Medicus*. It is enriched with supplementary material, particularly monographs. The machine-readable version of this bibliography is one of the MEDLARS databases available for online searching from the National Library of Medicine under the title HISTLINE. While some of the references in the database go back to 1964, most date from 1970.

3. Billick, G., ed. "References for the History of Human Nutrition in America, 1600 to the Present: A Selected Bibliography." **Journal of the NAL Associates** 5 (January/June 1980): 45-58.
    This bibliography lists 399 references, most with brief annotations.

4. **Dictionary of Scientific Biography**. Edited by Charles Coulston Gillespie. New York: Scribner, 1970-1980. 16v.
    A major source of biographical material for "dead and noted" scientists in all fields, including nutrition. Entries include useful bibliographies. Volume 16 is the supplement and index to the set.

5. Fruton, Joseph Stewart. **A Bio-bibliography for the History of the Biochemical Sciences since 1800**. Philadelphia, Pa.: American Philosophical Society, 1982. 885p. ISBN 0871699834.
    An extensive bibliography of biographical information on scientists who have made contributions to the field of biochemistry since 1800, including many greats in the field of nutrition. Arrangement is alphabetical by name. A key to

abbreviations of sources cited is included. A supplement to this bibliography was issued in 1985.

6. **ISIS Cumulative Bibliography; A Bibliography of the History of Science Formed from the ISIS Critical Bibliographies 1-90, 1913-1965.** Edited by Magda Whitrow. London: Mansell, in conjunction with the History of Science Society, 1971-1982. 5v.

The major bibliography on the history of science. Volume 1, *Personalities and Institutions: Personalities A-J.* Volume 2, *Personalities and Institutions: Personalities K-Z; Institutions.* Volume 3, *Subjects.* Volume 4, *Periods and Civilizations. Prehistory—Middle Ages.* Volume 5, *Periods and Civilizations. Fifteenth—Nineteenth Centuries.* Volume 6, *Author Index.*

7. **ISIS Cumulative Bibliography 1966-1975: A Bibliography of the History of Science Formed from ISIS Critical Bibliographies 91-100, Indexing Literature Published from 1965 through 1974.** Edited by John Neu. London: Mansell, in conjunction with the History of Science Society, 1980- .

A supplement to the *ISIS Bibliography 1913-1965.* Volume 1, *Personalities and Institutions.* Volume 2, *Subjects, Periods and Civilizations.*

8. McCay, Clive Maine. **Notes on the History of Nutrition Research.** Edited by F. Verzbar. Berne, Switzerland: Hans Huber, 1973. 234p. ISBN 3456002777.

Of particular note is the chapter entitled "Finding Your Way in the Nutrition Literature," which is divided into two major sections dealing with literature prior to 1800 and early nineteenth-century literature.

9. **Nutrition Abstracts and Reviews.** Vol. 1- . Farnham Royal, England: Commonwealth Agricultural Bureaux, 1931- . monthly. ISSN 0029-6619.

See entry 57.

10. Sharrer, G. Terry. **1001 References for the History of American Food Technology.** Davis, Calif.: Agricultural History Center, University of California, 1978. 103p.

A cooperative project by the Agricultural History Branch, Economic Research Service, U.S. Department of Agriculture and the Agricultural History Center, this bibliography lists books, periodical articles, reports, pamphlets, and other types of publications on all aspects of the history of the food industry in the United States. Arranged alphabetically by author and contains a subject and title index.

SELECTED REFERENCES

Bailey, Herbert. *The Vitamin Pioneers.* Emmaus, Pa.: Rodale, 1968. 329p.

Barber, Mary I., ed., *History of the American Dietetic Association, 1917-1959.* Philadelphia, Pa.: Lippincott, 1959. 328p.

Beeuwkes, Adelia M., E. N. Todhunter, and Emma S. Weigley, comps. *Essays on History of Nutrition and Dietetics.* Chicago: American Dietetic Association, 1967. 291p.

Carpenter, Kenneth J. *The History of Scurvy and Vitamin C.* Cambridge, N.Y.: Cambridge University Press, 1986. 288p. ISBN 0521320291.

Chichester, C. O., and William J. Darby. "The Historical Relationship between Food Science and Nutrition." *Food Technology* 29 (January 1975): 38-42.

Chick, Hariette. "The Discovery of Vitamins." *Progress in Food and Nutrition Science* 1 (1975): 1-20.

Coppock, John B. M. "The Evolution of Food Science and Technology in the United Kingdom." *Chemistry and Industry* 10 (19 May 1973): 455-60.

Darby, William J. *Nutrition Science: An Overview of American Genius.* Washington, D.C.: Government Printing Office, 1976. 39p. A77.10:D 24. (Also in *Nutrition Reviews* 34 [1976]: 33-38).

Galdston, Iago, ed. *Human Nutrition, Historic and Scientific.* New York: International Universities Press, 1960. 321p.

Goldblith, Samuel A., and Maynard A. Joslyn. *Milestones in Nutrition.* Westport, Conn.: AVI, 1964. 797p.

Guggenheim, Karl Y. *Nutrition and Nutritional Diseases: The Evolution of Concepts.* Lexington, Mass.: Callamore Press, 1981. 378p. ISBN 0669039500.

Haller, Albert von. *The Vitamin Hunters.* Translated from the German by Hella Freud Bernays. Philadelphia, Pa.: Chilton, 1962. 307p. [Translation of *Die Küche unterm Mikroskop.*]

Harris, Leslie Julius. *Vitamins in Theory and Practice.* 4th ed. Cambridge, England: Cambridge University Press, 1955. 366p.

Hess, Alfred Fabian. *Scurvy, Past and Present.* New York: Academic Press, 1982. 279p. (The Nutrition Foundation Reprints). ISBN 0123452805.

King, Charles Glen. *A Good Idea: The History of the Nutrition Foundation.* New York: The Nutrition Foundation, 1976. 241p.

McCollum, Elmer Verner. *A History of Nutrition: The Sequence of Ideas in Nutrition Investigations.* Boston: Houghton Mifflin, 1957. 451p.

Oser, Bernard L. "The Impact of Analytical Chemistry on Food Science." *Food Technology* 29 (January 1975): 45-47.

Pike, Ruth L., and Myrtle L. Brown. "Historical Perspective." In *Nutrition, an Integrated Approach*, 3rd ed., 3-14. New York: Wiley, 1984.

Roe, Daphne A. *A Plague of Corn: The Social History of Pellagra.* Ithaca, N.Y.: Cornell University Press, 1973. 217p.

Thurne, Stuart. *The History of Food Preservation*. Cumbria, England: Parthenon Publishing, 1986. 184p. ISBN 1850701296.

Todhunter, E. N. "Historical Landmarks in Nutrition." In *Present Knowledge of Nutrition*, R. E. Olson, et al., eds., 871-82. New York: The Nutrition Foundation, 1976.

Todhunter, E. N. "Some Aspects of the History of Dietetics." *World Review of Nutrition and Dietetics* 18 (1973): 1-46.

Tremolières, J. "A History of Dietetics." *Progress in Food and Nutrition Science* 1 (1975): 65-114.

Williams, Robert Runnels. *Toward the Conquest of Beriberi*. Cambridge, Mass.: Harvard University Press, 1961. 338p.

3
Literature of the Field and Its Publishers

TYPES OF PROFESSIONAL AND RESEARCH LITERATURE

In nutrition and food science most information is communicated through books and periodicals; to a lesser extent through papers presented at conferences; and through patents, standards, and nonprint media such as audiovisuals, electronic data banks, and computer programs. The use of computers has made electronically transmitted information widely accessible to libraries and to professionals with microcomputers. In fact, the use of this type of information is increasing so rapidly that in 20 to 30 years online access will probably be the norm rather than the exception.

In nutrition and food science, as in other fields of scientific endeavor, a vast amount of information is generated each year. Much of this information is truly "new," but a substantial amount is not. The new information is considered primary source literature, usually published in primary source journals. It can also be transmitted through papers presented at conferences, and technical reports of research performed under grants, and through patents.

The information that is not new has already appeared in the literature and has merely been "repackaged" or "condensed" and then published in some other form. Primary source literature in major research journals is frequently "repackaged" to appear in industry-based trade magazines, newsletters, books, handbooks, food composition tables, articles in the lay press, and literature review or survey articles.

For the researcher, professional, and student, the primary source literature is qualitatively different from this "repackaged" or secondary literature. It is useful to visualize the literature of nutrition and food science as a pyramid with the primary source literature on top, moving downward toward the base as it is reviewed and incorporated into books, food composition tables, and the popular press. The researcher who "created" the information is at the top, and the lay public reading popular books and magazines is at the bottom. The farther down the information moves, the more time has elapsed. It takes anywhere from one to several years for this information to be synthesized into books aimed at the professional and researcher and much longer for it to appear in books aimed at the public.

Researchers in the field form their judgments about information on the basis of a careful reading of the original research report in a primary source publication. It is inconsistent with the canons of science to rely on someone else's interpretation of data contained in a book, a newsletter presenting summaries of new research, or a review article on the subject. In other words, secondary sources are good starting points, but not good stopping points. They are best at providing a quick overview of a topic as well as a bibliography of primary citations.

TYPES OF PUBLICATIONS

Print materials are divided into two categories: periodicals and books (also called monographs). Periodicals will be considered first.

Periodicals

The term *serial* is the broadest possible category of publications issued "serially" over a period of time, but this term is used almost exclusively by librarians. It encompasses both regularly and irregularly appearing publications, including newspapers, periodic conferences, scientific journals, and such series as Wurtman's *Nutrition and the Brain*. The term *periodical* is frequently used as a synonym, but is narrower in scope and includes primarily publications appearing at regular intervals. The *American Journal of Clinical Nutrition* and the *Annual Review of Nutrition* are periodicals.

The term *magazine* almost always refers to a popular periodical intended for the lay public, such as *American Health*, *Health*, and *Prevention*. Nutrition articles in these publications are usually written by journalists with or without formal training in nutrition or dietetics.

RESEARCH OR PRIMARY SOURCE JOURNALS

Research or primary source journals are also called professional journals. Their function is to publish original research in a particular discipline. Most appear monthly or quarterly. They are published by professional societies or commercial publishing houses. Examples of society-produced journals in nutrition and food science are *American Journal of Clinical Nutrition*, *Journal of the American Dietetic Association*, *Journal of Nutrition*, *Journal of Food Science*, and *Proceedings of the Nutrition Society*. In recent years commercially published research journals have begun to proliferate in newly emerging special-ties for which no society journals existed. Some examples of commercially published journals are *Nutrition and Behavior* and *Nutrition Research*.

Studies have shown that in the nutrition and food science literature, which includes literally thousands of journals, most articles appear in a relatively small number of core journals, and much of the rest of the literature in this area is widely scattered among journals in the biomedical sciences, agriculture, and other fields (Gryboski, 1973; Maheswarappa and Surya Rao, 1982).

TRADE PERIODICALS

Industry-based trade periodicals report new developments, contain survey articles, are heavily product oriented, and contain a large amount of advertising. Most are in the area of food science and technology. A good example is *Chilton's Food Engineering*. Such periodicals generally do not publish the results of new research, although they frequently summarize or interpret research published elsewhere. Some even contain abstracts of recent journal articles and references to new patents. One example of this type of periodical in the field of nutrition is *Nutrition Today*. Although published by the Nutrition Today Society, it nonetheless has a strong food industry orientation.

FOOD AND DRUG INDUSTRY PERIODICALS

These are periodicals produced by the food or drug industry for the nutrition professional. Most are so brief they are essentially newsletters. Examples are the *Dairy Council Digest* and *Dietetic Currents* (produced by Ross Laboratories). These publications can contain valuable information; however, users should keep in mind that the content could be biased in favor of the industry.

NEWSLETTERS

This category of periodical recently has been proliferating. Not only are there many newsletters aimed at professionals, such as *Nutrition and the M.D.*, but an increasing number are available for the layperson. The trend is for major health care institutions and universities to publish "health letters" for the general public. The success of such publications as the *Harvard Medical School Health Letter* has spawned many imitators, including the *Tufts University Diet & Nutrition Letter*, the *Mayo Clinic Health Letter*, and the *University of California, Berkeley, Wellness Letter*. Even the Center for Science in the Public Interest has changed the title of its magazine to *Nutrition Action Health Letter*.

REVIEW PERIODICALS

These periodicals contain only review or survey articles, which critique or evaluate the literature on a specific subject. They usually contain a large number of citations to the literature and are a good starting point for a literature search. Most appear annually, but some are more frequent.

CONFERENCE PROCEEDINGS

Conferences are a principal means of communicating results of new scientific and technical information. They are generally announced far in advance in meeting calendars of journals or in either *World Meetings: United States and Canada* or *World Meetings: Outside the United States and Canada*. Some conferences are held only once, but many are held every few years. Most are sponsored by professional organizations or government agencies. In some cases the sponsoring organization publishes the proceedings of these conferences; in others, they are published by commercial publishing houses.

A significant number of papers presented at conferences are never published. Some are published in the proceedings of the conference as late as one to several years after the event. Others may be published individually in various journals. Some are even published as a group, taking up an entire issue or supplement to a journal..

Citations to unpublished conference papers usually do not include a publisher or an editor or pagination. If page numbers are given, they usually are not continuous; for example, the entry will have "10p." rather than "pp. 20-30" which would indicate that the paper was part of a volume. To determine if the proceedings or papers of a conference have been published, consult issues of the *Directory of Published Proceedings*. If a paper is unpublished, it can usually be requested from the author or the sponsoring society. Following are some of the major periodic conferences in nutrition and food science:

International Congress of Nutrition

Western Hemisphere Nutrition Congress

Swedish Nutrition Foundation Symposia

International Congress of Food Science and Technology

Monographs

The term *monograph* is library parlance for books. It refers to single works by one or more authors. They are usually not continued, and if they are, they will be completed in a specified number of volumes. This is in contrast to periodicals, which are expected to continue indefinitely. For research purposes books can provide background information, but because they may take many years to write and publish, they never contain the "cutting edge" of information that is found in research journals.

REFERENCE BOOKS

This category of books is defined by how it is used. A reference book is almost never read from cover to cover, and is only referred to when specific data are needed. These valuable compilations of information include, among other forms, handbooks and manuals, encyclopedias, dictionaries of specialized terms, and food composition tables.

Dictionaries

The purpose of a dictionary is to define terminology. There are many specialized dictionaries which define terminology not contained in standard dictionaries and terminology which deviates from standard usage. Some of these provide English-language equivalents for foreign terms, and vice versa.

Encyclopedias

Encyclopedias are compendia of concise, basic information arranged alphabetically. The treatment of individual subjects is much more extensive than that provided by the typical dictionary. Encyclopedias are a good starting point for material on an unfamiliar subject. Many provide references to relevant books or articles on a subject. As a general rule, they contain detailed indexes.

Handbooks, Manuals, and Other Data Compilations

The ideal handbook or manual should encompass most of the fundamental data a practitioner or a researcher refers to on a routine basis. Usually this includes basic principles, methods, formulas, etc. Handbooks or manuals are usually aimed at practitioners or researchers in a subject field or subfield. Sometimes the information presented in handbooks and manuals is similar to that contained in encyclopedias. The scope, however, is usually narrower. The arrangement is similar to that of most books. Chapters deal with specific subjects, arranged in logical, not alphabetical, order.

Directories

There are many types of directories; some provide information on individuals, some on organizations, institutions, academic programs, and manufacturers and/or products. Some directories, such as the *National Faculty Directory*, provide only names and addresses, whereas others such as *American Men and Women of Science*, provide more detailed biographical information.

Standards and Regulations

Standards and regulations, together with food inspection, are ways of ensuring the quality and safety of our food supply. Standards may be issued by national and international government agencies, and by professional or trade organizations. Some are voluntary and some have the force of law. They are discussed in chapter 21.

Bibliographies

Bibliographies are lists of references, most often to periodicals and books, but also to audiovisual aids or computer software. Many bibliographies are one-time publications. They list references on a subject for a specific period of time, and quickly become out-of-date unless the author produces a revised edition. An example of a one-time bibliography is *Nutrition References and Book Reviews*, published by the Chicago Nutrition Association. Other bibliographies are essentially periodicals, listing new literature on a continuing basis. An example of this type of bibliography is the *Bibliography of Agriculture*. Bibliographies can be either annotated (having descriptions) or unannotated.

Guides to the Literature

These guides are special types of bibliographies, usually annotated, that are designed to introduce the reader to the literature of a specific field. They are somewhat like road maps that point the reader to suitable reference sources for specific types of information.

Indexing/Abstracting Services

These can be subject and author indexes to periodicals such as *General Science Index* and *Index Medicus*, which are published monthly and are cumulated at regular intervals, or they can be abstracting services (sometimes just called abstracts) such as *Nutrition Abstracts and Reviews*, which perform all of the above functions, but index a much larger selection of journals, include conferences and other literature, and provide summaries or abstracts of the items listed.

SOURCES OF PROFESSIONAL AND RESEARCH LITERATURE

In nutrition and food science the bulk of information is published by commercial publishers, professional organizations, trade or industry groups, and national or international governmental agencies. Sometimes state and local health care agencies, hospitals, and organizations also issue relevant publications. Relative to other fields in science and technology a high percentage of material in this field comes from professional, trade, and industry groups. These publications generally are not available through the regular book trade distribution channels or in book stores. They must be ordered directly from the source.

Commercial Publishers

Books and journals in nutrition and food science are published by a large number of commercial publishers. Of these, only a handful concentrate on food science and nutrition materials:

AVI Publishing Company, Inc.
(250 Post Rd. E., P.O. Box 831, Westport, CT 06881)

Food and Nutrition Press
(265 Post Rd. W., Westport, CT 06880)

George Stickley Co.
(210 Washington Square, Philadelphia, PA 19106)

Elsevier Applied Science, formerly Applied Science Publishers
(22 Rippleside Commercial Estate, Ripple Rd., Barking, England 1G11
OSA-T:5952121. U.S. customers should apply to Elsevier Science Publishing in New York City for information).

Students and professionals will find it useful to get on their mailing lists for catalogs and book announcements.

Professional Organizations

Many of the major organizations publishing in the field limit themselves to the publication of professional or research journals. Some also sponsor and publish conferences and issue newsletters. Others, like the American Dietetic Association, have extensive publication programs.

Some of the major professional societies in nutrition, dietetics, and food science and technology are

American College of Nutrition (ACN)

American Dietetic Association (ADA)

American Institute of Nutrition (AIN)

American Society for Clinical Nutrition (ASCN)

American Society for Parenteral and Enteral Nutrition (ASPEN)

Center for Science in the Public Interest (CSPI)

Community Nutrition Institute (CNI)

Food and Nutrition Board, National Research Council, National Academy of Sciences (FNB)

Institute of Food Technologists (IFT)

International College of Applied Nutrition

National Nutrition Consortium (NCC)

Nutrition Foundation (NF)

Society for Nutrition Education (SNE)

The types of publications issued by most of these organizations are described below.

The American College of Nutrition (ACN) is a small organization of research scientists, physicians, and dietitians working toward better patient care through an exchange of information between nutrition scientists and physicians. In addition to its quarterly journal, the *Journal of the American College of Nutrition*, the ACN sponsors an annual meeting, the proceedings of which, when published, appear in its monograph series.

The American Dietetic Association (ADA) has an impressive output of publications and audiovisual materials, including video and audio cassette series and study kits intended for continuing education. In addition to its more specialized materials, the ADA issues a substantial number of publications aimed at the consumer. The organization is now raising funds for a National Center for Nutrition and Dietetics which is expected to serve as a repository for nutrition information.

The American Institute of Nutrition (AIN) is a professional society of researchers in nutrition. It publishes the *Journal of Nutrition* and copublishes the *American Journal of Clinical Nutrition* with the American Society of Clinical Nutrition, its clinical nutrition arm. It has sponsored or cosponsored many symposia and congresses, including the *Western Hemisphere Nutrition Congress* and some of the congresses in the *International Congress of Nutrition* series of publications. The AIN annual meeting is held in connection with the meeting of the Federation of American Societies for Experimental Biology. Many of the symposia sponsored by ASCN are published as special issues or supplements to the *American Journal of Clinical Nutrition.*

The Center for Science in the Public Interest, a consumer advocacy group, is an organization which has made food its major focus. In addition to its *Nutrition Action Health Letter*, it has published numerous books and pamphlets on nutrition and food safety.

The Community Nutrition Institute (CNI) is a group of "citizen advocates" concerned with food and nutrition issues including food programs, hunger, food quality and safety, nutrition education, food labeling, and marketing. It conducts the annual National Food Policy Conference. Its newsletter, *Nutrition Week*, keeps members informed about changes in government agencies or policies relevant to food and nutrition.

The Food and Nutrition Board (FNB) in the National Research Council, National Academy of Sciences, is a major source of authoritative materials on nutrition and food safety. The National Academy of Sciences (NAS) is a "private, self-perpetuating society of distinguished scholars in scientific and engineering research dedicated to the furtherance of science and its use for the general welfare." Although it is funded by the U.S. government, it is *not* a government agency. Its operating arm is the National Research Council, with its eight major units. The FNB "resides" in one of these subdivisions, the Commission of Life Sciences. Its most important publication is *Recommended Dietary Allowances*, revised at approximately five-year intervals and issued by its Committee on Dietary Allowances.

The Institute of Food Technologists (IFT) produces two major periodicals: the *Journal of Food Science*, its research journal and *Food Technology*, a general periodical containing articles of current interest, book reviews, news, conference announcements, and information on new patents. The IFT issues numerous conference publications, many through commercial publishers. It is one of the founding organizations of the International Food Information Service (IFIS).

The Nutrition Foundation (NF) is an industry-sponsored organization devoted to fostering basic research and education in nutrition by making grants to universities and other institutions for symposia, workshops, and monographs. The foundation is the publisher of the review journal, *Nutrition Reviews*. At approximately five-year intervals the NF publishes revised editions of its literature review monograph, *Present Knowledge in Nutrition*, an extremely useful survey publication.

The Society for Nutrition Education (SNE) has a modest publication program. In addition to the *Journal of Nutrition Education*, it publishes a series of bibliographies aimed at the lay public and professionals. Of particular interest to nutrition educators are those bibliographies dealing with teaching materials listing both print and nonprint media. The SNE maintains a resource center which distributes informational materials and films.

The National Nutrition Consortium (NCC), is a federation of major nutrition organizations formed to provide information on food, nutrition, and health to the general public and to furnish leadership and coordination in the nutrition community on questions of food and nutrition policy. It has produced a handful of practical publications on such subjects as vitamin toxicity and nutrition labeling.

Industry-wide Trade Organizations

Industry-wide trade organizations exist in almost every field, from the American Institute of Baking to the United Fresh Fruit and Vegetable Association. These organizations can be valuable sources of information. Most organizations publish industry-based trade periodicals. Many issue directories and statistics for the industry. Some produce extensive works of reference containing information that is not easily accessible elsewhere. Of course, their nutrition information should be evaluated with an eye to the vested interests they represent.

International and Foreign Organizations

There are few international nongovernmental organizations issuing publications in nutrition and food science. Their activities are overshadowed by governmental bodies such as the Food and Agriculture Organization (FAO) and the World Health Organization (WHO).

The International Union of Nutritional Sciences (IUNS) is an association of national and regional nutrition organizations founded in 1946 to promote cooperation in the scientific study of nutrition, to encourage research, and to facilitate the exchange of scientific information. It sponsors international congresses and publishes the reports of its commissions and committees. The Group of European Nutritionists is an affiliate organization of IUNS. Its conferences are published chiefly in the series Bibliotheca Nutritio et Dieta.

The International Union of Food Science and Technology (IUFoST) is the major international organization promoting cooperation among food scientists and technologists. It is made up of national organizations in over 43 countries. It sponsors the International Congress of Food Science and Technology and many other conferences and symposia and publishes a newsletter of activities.

In addition to professional societies, many countries have active organizations similar to the Nutrition Foundation in the United States. The foundations in England, Sweden, the Netherlands, Switzerland, and Italy form the International Group of Nutrition Foundations. Their common objectives are to promote research, professional, and general education, and to act in a public advisory role. A few of them publish materials in English.

Government Agencies

National and international government agencies are responsible for generating a significant share of the nutrition and food literature. Both the U.S.

government and the Food and Agriculture Organization of the United Nations are major publishers responsible for a large number of publications. Chapters 8 and 21 provide detailed information on the types of publications and their availability, as well as the issuing agencies.

SELECTED REFERENCES

De Bakey, Lois. *The Scientific Journal: Editorial Policies and Practices: Guidelines for Editors, Reviewers and Authors.* St. Louis, Mo.: C. V. Mosby, 1976. 128p. ISBN 0801612233.

Frank, Robyn C. "Information Resources for Food and Human Nutrition." *Journal of the American Dietetic Association* 80 (1982): 344-49.

Green, Syd. *Keyguide to Information Sources in Food Science and Technology.* London, New York: Mansell, 1985. 231p. ISBN 0720117488.

"International Union of Nutritional Sciences." *American Journal of Clinical Nutrition* 30 (1977): 1403-7.

King, Donald W., Dennis D. McDonald, and Nancy K. Roderer. *Scientific Journals in the United States: Their Production, Use and Economics.* Stroudsburg, Pa.: Hutchinson Ross; distr., New York: Academic Press, 1981. 319p.

Leitch, Isabella. "The Collection and Dissemination of Information on Nutrition Science with Special Reference to the United Kingdom." *Progress in Food and Nutrition Science* 2 (1976): 59-79.

Lowry, Charles D., and Robert Cocroft. "Literature Needs of Food Scientists." *Journal of Chemical Documentation* 8 (1968): 228-30.

Mann, E. J. *Evaluation of the World Food Literature: Results of an International Survey.* Farnham Royal, England: Commonwealth Agricultural Bureaux, 1967. 181p.

Mann, E. J. "Report on International Survey of the World Literature on Food Science and Technology." *Dairy Science Abstracts* 28 (1966): 603-6.

"Medical Advice That Comes in the Mail." *Changing Times* 40 (July 1986): 27-41.

Morton, L. T., ed. *Use of Medical Literature.* 2nd ed. London, Boston: Butterworths, 1977. 462p. ISBN 0408709162.

Nelson, Carnot E., and Donald K. Pollock, eds. *Communication among Scientists and Engineers.* Lexington, Mass.: D. C. Heath, 1970. 346p.

Rolander-Chilo, Brita, ed. *International Research in Nutrition*. Oxford, New York: Pergamon Press, 1979. 114p. ISBN 0080243991.

Strickland-Hodge, Barry, and Barbara C. Allan. *Medical Information: A Profile*. London, New York: Mansell, 1986. 145p. ISBN 0720117771.

"Symposium: Information and Documentation in the Food Industry: Six Papers Presented during This Symposium at IFT [Institute of Food Technology] 35th Annual Meeting Held June 8-11, 1975 in Chicago." *Food Technology* 30 (May 1976): 54-84.

United States Congress. Office of Technology Assessment. *Food Information Systems: Summary and Analysis*. Washington, D.C.: Government Printing Office, 1976. 85p. (OTA-F-35). Y3.T22:2F73/2.

Warren, Kenneth S., ed. *Coping with the Biomedical Literature: A Primer for the Scientist and the Clinician*. New York: Praeger, 1981. 233p. ISBN 0030570360.

Woodward, Anthony M. "The Roles of Reviews in Information Transfer." *Journal of the American Society for Information Science* 28 (May 1977): 175-79.

NOTES

Gryboski, Helen. (1973). Human nutrition. In *Fundamentals of Documentation: Students' Papers*, T. D. Wilson and E. Herman, eds., 138-56. College Park, Md.: School of Library and Information Services, University of Maryland.

Maheswarappa, B. S., and K. Surya Rao. (1982). Journal literature of food science and technology: A bibliometric study. *Annals of Library Science and Documentation*, *29*, 126-34.

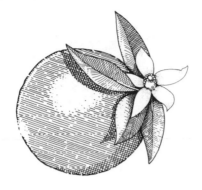

Part II

USING THE
LITERATURE

4
Locating Research
Indexing/Abstracting Services

This chapter discusses the function of indexing/abstracting services and how they can help in locating published research on a topic. It describes general and interdisciplinary indexing/abstracting services in the area of food and health science. More specialized indexing/abstracting services relating to nutrition, nutrition education, food science, food service, etc., are discussed in the chapters dealing with these fields.

Indexing/abstracting services include the following three types of continuing publications: periodical indexes, such as *Index Medicus*, which simply list periodical articles by subject; abstracting services, which index periodical articles and other literature by subject, but also provide summaries or abstracts of individual items indexed; and continuing bibliographies, which are similar to abstracting services in that they provide references to new literature on an ongoing basis, but frequently do not provide abstracts.

Most disciplines have services that provide indexed access to articles in periodicals reporting new research; these services may also include the following types of publications depending on their importance in the field: conference papers, selected government publications, patents, regulations, and standards. A few also index popular level materials which may be useful to nutrition educators or practitioners who counsel clients.

Literature searches for term papers, theses, dissertations, research proposals, and publications require a search of all the recent literature in English. In most instances the use of an indexing/abstracting service or an equivalent computer search service is the only way of searching the literature systematically.

Most databases used to produce indexing/abstracting services are now available for online searching. Descriptions included here of specific indexing/abstracting services list the names of the online database equivalents which can be searched in libraries or by individuals with microcomputers.

ABSTRACTING SERVICES

The citations in abstracting services are usually accompanied by an abstract which summarizes the subject content of the time, hence the term *abstracting service* and the name *abstract* in *Nutrition Abstracts and Reviews*, *Chemical Abstracts*, *Biological Abstracts*, etc.

Most abstracting services are published on a monthly or semi-monthly basis. Each reference is identified by an item or abstract number, arranged in continuous sequence from issue to issue within a given volume or year. Subject and author indexes generally appear at the end of each issue and are cumulated every six months or once a year. Entries in the index usually refer to the sequential item numbers in the individual issues.

The field of nutrition has a number of abstracting services which index relevant publications. The major one is *Nutrition Abstracts and Reviews*, but there are a number of others, such as *Biological Abstracts*, *Chemical Abstracts*, and *Food Science and Technology Abstracts*, which are not chiefly devoted to nutrition, but place varying degrees of emphasis on covering nutrition and food science materials.

PERIODICAL INDEXES

Periodical indexes provide access to current articles in periodicals on an ongoing basis. Usually the indexing is by subject, but frequently also by author. Individual issues, published monthly or sometimes quarterly, are cumulated into permanent annual volumes. In most instances no abstracts or summaries are provided. A good example of a periodical index is *Index Medicus*, the major periodical index in medicine.

CONTINUING BIBLIOGRAPHIES

Continuing bibliographies function essentially the same way as do indexing/abstracting services. They provide access to the literature on a periodic basis. They may or may not contain abstracts or summaries with the citations. The *Bibliography of Agriculture* is an excellent example of this type of publication.

BIBLIOGRAPHIES AND GUIDES TO INDEXING/ABSTRACTING SERVICES

11. **Abstracting and Indexing Services Directory.** Nos. 1-3. Edited by John Schmittroth. Detroit: Gale Research, 1982-1983. ISBN 0810316498.

This bibliography is complete in three issues. It contains over 1,700 detailed listings of indexes, abstracting services, bibliographies, digests, and catalogs. There is a cumulative index in the last issue which provides access by keywords, titles, former titles, variant titles, and acronyms. An address directory is included.

12. Owen, Dolores B. **Abstracts and Indexes in Science and Technology: A Descriptive Guide**. 2nd ed. Metuchen, N.J.: Scarecrow Press, 1985. 235p. ISBN 0810817128.

Descriptions of over 200 indexing and abstracting services in all fields of science and technology, including general and interdisiplinary titles, are included here. Sections of principal interest to those in food and nutrition fields are on the biological sciences, agricultural sciences, and health sciences. Information in each entry includes title, arrangement, coverage, scope, type of abstracts and indexes included, and equivalent databases. "An excellent access point to indexes and abstracts in the area of science and technology" (*Medical Reference Services Quarterly* 5 [1985]: 87-88).

GENERAL AND INTERDISCIPLINARY INDEXING/ABSTRACTING SERVICES

13. **Agrindex**. Vol. 1- . Rome: AGRIS Coordinating Centre, Food and Agriculture Organization of the United Nations, 1975- . monthly. ISSN 0254-8801.

This index is the product of AGRIS (International Information System for Agricultural Sciences and Technology), an international network of 130 cooperating centers which collect and index the current agricultural literature from abroad.

Coverage of nutrition and food science and technology materials is limited. Items included tend to focus on developing countries. This index has one noteworthy feature—a special section on food composition which lists literature separately by commodity. This approach makes it simpler to access this type of information without looking in an index for all entries relating to a food or a specific nutrient.

Included in each issue are indexes to personal authors, corporate entries, reports and patents, and commodities, as well as a geographical index in two sections: political geography and marine areas and physical geography.

Online Equivalent: AGRIS INTERNATIONAL.

Cumulative Indexes: A paper cumulative index is available for the years 1975-1977. Microfiche cumulations are now issued.

14. **Bibliography of Agriculture**. Vol. 1- . Phoenix, Ariz.: Oryx Press, 1942- . monthly. ISSN 0006-1530.

This is an interdisciplinary bibliography of citations on all aspects of food and agriculture, including food science and technology and human nutrition. Produced commercially from indexing done at the National Agricultural Library, it now contains over 120,000 citations a year from some 4,000 periodical titles, as well as USDA publications, publications of the state agricultural experiment stations and extension services, FAO publications, and foreign document materials, reports of research institutes, conference proceedings, and pamphlets.

Online Equivalent: AGRICOLA.

Arrangement: Continuously numbered citations without abstracts are arranged in broad subject categories with more detailed subject groupings within these categories.

Indexes: Each monthly issue has the following indexes: geographic, corporate author, personal author, and subject. These are cumulated annually.

Through 1984 the subject index was really a title keyword index (all the important words in titles) with some enrichments such as genera and species of plants and animals, geographic names, and explanatory remarks where titles were not descriptive enough. Since 1985, the subject index has been done using the *CAB Thesaurus*, the vocabulary used to index material in all of the CAB International abstracting services. This means that subject terms for the *Bibliography of Agriculture* will correspond to those now found in *Nutrition Abstracts and Reviews*. Where relevant, CAB geographic descriptors are also used. Genera and species of plants and animals are indexed under both common and scientific names.

Supplements: Supplementary volumes have been issued for some recent years. These include their own indexes.

Comments: The coverage of human nutrition material parallels that of the *Food and Nutrition Quarterly Index.* Although the Food and Nutrition Information Center at USDA provides food- and nutrition-related indexing for the *Bibliography of Agriculture*, the useful FNIC abstracts and FNIC index terms are not reproduced in the *Bibliography of Agriculture*. They do remain intact in its online version. Indexing of materials on the processing of agricultural commodities is limited to primary processing.

15. **Biological Abstracts**. Vol. 1- . Philadelphia, Pa.: BioSciences Information Service, 1926- . semi-monthly. ISSN 0006-3169.

Biological Abstracts (*BA*) is the major indexing/abstracting service covering the world's biological sciences literature, both pure and applied. Coverage ranges from botany, zoology, and agriculture to physiology, biochemistry, nutrition, food science and technology, and fisheries. *BA* now covers over 9,000 periodical titles. It indexes and abstracts literature in the following subjects relevant to nutrition and food science and technology: biochemistry, physiology, metabolism, digestive system, food and industrial microbiology, food technology, and nutrition science. This last section covers carbohydrates, dietary studies, therapeutic diets, general studies of nutritional status, lipids, malnutrition, minerals, proteins, peptides and amino acids, fat-soluble vitamins, and water-soluble vitamins.

Online Equivalent: BIOSIS Previews.

Arrangement: Continuously numbered abstracts are arranged in 84 broad subject categories.

Indexes: Author, subject, biosystematic, and generic indexes appear in each semi-monthly issue and are cumulated on a semi-annual basis.

Comments: The subject index found in *BA* is not a true subject index, but a keyword-in-context (KWIC) index based on title keywords, which lists every significant word in the title of an article in the context of adjacent words. This adjacency provides clues on the content and scope of an article that simple keyword indexing alone cannot provide.

To make the indexing less ambiguous, keywords are enriched by the addition of explanatory terms where relevant. These can include the name of the organism, organ systems and tissues, drugs, chemical names, enzyme names and numbers, disease names, apparatus and instrumentation used, etc. Another feature of the subject indexing is the abbreviation of terms for chemicals and enzymes, for example, *DNA* instead of *deoxyribonucleic acid* and *ATP* instead of *adenosine triphosphate*. A list of the commonly used abbreviations appears in the back of each issue.

The subject index is one of the most frequently used parts of the index and is the only one that provides indexing of subject content in sufficient detail to be useful in most searches. The point to keep in mind about this index is that it requires thought and imagination to look under every possible keyword that might have been used by an author in the title of an article. The taxonomic categories in the biosystematic index are too broad to be useful to most searchers, but the generic index, which has been available since 1974, is clearly a vital access point. It lists plants and animals and their products by genus and identifies them by species. It also provides abbreviated subject categories to describe the subject content of references.

List of Periodicals Indexed: A list of periodicals indexed is issued annually under the title *Serial Sources for the BIOSIS Data Base.* It lists abbreviated periodical titles as cited in *Biological Abstracts* with full title equivalents so that they can be located in library catalogs and periodical holdings lists. It also contains publishers' addresses, new serial titles, and ceased or changed titles.

16. **Biological Abstracts: RRM**. Vol. 1- . Philadelphia, Pa.: Biosciences Information Service, 1965- . ISSN 0192-6985.

Formerly titled *Bioresearch Index, Biological Abstracts: RRM* is a companion publication to *Biological Abstracts.* It contains the same types of indexes, with the same arrangement, minus the abstracts. Instead there are "content summaries," meaning that the index terms are printed following the citation. Although billed by BIOSIS as citations to reports, reviews, and meetings, *Biological Abstracts: RRM* also contains citations to some important journal literature. Students and researchers should use both *Biological Abstracts* and *Biological Abstracts: RRM* if they do not want to miss important literature.

Online Equivalent: BIOSIS Previews. This database includes both *Biological Abstracts* and *Biological Abstracts: RRM.*

Comment: Covers not only conference publications, but also edited books containing papers by various authors.

17. **Chemical Abstracts: Key to the World's Chemical Literature**. Vol. 1- . Columbus, Ohio: Chemical Abstracts Service, 1907- . weekly. ISSN 0009-2258.

This weekly abstracting service summarizes and indexes the world's new chemical literature. The following subject sections appear on alternate weeks: biochemistry and organic chemistry (including nutrition); and macromolecular chemistry, applied chemistry and chemical engineering, physical, inorganic, and analytical chemistry.

Subsection 18 in the biochemistry section contains the abstracts of the literature on animal nutrition, which includes nutritional studies of all animal species except protozoa. This section includes about 4,000 to 5,000 abstracts annually.

Subsection 17 "includes food and feed components and methods for their determination, additives, contaminants, toxicology, packaging and preservation systems, government regulations, and nutritive value evaluations in nontarget organisms or in vitro." Chemical substances are accompanied by chemical registry numbers, unique identifying numbers for chemical elements or compounds.

Online Equivalent: CA Search.

Indexes: Each issue has a keyword index, based on title words, for quick retrieval of current information. This bears little relationship to the standardized terminology used in the cumulative indexes. In addition, there are patent and author indexes.

Cumulative Indexes: The following types of indexes are issued semi-annually: author, general subject, chemical substances, formula, and patent. The chemical substances index indexes the literature by names of specific chemical substances (elements or compounds). For example, *L-arginine, ascorbic acid,* and *L-tryptophan* (filed under "t", not "l") are named chemical substances. The general subject index indexes classes of chemical compounds, such as amino acids and fatty acids, incompletely defined materials, reactions, concepts, phenomena, apparatus, and common or scientific names of plants or animals.

Collective Indexes: Collective indexes are indexes covering multiple years. The tenth or last collective index cumulates the semi-annual indexes for 1977-1981. These were formerly called decennial indexes because they cumulated ten years of semi-annual indexes at a time.

Index Guide: Chemical Abstracts follows the rules for naming chemical compounds set forth by the International Union of Pure and Applied Chemistry (IUPAC), a system that nonchemists almost always find difficult to use. The "Index Guide" which appears with *CA* is a guide to the correct chemical nomenclature for some of the compounds in the cumulative chemical substances indexes. It refers the user from alternative names of a substance to terminology actually used. For example, it refers from *palmitic acid* to *hexadecanoic acid,* the actual term used in indexing, and provides chemical registry numbers to identify compounds. If the numbers match, the compound is the same. Appendixes include detailed information on how the indexes are prepared to help the user who has questions about their use and arrangement.

18. **Consumer Health & Nutrition Index**. Vol. 1- . Phoenix, Ariz.: Oryx Press, July 1985- . quarterly. ISSN 0883-1963.

Consumer Health and Nutrition includes articles in 35 popular level health and nutrition magazines and newsletters. Covered are *American Health, Environmental Nutrition Newsletter, Harvard Medical School Letter, Mayo Clinic Health Letter, Medical Self Care, Nutrition Today, Tufts University Diet and Nutrition Letter, University of California, Berkeley, Wellness Letter,* and numerous other titles. Many of these periodicals are not indexed elsewhere.

There is a subject index with terms based on the National Library of Medicine's *Medical Subject Headings (MeSH),* and a book review index. Though it is aimed at a lay audience and is intended for public library users, high school and college students, health maintenance organizations, clinics, and other health facilities, *Consumer Health & Nutrition Index* may be of interest to nutrition practitioners because it indexes major newsletters.

19. **Index Medicus**. Vol. 1- . Bethesda, Md.: National Library of Medicine, 1961- . monthly. ISSN 0019-3879.

Not counting an occasional hiatus, *Index Medicus* has existed in various forms for more than a century. It is a monthly subject and author index to over 2,700 journals in clinical medicine and the biomedical sciences, including 40 to 50 nutrition journals. The journals selected for indexing are those most directly relevant to clinical medicine. Some major journals, such as *Ecology of Food and Nutrition* and the *Journal of Nutrition Education,* are omitted. Editorials, letters, biographical materials, and obituaries are indexed.

The indexing is done according to the defined list of terms published in *Medical Subject Headings (MeSH). MeSH* appears annually as a separate publication. It is also issued as a part of the *Cumulated Index Medicus.* To index an article, indexers assign as many *MeSH* terms as necessary to describe its content. In the printed *Index Medicus*, however, the article appears only under the most important subject(s) because of space limitations. In MEDLINE (Medical Literature Analysis and Retrieval System Online), its computer-searchable equivalent, searching is possible under all of the assigned terms as well as keywords from the titles and abstracts of papers.

Online Equivalent: MEDLINE.

Cumulations: A cumulated version is issued annually under the title *Cumulated Index Medicus*.

Comments: Because indexers are instructed to be as specific as possible in their choice of *MeSH* terms, articles on thiamin, riboflavin, or pyridoxine, for instance, are indexed under those specific names rather than under the more general terms *vitamin B complex* or *vitamins*. Occasionally the more general terms will yield successful results when there is little material on a specific subject. In most cases, however, the literature is so plentiful that it is not useful to expand a search to a more general term. *MeSH* and *Index Medicus* both refer the user from terms not used to those which are a part of the *MeSH* vocabulary. For instance, there are *see* references from *vitamin B-1* to *thiamin*, from *vitamin B-2* to *riboflavin*, and so on.

Using MeSH: To use *Index Medicus* effectively it is necessary to use *Medical Subject Headings* (*MeSH*) to locate the appropriate terms for a subject. *MeSH* is essentially a record of all index terms and their interrelationships. It is divided into two parts: the "alphabetical list" and the "tree structures." The alphabetical list consists of *MeSH* terms with appropriate *see*, *see also*, *see under*, and *see related* references. A *see* reference directs the user from a term which is not used to one that is, while a *see under* directs the user from a specific term which does not appear in *Index Medicus* to a more general term which includes material on that subject. Terms with *see under* references attached are considered minor descriptors and cannot be searched directly in *Index Medicus*. However, they can be searched in MEDLINE. Obvious cross-references, for instance from an organ to its diseases, are avoided.

Topical subheadings listed in the front of *MeSH* are extremely useful in helping the user focus on specific aspects of a subject. For example, under the *MeSH* term *pyridoxine*, the most general articles are listed first. These are followed by references listed under the following topical subheadings: "Administration and Dosage," "Adverse Effects," "Analogs and Derivatives," "Analysis," "Antagonists and Inhibitors," "Biosynthesis," "Blood," "Diagnostic Use," "History," "Immunology," "Isolation and Purification," "Metabolism," "Pharmacodynamics," "Physiology," "Poisoning," "Standards," and "Therapeutic Use."

For information on the adverse effects of pharmacological doses of pyridoxine, the user may need to scan several of these topical subheadings.

The "tree structures" part of *MeSH* is very aptly named, because it suggests a broad trunk with various levels of branches, some larger, some smaller. Visualizing each of the 15 major subject categories as a tree trunk with many levels of branches representing more specific related subjects facilitates use of this part of *MeSH*. As illustrated by figure 1, all the chemicals and drugs are grouped in "tree" D, with growth substances, pigments, and vitamins listed in subcategory D11. The "trees" are used to ensure that the search is made under the most specific *MeSH* heading available and to make it possible to locate either more general, more specific, or related *MeSH* headings.

MEDICAL SUBJECT HEADINGS
ALPHABETIC LIST

MeSH Heading ——— **PYRIDONES**
D3.383.725.791+

Year this term ——— 68; was PYRIDINONES 1966-67
was first used   X PYRIDINONES
                              XU MIMOSINE

Previous term

Indicates reference
under Mimosine to
"see under" Pyridones
as more general term

+Indicates more
specific terms
indented under
this number in
Tree Structures

PYRIDOSTIGMINE BROMIDE
D3.383.725.762.740   D8.373.275.829
D16.698.410.778
65: PYRIDOSTIGMINE was see under PARASYMPATHOMIMETICS
1963-64

PYRIDOXAL
D3.383.725.676.635+   D11.786.708.704
74

PYRIDOXAL KINASE see under PHOSPHOTRANSFERASES, ATP ——— Reference from
  X   PYRIDOXAMINE KINASE   specific term
  X   PYRIDOXINE KINASE   Pyridoxal Kinase
                                                             to "see under"
PYRIDOXAL PHOSPHATE   more general term
D3.383.725.676.635.600   D8.176.740   Phosphotransferases,
                                                             ATP
PYRIDOXAMINE
D3.383.725.676.760   D11.786.708.733
74

PYRIDOXAMINE KINASE see PYRIDOXAL KINASE

PYRIDOXAMINEPHOSPHATE OXIDASE see under AMINE
OXIDOREDUCTASES
  X   PYRIDOXINEPHOSPHATE OXIDASE

PYRIDOXIC ACID see under ISONICOTINIC ACIDS
  X   PYRIDOXINECARBOXYLIC ACID

MeSH Heading ———**PYRIDOXINE**

       D11.786.708.762 ——— Tree Structures

This term not used. ———⟶ X VITAMIN B 6   number
There is reference
under Vitamin B 6
to "see" Pyridoxine

PYRIDOXINE DEFICIENCY
    C18.654.223.133.699.635
    see related
Reference to Anemia,   ANEMIA, SIDEROBLASTIC
Sideroblastic as a   XR ANEMIA, SIDEROBLASTIC
related term

Reference from Anemia, **PYRIDOXINE KINASE see PYRIDOXAL KINASE**
Sideroblastic to
Pyridoxine Deficiency **PYRIDOXINECARBOXYLIC ACID see PYRIDOXIC ACID**
as a related term
PYRIDOXINEDISULFIDE see PYRITHIOXIN

PYRIDOXINEPHOSPHATE OXIDASE see PYRIDOXAMINEPHOSPHATE
    OXIDASE

PYRIDYLCARBINOL see NICOTINYL ALCOHOL ——— "See" reference
                                      from term not
PYRILAMINE see under AMINOPYRIDINES   used to correct
    X MEPYRAMINE   MeSH Heading
    X PYRANISAMINE

PYRIMETHAMINE
    D3.383.742.675   D21.370.286.635

PYRIMIDINE DIMERS
    D13.695.578.424.600   D13.695.740.600
    77
    X THYMINE DIMERS
    XR DNA REPAIR

Fig. 1a. *MeSH* alphabetical list.

MEDICAL SUBJECT HEADINGS

TREE STRUCTURES

D11 – CHEMICALS AND DRUGS–GROWTH SUBSTANCES, PIGMENTS, VITAMINS

GROWTH SUBSTANCES, PIGMENTS, VITAMINS (NON MESH)

Term	Tree number				
VITAMINS	D11.786				
ASCORBIC ACID	D11.786.100	D2.241.81.			
DEHYDROASCORBIC ACID •	D11.786.100.260	D2.241.511.	D2.540.260	D9.203.811.	D9.203.811.
		D2.241.81.			
BIOFLAVONOIDS	D11.786.170	D9.203.408.			
ESCULIN •	D11.786.170.264	D9.203.408.			
FLAVONES	D11.786.170.381	D3.438.150.			
QUERCETIN •	D11.786.170.381.636	D3.438.150.			
HESPERIDIN •	D11.786.170.516	D9.203.408.			
RUTIN	D11.786.170.804	D9.203.408.			
VITAMIN A	D11.786.652	D2.455.849.	D11.557.261.		
VITAMIN B COMPLEX	D11.786.708				
AMINOBENZOIC ACIDS	D11.786.708.54	D2.241.223.			
P-AMINOBENZOIC ACID •	D11.786.708.54.75	D2.241.223.	D26.368.878.		
BIOTIN	D11.786.708.118	D8.176.96			
CARNITINE	D11.786.708.168				
ACETYLCARNITINE •	D11.786.708.168.90				
PALMITOYLCARNITINE •	D11.786.708.168.700				
FOLIC ACID	D11.786.708.328	D2.241.81.			
PTEROYLPOLYGLUTAMIC ACIDS •	D11.786.708.328.700	D3.438.733.	D12.125.119.	D19.461.543.	
FORMYLTETRAHYDROFOLATES •	D11.786.708.350				
CITROVORUM FACTOR	D11.786.708.350.220	D8.176.840.			
INOSITOL	D11.786.708.415	D9.203.853.	D10.642.441	D2.33.800.	
LIPOIC ACID	D11.786.708.469	D8.176.515			

NICOTINIC ACIDS	D11.786.708.547	D3.66.515	D3.383.725.
NIACIN	D11.786.708.547.500	D3.66.515.	D3.383.725.
NICOTINAMIDE	D11.786.708.547.565	D3.66.515.	D3.383.725.
6-AMINONICOTINAMIDE •	D11.786.708.547.565.50		
PANGAMIC ACID •	D11.786.708.596		
PANTOTHENIC ACID	D11.786.708.625		
PYRIDOXAL	D11.786.708.704	D3.383.725.	
PYRIDOXAMINE	D11.786.708.733	D3.383.725.	
PYRIDOXINE	D11.786.708.762		
RIBOFLAVIN	D11.786.708.806	D11.557.405.	
THIAMINE	D11.786.708.887		
THIAMINE MONOPHOSPHATE •	D11.786.708.887.600		
THIAMINE PYROPHOSPHATE	D11.786.708.887.702	D8.176.878	
THIAMINE TRIPHOSPHATE •	D11.786.708.887.900		
VITAMIN B 12	D11.786.708.950	D19.461.543.	
COBAMIDES	D11.786.708.950.270	D8.176.175	
HYDROXOCOBALAMIN	D11.786.708.950.560	D19.461.543.	
TRANSCOBALAMINS	D11.786.708.950.900	D12.776.124.	D12.776.157.	D12.776.377.
VITAMIN D	D11.786.763		
CHOLECALCIFEROLS	D11.786.763.196	D4.808.247.	D4.808.247.	D4.808.812.
		D10.516.851.	

Note hierarchical structure:

D = Chemicals and Drugs
D11 = Growth Substances, Pigments, Vitamins
D11.786 = Vitamins (as a general category)
D11.786.708 = Vitamin B Complex
D11.786.708.887 = Thiamine

*Indicates minor descriptors not found in Index Medicus.

Tree Structures numbers in smaller type are alternate locations of the term in other parts of "Tree Structures" list.

Fig. 1b. *MeSH* tree structures.

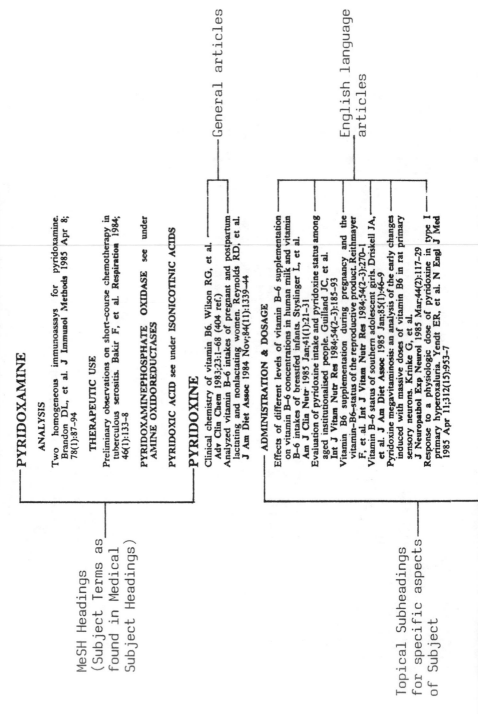

CUMULATED INDEX MEDICUS

PYRIDOXAMINE

ANALYSIS

Two homogeneous immunoassays for pyridoxamine. Brandon DL, et al. J Immunol Methods 1985 Apr 8; 78(1):87–94

THERAPEUTIC USE

Preliminary observations on short-course chemotherapy in tuberculous serositis. Bakir F, et al. Respiration 1984; 46(1):133–8

PYRIDOXAMINEPHOSPHATE OXIDASE see under AMINE OXIDOREDUCTASES

PYRIDOXIC ACID see under ISONICOTINIC ACIDS

PYRIDOXINE

Clinical chemistry of vitamin B6. Wilson RG, et al. Adv Clin Chem 1983;23:1–68 (404 ref.)
Analyzed vitamin B-6 intakes of pregnant and postpartum lactating and nonlactating women. Reynolds RD, et al. J Am Diet Assoc 1984 Nov;84(11):1339–44 — General articles

ADMINISTRATION & DOSAGE

Effects of different levels of vitamin B-6 supplementation on vitamin B-6 concentrations in human milk and vitamin B-6 intakes of breastfed infants. Styslinger L, et al. Am J Clin Nutr 1985 Jan;41(1):21–31
Evaluation of pyridoxine intake and pyridoxine status among aged institutionalised people. Guilland JC, et al. Int J Vitam Nutr Res 1984;54(2–3):185–93
Vitamin B6 supplementation during pregnancy and the vitamin-B6-status of the reproductive product. Reithmayer F, et al. Int J Vitam Nutr Res 1984;54(2–3):270–1
Vitamin B-6 status of southern adolescent girls. Driskell JA, et al. J Am Diet Assoc 1985 Jan;85(1):46–9
Pyridoxine megavitaminosis: an analysis of the early changes induced with massive doses of vitamin B6 in rat primary sensory neurons. Krinke G, et al. J Neuropathol Exp Neurol 1985 Mar;44(2):117–29
Response to a physiologic dose of pyridoxine in type I primary hyperoxaluria. Yendt ER, et al. N Engl J Med 1985 Apr 11;312(15):953–7 — English language articles

MeSH Headings
(Subject Terms as found in Medical Subject Headings)

Topical Subheadings for specific aspects of Subject

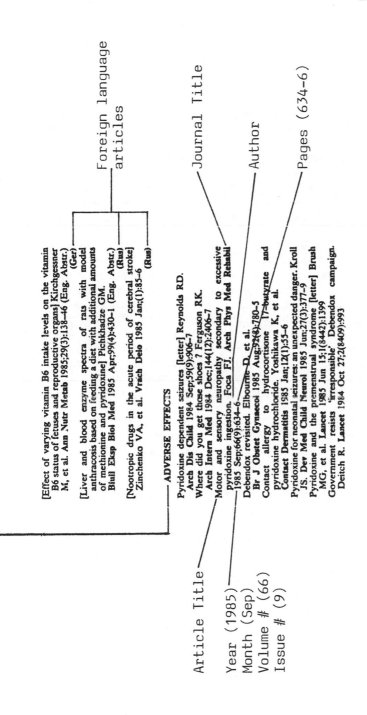

Fig. 1c. *Cumulated Index Medicus.*

Bibliography of Medical Reviews: This is a separate subject index to articles which survey or review the literature. It appears in the front of each monthly issue and in the *Cumulated Index Medicus*. These same articles also appear in *Index Medicus* proper. However, it is sometimes useful to be able to access them separately when starting a literature search or when there is so much literature on a subject that there is time to read only reviews.

List of Journals Indexed in Index Medicus: This list is published separately and in the front of the *Cumulated Index Medicus*. In addition to providing an abbreviations key to decode the abbreviated journal citations in *Index Medicus*, this list also has full title, subject, and geographic sections.

Literature Searches: The National Library of Medicine publishes numerous literature searches of its databases on topics of current interest. They are announced in monthly issues of *Index Medicus*, and may be obtained free of charge from NLM. Many libraries make them available.

20. **Science Citation Index**. Vol. 1- . Philadelphia, Pa.: Institute for Scientific Information, 1964- . ISSN 0036-827X.

A citation index provides information on who cited a certain book or article and where. It is designed to exploit the subject relationship between a scientific work (mostly articles, but also books) and the references or citations it contains to buttress its argumentation. Thus, with a relevant citation, the user can search the *Science Citation Index* to locate articles on the same subject (articles citing the original reference), without using an index term or a keyword. This is a way of doing a traditional literature search from the references in one article to the references in another article and so on, but instead of moving backward in time, one moves forward, searching all years subsequent to the publication of the original reference.

The *Science Citation Index* now consists of four major parts:

Citation Index: This is the entry point for a citation search. It is an alphabetical author index to the references that are cited in about 3,300 basic science and technology journals, with heavy emphasis on the biomedical sciences. Under each cited author's name there is a chronological listing of who referred to the original article and where. Because the actual article titles are omitted from this information, it is necessary to consult the *Source Index* to obtain complete information on the citing article.

Source Index: This is an author list of articles in the 3,300 basic science and technology journals covered. It indexes the citing authors for each year. The Institute for Scientific Information then indexes the references in these articles, arranges them in alphabetical order by cited authors, and produces the *Citation Index* mentioned above.

Permuterm Subject Index: This index provides access by title keywords. Every significant word in the title of a paper is paired once with every other significant word. This is very different from the KWIC, or keyword-in-context index in *Biological Abstracts*, which indexes keywords in the context of adjacent words. In the *Permuterm Subject Index* the arrangement is by primary term, and within that by co-term. The user is referred to the author of a paper in the *Source Index* and there retrieves complete information about the reference.

Corporate Index: This index has a geographic section and an organizations section. In the geographic section, items represented in the *Source Index* are arranged alphabetically by state and city for U.S. entries, and following that by country and city for foreign entries. The organization section simply indicates where in the geographic section a particular institution can be found. For complete information on articles in the geographic section, consult the *Source Index*. The *Corporate Index* is useful for finding out what kind of research is being done by a particular institution.

Guide and List of Periodicals Indexed: A complete guide on how to use *SCI* and a "List of Source Publications" appears with the *Source Index*. It is also issued as a separate publication and includes a publishers' address directory.

Comments: The *SCI* has so many virtues that it is best to maintain a sense of perspective and bear in mind that as seductive as it is, it indexes only 26 or so nutrition journals and about 40 food science and technology journals. On the other hand, if the information sought is likely to be scattered throughout the biomedical literature, or if there are problems with indexing terminology, the *SCI* can be helpful.

SCI invites imaginative approaches to literature searching. If a key reference is not available, the user should consult the *Permuterm Subject Index* and the *Source Index* to locate a reference, then use the *Citation Index* to determine where it was cited. Cycling is another way to maximize the use of this index. The user locates a known reference in the *Citation Index*, determines where it has been cited, and then uses the bibliographies of the citing papers as additional entry points. (See figure 2.)

As of 1982, *SCI* has greatly curtailed its indexing of books. It retains coverage of 250 important monographic series. Books are now covered in a separate index, *Index to Scientific and Technical Proceedings and Books* (ISI/ISTP&B), available in printed form and online.

DOING A CITATION SEARCH IN SCIENCE CITATION INDEX

1) Start with a known reference on the subject

The American Journal of Clinical Nutrition
36: NOVEMBER 1982 pp986–1013

Calcium nutrition and bone health in the elderly[1]

Robert P Heaney,[2] MD, JC Gallagher,[3] MD, CC Johnston,[4] MD, Robert Neer,[5] MD, A Michael Parfitt,[6] MB, BChir, and G Donald Whedon,[7] MD

Adult calcium intake

Calcium intake in the United States has been stu... ...tensively for the ...t 25 yr. Nor... ...blic Healt...

and the FCS data. Males have both higher intakes and a broader range of intakes than do females, with 60 to 70% exhibiting intakes on an... ... day above th... ...mended ... (RD... ...om

2) Use the Citation Index to locate articles citing this reference

Cited Author

HEANEY RP					
62 AM J MED 33 188					
MAYNARD FM	ARCH PHYS M		67	41	86
MCDONALD R	ACS SYMP S	R	294	87	86
STEPANIA.PC	AVIAT SP EN		57	174	86
65 AM J MED 39 877					
NORDIN BEC	CLIN ORTHOP			181	85
73 BIOL MINERALIZATION 329					
CHARLES P	J CLIN INV		76	2254	85

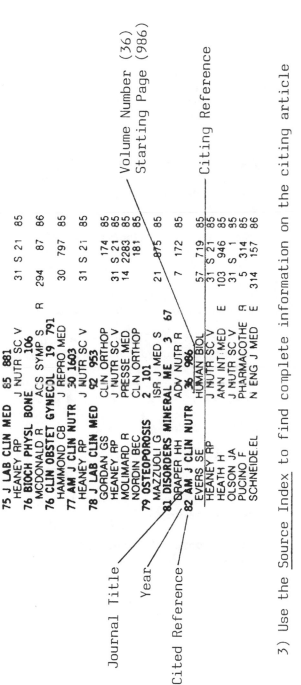

3) Use the Source Index to find complete information on the citing article

Fig. 2. Reprinted with permission from the *Science Citation Index*®. 1986 Annual. Copyright © 1985 by the Institute for Scientific Information® (Philadelphia, PA, USA) and with permission from *American Journal of Clinical Nutrition*, © 1982 American Society for Clinical Nutrition.

SELECTING AN
INDEXING/ABSTRACTING SERVICE

The indexing/abstracting service chosen will depend on the subject searched and the type of material likely to contain the needed information. First, it is necessary to categorize the search by broad subject and examine specific sources that cover the subject.

If the subject is:	Use:
nutrition science generally	*Nutrition Abstracts and Reviews, Index Medicus, Food and Nutrition Quarterly Index, Chemical Abstracts, Biological Abstracts*
biochemistry	*Chemical Abstracts, Biological Abstracts, Index Medicus, Nutrition Abstracts and Reviews*
dietetics	*Index Medicus, Nutrition Abstracts and Reviews, Hospital Literature Index*
food science and technology	*Food Science and Technology Abstracts, Chemical Abstracts, Biological Abstracts, Bibliography of Agriculture*
analytical methods	*Analytical Abstracts, Chemical Abstracts*
food chemistry	*Chemical Abstracts*
food composition	*Food Science and Technology Abstracts, Chemical Abstracts, Agrindex*
food microbiology	*Food Science and Technology Abstracts, Biological Abstracts*
health related	*Index Medicus, Nutrition Abstracts and Reviews*
social or behavioral	*Psychological Abstracts, Social Sciences Citation Index, Nutrition Planning, Sociological Abstracts*
economics	*World Agricultural Economics and Rural Sociology Abstracts*
education related	*Food and Nutrition Quarterly Index, Current Index to Journals in Education, Resources in Education, Nutrition Abstracts and Reviews*

food service   *Food and Nutrition Quarterly Index, Bibliography of Hotel and Restaurant Administration, Bibliography of Agriculture, Hospital Literature Index*

Next, consider the kind of literature or material most likely to contain information on the subject and determine if the above sources cover this type of material:

research journals

conference publications

practice-oriented materials

books

audiovisual materials

review articles

foreign literature

standards

patents

industry-based trade periodicals

popular magazines and newsletters

government publications

Other points to consider:

1. How extensive is the coverage of the subject? Is it central or peripheral?

2. Does it cover the period of time you need to search?

3. Is indexing terminology adequate to retrieve material on the subject?

4. Is indexing terminology in the field well or poorly defined?

STEPS IN USING
AN ABSTRACTING SERVICE

1. Read the directions for use included in the publication.

2. Use available vocabulary or terminology lists, such as the *Index Guide* to *Chemical Abstracts* to locate terms used to index the subject.

3. Start with the most recent cumulated index or volume and work back, saving the most recent issues for last.

4. Locate the appropriate subject alphabetically in the cumulated index. Sometimes cumulated indexes appear every six months, sometimes once a year. If they are not too bulky, these indexes are bound into the back of the volume containing the individual issues indexed. If they are bulky, they are usually bound separately.

5. Scan entries listed under the subject for relevant items.

6. Copy numbers of relevant references.

7. Follow up abstract numbers in monthly (semi-monthly or weekly) issues. Most likely, these issues are already bound into one volume and abstract numbers are arranged sequentially from issue to issue. Very often the spine of a bound volume indicates the numbers it contains.

8. Accurately copy the full citation on cards, or simply photocopy the page and cut apart if that seems more convenient. The citation usually consists of the following:

   author or authors

   title of article

   periodical or journal abbreviation or title

   volume number of periodical

   issue number within that volume

   month or date

   year

   pages

   source of reference (e.g., Biol. Abst. v.82 #16054)

9. If the periodical title is given in abbreviated form, locate the full title by using the list of periodicals published with or in the abstracting service.

10. To determine if the library has the title, locate the periodical title in the library's list of current periodicals, in the online catalog, in the microfilm or microfiche catalog, or in the card catalog. Ask a librarian which source is most likely.

11. Carefully copy down the location and/or call number for the periodical and check the stacks for the item.

STEPS IN USING *INDEX MEDICUS*

1. Read directions for use.

2. Use *MeSH* to locate correct subject term.

3. Locate subject term in the *Subject Index*.

4. Scan topical subheadings and titles to find relevant articles.

5. Accurately copy down full citation or photocopy, as outlined in step 8 above. Note that in *Index Medicus* title is given first.

6. Identify periodical abbreviation in *Journals Indexed in Index Medicus*.

7. Follow steps 10 and 11 above to locate the item in the library.

IDENTIFYING PERIODICAL ABBREVIATIONS

Often it will be necessary to identify abbreviated periodical titles from another source because it is difficult or impossible to locate abbreviated titles in a library periodicals list or catalog. The following periodical lists are especially useful in identifying periodical abbreviations in nutrition, dietetics, and food science:

21. Alkire, Leland G., comp. **Periodical Title Abbreviations: Covering Periodical Title Abbreviations in Science, the Social Sciences, the Humanities, Law, Medicine, Religion, Library Science, Engineering, Education, Business, Art, and Many Other Fields**. 5th ed. Detroit: Gale Research, 1986. 2v. ISBN 0810305313 (vol. 1); 0810305321 (vol. 2).
Kept up-to-date by annual supplement: *New Periodical Title Abbreviations*. This edition has been expanded to include approximately 80,000 periodical title abbreviations and periodicals. A useful source for decoding abbreviated periodical citations. Volume 1 lists periodicals by abbreviation. Volume 2 lists periodicals by title, with abbreviations given.

22. American Chemical Society. Chemical Abstracts Service. **Chemical Abstracts Service Source Index**. Columbus, Ohio: American Chemical Society, 1975- . quinquennial. ISSN 0001-0634.
This list is also called *CASSI*. It is kept up-to-date by quarterly supplements which are cumulated annually. This is now one of the most extensive periodicals lists available.

23. BioSciences Information Service of Biological Abstracts. **Serial Sources for the BIOSIS Data Base**. Philadelphia, Pa.: BioSciences Information Service, 1978- . annual. ISSN 0162-2048.
Serial Sources continues *BIOSIS List of Serials with Coden, Title Abbreviations, New, Changed and Ceased Titles*. Useful for all pure and applied biological science fields including food science and nutrition.

24. United States. National Library of Medicine. **Index of National Library of Medicine Serial Titles**. 1st ed.- . Bethesda, Md.: National Library of Medicine, 1972- . annual. ISSN 0162-6639.
This is a keyword listing of current NLM periodicals.

This chapter has been designed to acquaint the user with the major interdisciplinary indexing/abstracting services available in food and nutrition and to provide general instructions on how to use them. Information on more specialized indexing/abstracting services is provided in sections pertaining to specific topics.

SELECTED REFERENCES

Beatty, William K. "Libraries and How to Use Them." In *Coping with the Biomedical Literature*, Kenneth S. Warren, ed., 199-225. New York: Praeger, 1981. ISBN 0030570360. (Explains how to use *Index Medicus*.)

Bottle, R. T., ed. *Use of Chemical Literature*. 3rd ed. London, Boston: Butterworths, 1979. 306p. ISBN 0408384522.

Cummings, Martin M. "The National Library of Medicine." In *Coping with the Biomedical Literature*, Kenneth S. Warren, ed., 161-81. New York: Praeger, 1981. ISBN 0030570360.

Davis, Elisabeth B. *Using Biological Literature: A Practical Guide*. New York: Marcel Dekker, 1981. 286p. ISBN 0824713745.

Garfield, Eugene. *Citation Indexing, Its Theory and Application in Science, Technology, and Humanities*. New York: Wiley, 1979; repr., Philadelphia, Pa.: ISI Press, 1983. 274p. ISBN 0471025593.

Garfield, Eugene. "How to Use Science Citation Index." In *Essays of an Information Scientist*, Eugene Garfield, vol. 6, 53-57. Philadelphia, Pa.: ISI Press, 1984. ISBN 0894950320.

Garfield, Eugene. "The Institute for Scientific Information." In *Coping with the Biomedical Literature*, Kenneth S. Warren, ed., 183-98. New York, Praeger, 1981. ISBN 0030570360.

Kirk, Thomas G. *Library Research Guide to Biology: Illustrated Search Strategy*. Ann Arbor, Mich.: Pierian Press, 1978. 79p. ISBN 087650098X.

Poyer, R. K. "Journal Article Overlap among Index Medicus, Biological Abstracts and Chemical Abstracts." *Bulletin of the Medical Library Association* 72 (1984): 353-57.

Skolnik, Herman. *The Literature Matrix of Chemistry*. New York: Wiley, 1982. 297p. ISBN 0471495453.

Smith, Roger C., W. Malcolm Reid, and Arlene E. Luchsinger. *Smith's Guide to the Literature of the Life Sciences*. 9th ed. Minneapolis, Minn.: Burgess Publishing Co., 1980. 223p. ISBN 0808735764.

Strickland-Hodge, Barry. *How to Use Index Medicus and Excerpta Medica*. Brookfield, Vt.: Gower, 1986. 60p. ISBN 0566035324.

5
Letting a Computer Do the Work
Online Databases

This chapter provides background information on online searching and discusses databases relevant to more than one of the major topics discussed in this book. For a description of the more specialized databases, consult chapters on the individual topics. This section is intended as a brief introduction to principles of online searching that will enable the user to be more successful in negotiating a search request. It is not intended to turn the user into an online searcher.

Online databases are made available to libraries through commercial database vendors or directly from the indexing/abstracting services producing them. The major database vendors in the United States are DIALOG Information Services, Inc. (Palo Alto, Calif.), SDC Information Services (Santa Monica, Calif.), and BRS (Latham, N.Y.). The National Library of Medicine is both a producer and a major vendor of MEDLINE and other databases.

Almost all indexing/abstracting services have their computer-searchable online counterparts, though these databases often have different names from the printed versions. A few databases have no printed equivalent.

Generally, online databases are structured to parallel the printed indexing/abstracting services, but usually many more elements are searchable. Even databases with structured indexing vocabularies, for instance, allow the option of searching by text words from a title or abstract in addition to the officially used vocabulary. In addition, the subject category codes or numbers used in the arrangement of the printed product are usually searchable, as are author names and language codes for the language of publication.

Before requesting a search, consider whether it is truly cost-effective and less time consuming than manual searching. Whether the search is cost-effective depends on the complexity of the search strategy and the number of years searched. For example, a simple single-term search for a period of three to four years in *Index Medicus* is faster than a computer search—if pages from *Index Medicus* are simply photocopied. To have a computer search done a user needs to fill out a request form, discuss the information needed with the searcher, wait for the search to be done, and pick it up and pay for it. Even if the cost is reasonable, it is probably at least 10 to 15 times higher than photocopying.

HOW ONLINE SEARCHES ARE DONE

The process of online searching involves searching the database for any term, usually assigned subject terms, categories, or words from the title or abstract, creating sets of references with the retrieval, and manipulating these sets of references by the use of the logical connectors (also called Boolean operators) *and*, *or*, and *and not*, to create new sets.

This chapter uses MEDLINE to illustrate how a search works, but the basic logic of the search applies to all online databases. The topic searched is dietary calcium and hypertension.

The searcher formulates the search, deciding on a specific search strategy which will retrieve the desired citations. This includes the selection of appropriate subject *MeSH* terms from the *Medical Subject Headings* list, and how these are to be logically connected to achieve the desired results. The searcher sits down at a computer terminal or a microcomputer, dials the local Telenet or Tymnet number, is connected to the National Library of Medicine Computer, and selects a particular file of references. Since recent information is desired, the file selected is MEDLINE, which contains the most current references found in *Index Medicus* as well as some that have not yet been printed in this index.

Imagine a large rectangular box containing the entire universe of current references to the medical literature. Searches are done by pulling sets of references out of this box, setting them aside, and manipulating them with the logical connectors *and*, *or*, and *and not*.

Example No. 1

The searcher enters the universe of citations and instructs the computer to retrieve all citations on the subject of dietary calcium. The system responds that there are 276 citations in the database. These are held aside as Set Number 1, also called Search Statement Number 1.

The searcher then searches this same "box" of citations for references on hypertension. The system responds that there are 9,602 items in the database dealing with this subject. These are held aside as Set Number 2. (See figure 3a.)

Example No. 1

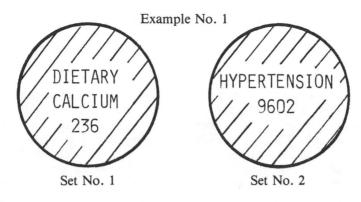

Set No. 1   Set No. 2

Fig. 3a.

The searcher then specifies that he or she wants only citations dealing with both of these subjects by linking them together with the logical connector *and*. This operation is phrased very simply as "1 and 2," and it produces a third set of citations in which each reference deals with both dietary calcium and hypertension—Set Number 3. This set contains only 32 citations; however, most of them will deal directly with the subject. The use of the logical *and* greatly reduced the retrieval, and as a general rule, the more *ands* are used, the fewer citations are retrieved. As demonstrated in figure 3b, the area where the circles (sets) intersect is the area of overlap between the two sets of references and represents Set Number 3, the set dealing with both dietary calcium and hypertension.

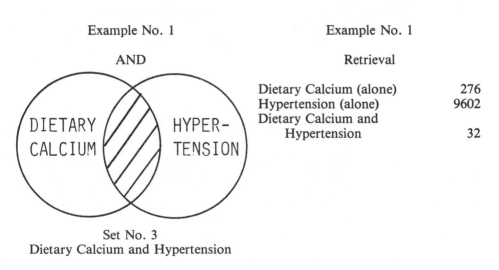

Example No. 1

AND

Set No. 3
Dietary Calcium and Hypertension

Fig. 3b.

Example No. 1

Retrieval

Dietary Calcium (alone)	276
Hypertension (alone)	9602
Dietary Calcium and Hypertension	32

Example No. 2

The logical connector *or*, on the other hand, increases retrieval. Unless the items linked are carefully chosen, the search can result in far too many items being retrieved. In the above search there are 276 citations on dietary calcium, but if the searcher wants to expand the above search to include literature on milk intake as related to hypertension, the logical *or* can be used to create a set of references that have to do with either dietary calcium or milk. There are 1,492 references on milk. The logical *or* greatly increased the number of citations retrieved. It is important to note, however, that the set dealing with either dietary calcium or milk is smaller than the sum of the two individual sets. This is because some references deal with both of these subjects and these duplicate citations are eliminated in the set that has been linked by *or*. Figure 4 shows this small area of overlap in the center.

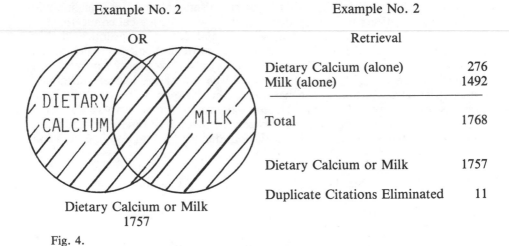

Example No. 2

OR

Dietary Calcium or Milk
1757

Fig. 4.

Example No. 2

Retrieval

Dietary Calcium (alone)	276
Milk (alone)	1492
Total	1768
Dietary Calcium or Milk	1757
Duplicate Citations Eliminated	11

Example No. 3

The searcher is interested in dietary calcium, but wants to exclude references that also deal with sodium. In MEDLINE the searcher uses the *and not* connector to create a set of references which deal with dietary calcium, but not sodium. In other online search systems, this connector is often just *not*. A diagram of the search is presented in figure 5. Note that, as before, the shaded area represents the desired retrieval. The area where the circles (sets) intersect represents the citations which have to do with both dietary calcium and sodium. These overlapping citations are eliminated from the final set because they deal with both subjects and the searcher has instructed the system to eliminate any references dealing with sodium. Knowledgeable searchers do not use the *and not* connector often because it eliminates desirable citations just because they also happen to contain some material on the undesirable subject. In other words, it takes a bite out of the apple. The reasoning is usually that it is better to get a few less pertinent citations than to eliminate some that could be important, leaving the apple intact.

Example No. 3

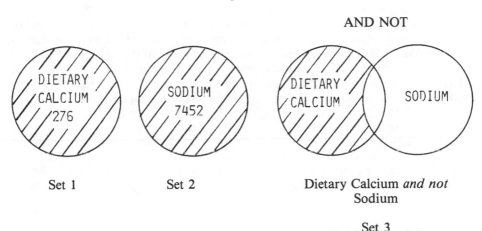

Set 1   Set 2   Dietary Calcium *and not* Sodium

Set 3

Example No. 3

Retrieval

Dietary Calcium (alone)   276
Sodium (alone)   7452
Dietary Calcium *and not* Sodium   267
Citations Lost by *and not*   9

Fig. 5.

GENERAL DATABASES IN FOOD AND NUTRITION

MEDLARS: The NLM Databases

The acronym MEDLARS stands for Medical Literature Analysis and Retrieval System, a computerized indexing and retrieval system for the health sciences literature available from the National Library of Medicine at Bethesda, Maryland. The system now consists of a number of databases with some files containing data rather than bibliographic references.

Searches of these databases are available through a network of 1,900 MEDLINE search centers in university and medical libraries, medical schools, government agencies, and businesses throughout the country. Of the individual databases in the system, the following are most useful for topics dealing with food and nutrition:

25. MEDLINE

The acronym MEDLINE stands for MEDLARS online. It includes references from approximately 3,200 current journals from about 70 countries in all fields of biomedicine. The database usually includes the current year and the two or three preceding years. MEDLINE and its backfiles now contain about 5,000,000 citations which can be searched online back to 1966. The MEDLINE database corresponds to the following printed indexes: *Index Medicus, Index to Dental Literature,* and *International Nursing Index.* In contrast to these printed indexes, MEDLINE includes abstracts for roughly half of the citations. The most recent month of the MEDLINE database is duplicated in a separate file called SDILINE. This is specifically designed for monthly searches to keep researchers and practitioners abreast of the most recent literature on a topic.

In addition to the more than 14,000 subject terms found in *Medical Subject Headings (MeSH)*, references in the database can be retrieved by text words, author, contract number, document type, journal title, language, year of publication, *Chemical Abstracts* registry numbers, and "check tags" such as animal or human, female or male, and age groups. These check tags allow a searcher to limit retrieval specifically to animal or human studies, by age groups from birth to the age of 65 or over, and by sex.

26. BIOETHICSLINE

This database is the online equivalent of the *Bibliography of Bioethics* produced by the Center for Bioethics, Kennedy Institute of Ethics, Georgetown University, Washington, D.C. It contains over 19,000 citations dealing with ethical questions relating to the biological and health sciences.

27. CANCERLIT

Formerly called CANCERLINE, this database is sponsored by the National Cancer Institute and contains over 500,000 references with abstracts dealing with all aspects of cancer. It covers over 3,000 domestic and foreign journals, books, conference proceedings, and other publications.

28. CATLINE

This database is the online version of the catalog of the National Library of Medicine. It provides cataloging information on books and periodicals in the health sciences. It can be searched like any library catalog to locate books by subject.

29. HEALTH PLANNING & ADMIN

This file is a database of over 328,000 citations on the management of health care facilities, primarily hospitals. It is produced by the National Library of Medicine in cooperation with the American Hospital Association and corresponds to *Hospital Literature Index*, with the addition of selected citations from MEDLINE. This is a useful database for topics such as hospital food and dietetic services.

30. HISTLINE

This history of medicine database consists of selected citations from MEDLINE with supplementary material in the form of books and journals outside the medical sciences. This is a useful database for subjects related to the history of diet and nutrition. Its printed equivalent is *Bibliography of the History of Medicine.*

31. TOXLINE

A database of over 1.6 million references to human and animal toxicity studies, TOXLINE citations with abstracts are taken from five major indexing/abstracting services in the sciences. TOXLINE is useful for searches related to the toxicity of food components or additives.

GENERAL DATABASES
IN RELATED FIELDS

32. AGRICOLA

Produced by the National Agricultural Library, this database consists of the *Bibliography of Agriculture* and the catalog of the National Agricultural Library. Food and nutrition materials are indexed at the Food and Nutrition Information Center at NAL. Although much of the AGRICOLA file deals directly or indirectly with food or agricultural commodities, indexing of food science and technology materials is limited to primary processing. The material indexed by FNIC deals chiefly with human nutrition, diet and disease, food service, nutrition education, domestic food programs, food policy, and home economics. The material indexed by FNIC includes abstracts, whereas other citations in the database do not. This database provides extensive coverage of the agricultural literature, regularly indexing some 4,000 journals as well as books, pamphlets, conference publications, and USDA and FAO publications. Approximately 120,000 new records are added to a database of over 2,000,000 references each year. The National Agricultural Library is paring its list of indexed periodicals to eliminate duplicate coverage of foreign materials also indexed in *Agrindex* and the AGRIS INTERNATIONAL database.

In addition to the text words and added index terms, over 30 elements are searchable, including publication type, subject category code, language, etc. This varies with the type of publication. From 1985 citations are indexed using the *CAB Thesaurus*, the same vocabulary list used to index material for all of the abstracting services published by CAB International. Among these are *Nutrition Abstracts and Reviews* and *Dairy Science Abstracts.*

33. AGRIS INTERNATIONAL

This file is the online equivalent of *Agrindex*, an international index to information dealing with all aspects of food and agriculture. All materials covered originate outside the United States. They are collected and indexed by 130 national and multinational centers throughout the world. Although the coverage of these fields is not extensive, it indexes materials on human nutrition, food science, and food composition. It is particularly strong in materials relating to the developing countries. Only a small number of the records in the database are accompanied by abstracts. AGRIS INTERNATIONAL currently contains over 850,000 citations, with roughly 3,000 to 4,000 items added each month. This database is now available in the United States through DIALOG Information Services, Inc.

34. BIOSIS Previews

This database corresponds to *Biological Abstracts* and *Biological Abstracts: RRM*. About 290,000 abstracts from over 9,000 journals and other types of publications are added annually to a database of over 4,500,000 records. Like *Biological Abstracts* and *Biological Abstracts: RRM*, BIOSIS Previews provides extensive coverage of the nutrition and food science literature. In addition to the indexing found in these printed products, BIOSIS Previews is searchable by concept codes representing broad subjects, journal name, language, and any combination of search elements found in the printed or online version.

35. CA Search

This database of over 7,000,000 records corresponds to weekly issues of *Chemical Abstracts*, its semi-annual cumulated indexes, and the *CA Index Guide*. In addition to all of the access points for manual searching (authors, general subjects, chemical substances, molecular formulas, and patent numbers), there are over 20 types of access points including the *Chemical Abstracts* registry numbers, journal title, and language.

36. SCISEARCH

Produced by the Institute for Scientific Information, SCISEARCH covers the whole spectrum of scientific and technical literature, but is particularly strong in the biomedical sciences. The database contains over 6,500,000 references and covers about 3,300 major scientific and technical periodicals, with roughly 58,000 items added each year. This file corresponds roughly to the *Science Citation Index* and the *Current Contents* current awareness services. It provides author and keyword access to articles in the source journals. It also provides citation searching by linking cited authors and articles and source journal citations.

END USER SEARCHING

The increased use of microcomputers by health professionals, faculty, and students is beginning to shift online searching from the library to the end user. More and more library users will use their microcomputers to do searches for themselves and librarians increasingly will act as consultants and perhaps even as trainers.

Thanks to a number of recent developments, end user searching is easier and cheaper than ever before. Two major database vendors now entice end users by offering cheaper after-hours rates. DIALOG Information Services, Inc., makes its most popular databases available in its Knowledge Index. BRS has initiated a similar service called BRS After Dark. Both of these services include MEDLINE, BIOSIS Previews, and AGRICOLA. Knowledge Index also includes CAB Abstracts, the file containing *Nutrition Abstracts and Reviews*. In addition to its "after hours only" services, BRS has initiated BRS/BRKTHRU, another service intended for the end user, available day or night. Though daytime rates are standard and nighttime rates are somewhat higher than for BRS After Dark, BRS/BRKTHRU provides access to more databases. For information and application forms, write to:

DIALOG Information Services, Inc.   BRS
3460 Hillside Avenue   1200 Route 7
Palo Alto, CA 94304   Latham, NY 12110

Because these services are aimed specifically at the end user, rather than the library market, search commands are simplified versions of the protocols used by librarians.

Another development which makes it easier for the user to do his or her own searching is the availability of front-end programs such as In-Search, Sci-Mate, and DIALOGLINK, which provide a simplified interface with the online system. In-Search was designed to be used with the DIALOG system. DIALOGLINK, though developed by DIALOG Information Services, can be used to search in other systems. The Sci-Mate Universal Online Searcher, produced by the Institute for Scientific Information in Philadelphia, Pennsylvania, interfaces with the MEDLARS databases, DIALOG, SDC, and BRS. Another part of the program, the Personal Data Manager, is available separately and manages files of bibliographic citations downloaded by the Universal Online Searcher or input locally. This program enables one to maintain personal bibliographic databases which can then be searched using the logical connectors or Boolean operators discussed earlier in this chapter. Downloading can be a sticky issue because databases are protected by copyright law just like books and other printed materials. Many database producers allow the user to download a small number of references for personal use. Others do not allow downloading without permission. Be sure to check with the database vendor or producer.

Until recently it was impossible for a library user to receive an ID number to search the MEDLARS databases without at least a five-day training program. Training is no longer required, but it is recommended. Shorter training programs specifically aimed at the end user are now being offered in some localities. Costs for searching are low. They are based on online connect time, telecommunication costs, and an algorithm for how much work the NLM computer does during a search.

Two recent developments have made life easier for the end user who wants to search MEDLINE. One is the development of PaperChase, a commercial search service using a menu-driven approach to searching MEDLINE (PaperChase, Beth Israel Hospital, 330 Brookline Avenue, Boston, MA 02215). Another is the debut of Grateful Med, the National Library of Medicine's own program for end user searching. It enables the search to be formulated offline on a single screen. The program includes a telecommunications package which dials NLM, does the search, and downloads it. After checking the retrieval and noting the subject terms assigned to the citations, the user may run the search again to increase or decrease retrieval.

There are advantages to end user searching. The user knows better than anyone else what information is needed, so nothing gets lost in conveying the exact nature of a subject to a librarian. The search can be done at the user's convenience, not the librarian's. And finally doing some online searching is bound to make the individual a more sophisticated user of the service, better able to analyze and phrase a search request when someone else does the searching.

But there are some disadvantages. The act of filling out a search request often helps one think through the subject more carefully. Also, discussing it with a librarian and taking advantage of his or her experience can help clarify what needs to be done. What is more, the librarian frequently knows from experience when a search request is phrased in terms that are too general or too specific. The books and articles below will help those who want to get started doing online searches for themselves.

SELECTED REFERENCES

Borgman, Christine L., Dineh Moghdam, and Patti K. Corbett. *Effective Online Searching: A Basic Text.* New York: Marcel Dekker, 1984. 201p. ISBN 0824771427.

Casbon, Susan. "Online Searching with a Microcomputer—Getting Started." *Online* 7 (November 1983): 42-46.

Feinglos, Susan J. *MEDLINE, a Basic Guide to Searching.* Chicago: Medical Library Association, 1985. 138p. (MLA Information Series). ISBN 0912176199.

Fenichel, Carol Hansen. "Using a Microcomputer to Communicate: Part I: The Basics." *Microcomputers for Information Management* 2 (April 1985): 59-76.

Frank, Robyn C. "Information Resources for Food and Human Nutrition." *Journal of the American Dietetic Association* 80 (1982): 344-49.

Garfield, Eugene. "Introducing Sci-Mate—A Menu-Driven Microcomputer Software Package for Online and Offline Information Retrieval. Part 2: The Sci-Mate Universal Online Searcher." In *Essays of an Information Scientist,* Eugene Garfield, vol. 6, 96-105. Philadelphia, Pa.: ISI Press, 1984. ISBN 0894950320.

Goldmann, Nahum. *Online Research and Retrieval with Micro-computers.* Blue Ridge Summit, Pa.: Tab Books, 1985. 193p. ISBN 083061947X.

Hawkins, Donald T., and Louise R. Levy. "Front End Software for Online Database Searching. Part 1." *Online* 9 (November 1985): 30-37.

Hawkins, Donald T., and Louise R. Levy. "Front End Software for Online Database Searching. Part 2: The Market Place." *Online* 10 (January 1986): 33-38.

Hawkins, Donald T., and Louise R. Levy. "Front End Software for Online Database Searching. Part 3: Product Selection Chart and Bibliography." *Online* 10 (May 1986): 49-58.

Haynes, R. B., et al. "Computer Searching the Medical Literature: An Evaluation of MEDLINE Searching Systems." *Annals of Internal Medicine* 103 (1985): 812-16.

Homan, J. Michael. "End-User Information Utilities in the Health Sciences." *Bulletin of the Medical Library Association* 74 (January 1986): 31-35.

Janke, Richard V. "Online after Six: End User Searching Comes of Age." *Online* 8 (November 1984): 15-29.

Jeremy, Joan Hewes. "Dialog: The Ultimate On-Line Library." *PC World* 1 (September 1983): 74-88.

Johnson, Diane E. P., and Susan Barnes. *Introduction to Online Computer Searching*. rev. ed. Los Angeles, Calif.: UCLA Biomedical Library, 1986. 25p.

Lisanti, Suzana. "The On-Line Search." *Byte* 9 (December 1984): 215-30.

Newlin, Barbara. *Answers Online: Your Guide to Informational Data Bases*. Berkeley, Calif.: Osborne/McGraw-Hill, 1985. 373p. ISBN 0881341363.

Ojala, Marydee. "End User Searching and Its Implications for Librarians." *Special Libraries* 76 (Spring 1985): 93-99.

Stout, Catheryne, and Thomas Marcinko. "Sci-Mate: A Menu Driven Universal Online Searcher and Personal Data Manager." *Online* 7 (September 1983): 112-16.

Tenopir, Carol. "Database Access Software." *Library Journal* 109 (1 October 1984): 1828-29.

Tenopir, Carol. "Online Searching with a Microcomputer." *Library Journal* 110 (15 March 1985): 42-43.

6
Using a Research Library

As in any other field, librarians and libraries have their own special language. Because librarians are so immersed in it, they often forget that library users don't speak it. This chapter contains most of the basic explanations for library use and is a foundation on which to build.

Research libraries are organized according to certain common patterns. Materials can be housed centrally in one building or scattered in smaller branch or departmental libraries. When there is a central library that houses most of the library's collections, services to users are frequently decentralized. There may be separate reference departments for the humanities, social sciences, and science and technology. Materials in science and technology are frequently segregated because they are more easily serviced by librarians who have specialized expertise. Documents of national and international governmental agencies are frequently housed in separate government documents collections. Other collections commonly segregated are special subject collections or collections focusing on a special geographic area.

Another common organizational pattern is to have a main library consisting primarily of humanities and social sciences materials with separate science and technology and/or biomedical libraries. As a general rule, medical and law libraries are separate. Some universities also have separate undergraduate libraries. However, the amount of scientific and technical material housed in undergraduate libraries is generally limited.

In the largest academic libraries, materials tend to be more scattered. There may be numerous departmental or branch libraries. Such libraries may be difficult to use because materials on a subject may be scattered among several buildings. The current trend is for more centralization and consolidation of small branch libraries to form larger units. For instance, physics, chemistry, mathematics, and engineering may be combined to form a physical science and engineering library or biology, medicine, public health, and nursing may be combined to form a biomedical library.

An unfamiliar library can be a perplexing place for anyone, including librarians not familiar with that institution. While there are some general principles on how materials are arranged, there are countless local idiosyncracies which can cause the new user problems. For instance, on what basis are decisions made on what is housed in a science library, a biomedical, or a health sciences library? If materials are divided between a main library and an undergraduate library, what types of materials are likely to be in each? By what classification system(s) are materials arranged? What hours are reference librarians available to assist patrons? What types of materials can be borrowed and for how long? Which collection or library has most of the nutrition and food science materials? Knowing the answers to the above questions will save time, enable the user to find more material, and make anyone a more efficient library user.

CLASSIFICATION SYSTEMS

It is common for medium- and large-sized academic libraries in the United States to use the Library of Congress Classification system. In general, this system is more suited to extensive collections and also greatly cuts down on the cost of processing new materials.

Health sciences libraries frequently use the National Library of Medicine Classification system for medical materials and another system, such as the Library of Congress Classification, for nonmedical materials. The National Library of Medicine Classification System uses the letters "QS"-"QZ" and "W." To avoid confusion, these are permanently excluded from the Library of Congress Classification system.

In the last three decades most academic libraries whose collections were cataloged in the Dewey Decimal System decided to convert to the Library of Congress system. Converting to the Library of Congress system, unfortunately, is a long-term endeavor requiring tremendous human and financial resources, and many libraries have been unable to carry it to completion. As a result, in some libraries older materials are still classed in Dewey, while newer materials are classed in the Library of Congress system.

The Library of Congress system is an alphanumeric classification scheme. There are 22 major classes, represented by letters of the alphabet. Within these 22 sequences there are further subject subdivisions by second letter and by number. It is unfortunate that in this system food science and nutrition materials are so widely scattered as to make access by browsing limited. These numbers reflect the broad scope of the field and remind us of its historical origins.

Figure 6 is an outline of the major classification numbers in the Library of Congress Classification system relating to food science and human nutrition.

Nutrition and Food Science in
the Library of Congress System

Q   Pure Science

QP	Physiology and Biochemistry
QP141-185.3	Nutrition and Metabolism
QP531-535	Minerals
QP551-562	Protein and Amino Acids
QP701-702	Carbohydrates
QP751-752	Lipids
QP771-772	Vitamins

R   Medicine

RA	Public Health
RA645.N87	Public Health Aspects of Nutrition
RC	Internal Medicine
RC620-632	Nutritional and Metabolic Diseases
RJ	Pediatrics
RJ53.D53	Diet Therapy for Infants and Children
RJ53.P37	Parenteral Nutrition for Infants and Children
RJ206-216	Nutrition and Feeding of Infants and Children
RJ360-400	Metabolic and Nutritional Diseases of Children and Infants
RK	Dentistry
RK281	Nutrition and Dentistry
RM	Therapeutics. Pharmacology
RM214-267	Diet Therapy and Special Diets

T   Technology and Engineering

TP	Chemical Technology
TP368-659	Food Processing and Manufacture
TS	Manufactures
TS1950-1981	Animal Products
TS2120-2159	Cereals and Grains. Milling Industry
TX341-641	Nutrition, Foods and Food Supply
TX645-840	Cookery

Fig. 6

RECORDS OF
BOOKS AND PERIODICALS

Unless there is some fairly easy and foolproof way to determine what books and periodical titles a particular library has, and what volumes or issues of periodicals have been received, even the most extensive collections of materials are impossible to use.

Libraries generally maintain extensive records that tell the staff and library users whether specific materials are in the collection. For information about books this record used to be the card catalog; but many institutions have found it too costly to maintain card catalogs. With library automation proceeding at a fairly steady pace, numerous institutions have ceased keeping up their card catalogs and are producing online catalogs that enable users to do their searching on computer terminals.

Some libraries have gone to computer-produced microfiche or microfilm catalogs (called COM or computer output microfilm catalogs) to serve as backups in case the online system is down or as interim measures before they are able to produce full-fledged online catalogs. Card or microfiche catalogs can be arranged in one alphabetical sequence A-Z. Such catalogs are called dictionary catalogs because the arrangement is similar to that of a dictionary. They can be divided into two or three alphabetical sequences — an author and title catalog with a separate subject catalog, or separate author, title, and subject catalogs. In the case of microfiche catalogs, there may be periodic updates before a completely new catalog is issued.

All this means that the days of the traditional card catalog are numbered. In many libraries they are not being maintained on a current basis. They are considered closed, rather than active, and therefore only serve as a valid record of older books and periodicals. In some cases, where cards for missing materials are not removed from the catalog, they may actually mislead the user into thinking that materials are available when they are not.

Since many libraries that are automating are actively working to convert records for older materials into machine-readable form, it is usually a good practice to check online or microfiche catalogs before checking the card catalog. Because catalogs are such basic finding tools, library users should familiarize themselves with the types available at a particular library and the periods or types of materials covered by each.

Card and microfiche catalogs provide essentially the same type of access to materials. Books are entered under authors (this includes organizations as well as individuals), titles, subjects, and series. Online catalogs have all these access points and much more. Most permit the user to search by keywords appearing in the titles of books. Some even allow author searches by individual words in the name of an organization, for instance, or individual words in subject headings consisting of more than one word. For example, the term *nutrition disorders* would be searchable under the word *nutrition* and under the word *disorders*.

Some online catalogs allow the user the flexibility of combining keywords, subject headings, or authors to retrieve single books on more than one subject, by more than one author, or any combination thereof. Limiting retrieval by date is another option available on some systems.

Whatever the type of catalog, medium- and large-sized libraries usually assign subject terms to describe the content of books and other materials from an enormous list published by the Library of Congress, the *Library of Congress Subject Headings* (*LCSH*), which is kept up-to-date by periodic supplements. Librarians and library users refer to this list when they need to know what specific terms to look under for material on a subject. These subject headings frequently do not correspond to the vocabulary used by specialists in the field, which changes rapidly. The *Library of Congress Subject Headings* tend to be more static. For instance, there is no subject heading specifically for nutrition assessment. Books on this subject may be entered under several different headings, including "Nutrition-Evaluation," "Nutrition Disorders," "Malnutrition-Diagnosis," or "Nutrition Surveys."

It is important to stress that the access to periodical titles provided by all types of catalogs is quite different from that provided for books. If periodicals appear in such catalogs, they are entered under title, issuing organization, and by subject of the entire periodical. For example, the *Journal of Nutrition* is entered under title, under "Nutrition-Periodicals," under "Diet-Periodicals," and under "American Institute of Nutrition" as issuing organization. *No entries for individual articles contained in issues of the periodical are made*, although separate entries may be made for supplements or special issues of periodicals on a selective basis.

RECORDS FOR PERIODICAL TITLES AND HOLDINGS

The fact that a library has some holdings of a given periodical title is often registered in the card, microfilm, microfiche, or online catalog. However, precisely what issues or volumes are held is generally not recorded there. There may be a separate list of periodical titles currently received in the library, in other words, a list of journals and other periodicals coming into the library either on a subscription basis or as gifts or exchanges.

This list may or may not duplicate the catalogs. Sometimes such lists are printed and sometimes they are produced on microfiche. These lists may or may not provide a record of which volumes or issues of a periodical the library has received. However, all libraries have behind-the-scenes records of such receipts. In some cases they are in or near periodical reading rooms and are available to the public. Sometimes, however, they are accessible only to the staff. Under the latter circumstances, library users should always ask librarians to check holdings for them if issues are not found in their proper location.

ARRANGEMENT OF MATERIALS

Reference Collections

Within a specific library or collection, books are arranged according to whatever classification system is used—usually the Library of Congress system. However, the user must be mindful of other ways of segregating groupings of materials. For example, materials which are labeled "reference" (frequently just "ref"), are segregated by use. They are materials which are frequently consulted for specific information and are generally not read from cover to cover like other books. For convenience, collections of reference materials are generally close to reference or information desks.

Large Format Materials

Another way of segregating materials is by size. To save space in stack areas, most libraries have special sections for large format books or periodicals called folios. This means that only a few shelves in the library need to be set at a height to accommodate the physically larger volumes.

Closed Shelves Materials

Every library has some materials that need securing. There may be a special rare books collection for very old and valuable materials, but many useful books that need securing are not particularly rare. They just need a little protection from the unscrupulous user. Most libraries have such areas. The user must request that materials from closed shelves areas be retrieved by a staff member.

Government Publications

Other types of materials that are frequently separated are publications of government agencies, particularly those from the U.S. government and the United Nations. U.S. government materials have traditionally been handled separately because they are usually arranged according to the Superintendent of Documents Classification system, which is by issuing agency. This is in contrast to other classification systems in which materials are arranged by subject.

Document materials are often excluded from card, microfiche, and online catalogs because they do not receive standard cataloging. It is best not to make assumptions; ask the librarian.

Microform Collections

The term *microforms* refers to all types of formats containing micro-images of printed material. It includes microfilm (transparent film on reels), microfiche (transparent film in sheets), and microcard or microprint (opaque cards or sheets). Collections of such materials are separate because there is no practical way of integrating them fully with print materials and because specialized equipment is required to read and duplicate them. Such collections are expanding rapidly as space becomes scarce in many libraries. They generally contain back-files of newspapers and periodicals as well as out-of-print materials and may include specialized collections such as the Human Relations Area Files and ERIC documents. The arrangement is generally in a numerical or alphabetical sequence. The materials may be recorded in the card, microfiche, or online catalogs, or in periodical lists or specialized lists of microform holdings.

Special Subject and Area Focus Collections

Medium- and large-sized libraries usually have many special collections of materials. Some focus on a specific subject, some on a particular geographic area, while others contain materials in specific languages. Many libraries have separate collections of state, local, or regional publications. Rare materials, manuscript collections, and valuable historical materials are frequently housed in separate collections.

Periodicals Collections

Many libraries have periodical rooms for general periodicals. Periodical rooms may contain only recent issues or they may contain full runs of periodicals. Sometimes periodicals are simply arranged alphabetically by title in a special section of the library or in a periodical room. Scientific and technical periodicals are usually found with the scientific and technical books. Some libraries give periodicals full cataloging, listing them by title, issuing organization, and subject (of the entire periodical) and they are assigned a unique number in whatever classification scheme is used. This makes it possible to arrange them on the shelves with books on the subject, a system preferred by many libraries with larger collections.

Most libraries provide some type of periodical display area for current issues of periodicals to make it easy for users to browse through new issues. Scientific, technical, and health science libraries or collections usually take special care to make these areas convenient and easy to use because they recognize that scientists and health professionals must browse to keep up with new literature.

SERVICES

Borrowing

It may seem too obvious to mention that most libraries allow patrons to borrow books. A few even allow very short-term borrowing of periodicals. However, there are some research libraries or special research collections which do not loan any of their materials. Materials marked reference generally do not circulate except by special arrangement. Usually brochures or pamphlets describing collections and services indicate what materials may be borrowed. Most questions relating to borrowing privileges (library cards, loan periods, recalls of books, and payment of fines) are handled by the circulation or loan desk. This department is entrusted with the very important function of keeping accurate records of the thousands of items that are out on loan, so that specific books can be accounted for or recalled when needed by another library user.

Reference Service

Most library users do not realize the extent to which reference librarians are prepared to assist them in locating or using materials. It is the job of the reference librarian to interpret library records of holdings to the user; to provide group or individual instruction in library use; to help students, faculty, and others use the materials available; to use the resources of the library to answer requests for specific information; to provide bibliographic assistance, such as helping users identify abbreviated periodical titles; to purchase new reference materials; and to suggest alternative sources of information when the required material is not available. Is it any wonder that reference librarians occasionally seem rushed? Still, a patron should never hesitate to ask for assistance, even if it is sometimes necessary to wait a moment to obtain the librarian's full attention. Keep in mind, though, that looking for information requires time and patience.

Interlibrary Loan

Not even the largest library has everything its users might need. And sometimes, even though library records indicate that a specific item is supposed to be available, it can be permanently missing from the library shelves.

Although it is frustrating to find that a book or journal is not available, there is hope in the form of interlibrary borrowing, usually called interlibrary loan. Any number of libraries in the country may have the needed item, but they will not loan it directly to an individual. They will loan it to a library for patron use. In the case of journal articles, photocopies are usually made. Charges incurred by the library in this process are generally passed on to the user. Depending on the distance the library must send to in order to locate the item and the backlog of requests at the fulfilling library, it may take several weeks to a month or more to provide the needed item.

ANGLO-AMERICAN CATALOGUING RULES

Cataloging that describes materials by stating the facts of publication so the identity of a specific item can be established is called descriptive cataloging. This is distinct from subject cataloging, which describes the content of the material by assigning subject terms and a subject classification number. Descriptive cataloging, however mystifying it might seem, is done according to a specific set of rules. In the United States, in Canada, and in the United Kingdom this set of rules is the *Anglo-American Cataloging Rules.*

A second edition of the *Anglo-American Cataloguing Rules* was finally implemented by the Library of Congress in 1982, and also necessarily by libraries using Library of Congress cataloging information. Some of the revisions in this edition were so far-reaching that it was viewed as a major disaster by the heads of library cataloging departments and processing operations.

What was so terrible about these changes and why do library users need to be concerned about them? The changes which affected libraries most were new rules for entering and formulating the names of persons, organizations, institutions, and government agencies. For example, under the old rules, material from the National Center for Health Statistics was entered under "U.S. National Center for Health Statistics." Under the new rules, it is entered directly under "National Center for Health Statistics (U.S.)."

Imagine the migraines across the country as heads of cataloging departments tried to assist library users by providing links from the old form of the name to the new form of the name and vice versa, so that someone looking in a card, microfiche, or microfilm catalog could locate all the books by a specific author or all of the conferences sponsored by an organization. Many libraries "closed off" their old catalogs and started new ones. Some libraries gave up on the card catalog altogether and went to online catalogs. Still others used computer output microfilm or microfiche (COM) catalogs as a stop-gap measure while working toward online systems.

Some heads of cataloging valiantly tried to provide *see also* references to alternative forms of the names and succeeded—for a while. In the meantime, backlogs of uncataloged materials reached gargantuan proportions and library users started to complain about the lack of availability of new materials. Some libraries gave up creating any kind of *see also* references to variant forms of names.

Slowly, libraries recovered, but quite a few library catalogs will never be the same again. As a result of these changes, library users should be cautious and avoid premature conclusions about the unavailability of materials. First, they should be sure they are checking in the right catalogs. For instance, if the library stopped adding new material to its card catalog in 1982, then a book published in 1983 is unlikely to be listed there. The user should check in whatever catalog lists newer materials. Also, it is always a good practice to check under all the permutations and variations of an organization's or agency's name or under the title and then head straight for the reference desk and ask a librarian to verify whether an item is available.

The changes in cataloging had a major impact on the way periodicals were treated. In the old system, journals that did not have distinctive titles, but were merely called the proceedings, bulletins, journals, or transactions of societies were cataloged under the name of the society or organization. The *Journal of the American Chemical Society* was listed under "American Chemical Society." *Proceedings of the Nutrition Society* was listed under "Nutrition Society," and so on. The new rules preserve the natural word order of the title as printed on the periodical itself. If the above titles were being cataloged today they would be entered under *Journal of the American Chemical Society* and under *Proceedings of the Nutrition Society*. The point is simply that they are *not* being cataloged today. Most libraries acquired them years ago, and as a result most libraries have listed them under the old form, whereas an analogous, but newly acquired title would be found under the new form. Library users must search under both forms to be sure they do not miss a title. A good rule of thumb is that if the periodical has the name of an organization appearing in the title, one should reverse the word order and look under both forms. To locate the *Journal of the American Dietetic Association*, for instance, look both under "Journal of the" and under "American Dietetic Association." And above all, never hestitate to ask questions.

To reiterate: large libraries are extremely complex. Not only are the catalogs and other records intricate, but just keeping track of millions of books and periodical issues, each addressed to a specific call number in the stacks, many in a perpetual state of flux—removed from the shelves and then reshelved—can be a monumental task. It is a minor miracle that most of the time books and periodicals are sitting in their rightful place.

The more a user learns about libraries in general and the idiosyncrasies of particular libraries, the more successful he or she is likely to be in locating specific materials or information. It is unfortunate that there are almost no books on using research libraries geared to the science user. Many of those in the list of references below are either too general or too specialized. Some are geared to the professional only. Nonetheless, there is material in all of them useful for specific purposes.

SELECTED REFERENCES

Carmel, Michael. *Medical Librarianship*. London: Library Association, 1981. 359p. ISBN 0853655022.

Cook, Margaret G. *The New Library Key*. 3rd ed. New York: H. W. Wilson, 1975. 264p. ISBN 0824205413.

Darling, Louise, ed. *Handbook of Medical Library Practice*. 4th ed. Chicago: Medical Library Association, 1982. 2v. ISBN 0912176121.

Dickinson, Isabel. *Self-Paced Library Instruction Workbook for the Sciences*. Riverside, Calif.: Library of the University of California, Riverside, 1980. 50p.

Gorman, Michael, and Paul Winkler, eds. *Anglo-American Cataloguing Rules*. 2nd ed. Chicago: American Library Association, 1978. 620p. ISBN 083893210X.

Hauer, Mary G., et al. *Books, Libraries and Research*. Dubuque, Iowa: Kendall/ Hunt Publishing Co., 1979. 125p. ISBN 0840319533.

Morton, Leslie T. *How to Use a Medical Library*. 6th ed. London: Heineman, 1979. 118p. ISBN 0433224517.

Mount, Ellis. *University Science and Engineering Libraries*. 2nd ed. Westport, Conn.: Greenwood press, 1985. 303p. ISBN 0313239495.

Picken, Fiona M., and Ann M. C. Kahn. *Medical Librarianship in the Eighties and Beyond: A World Perspective*. London: Mansell, 1986. 423p. ISBN 0720117763.

Ryans, Cynthia C., ed. *The Card Catalog: Current Issues: Readings and Selected Bibliography*. Metuchen, N.J.: Scarecrow Press, 1981. 334p. ISBN 081081417X.

Sewell, Winifred, ed. *Reader in Medical Librarianship*. Washington, D.C.: NCR Microcard Editions, 1973. 382p. ISBN 0910972273.

Warren, Kenneth S., ed. *Coping with the Biomedical Literature: A Primer for the Scientist and the Clinician*. New York: Praeger, 1981. 232p. ISBN 0030570360.

Whittaker, Kenneth. *Using Libraries: An Informative Guide for Students and General Users*. 3rd ed. London: Deutsch, 1972. 140p. ISBN 0233963588.

7
Government Publications

NATIONAL

The U.S. government is a major publisher of nutrition- and food-related materials. Much of the material published by federal agencies falls into the following categories: periodicals or series, information booklets on food preparation, handbooks, food composition tables, and the results of food consumption and nutrition surveys.

The locus of nutrition research and education activity has traditionally been in the U.S. Department of Agriculture, although a number of relevant nutrition and food publications originate in other agencies, particularly in the Department of Health and Human Services. Most of this material is centrally published and distributed by the U.S. Government Printing Office. The bulk of it is available to users in designated depository libraries throughout the country. There are now over 1,300 selective depository libraries and over 50 regional depository libraries throughout the country. Whereas the selective depositories can choose which materials to add to their collections, the regional depositories must make available at least one copy of every depository item to the public. Many of the regional depositories are at university libraries.

United States Department of Agriculture
(USDA)

Nutrition activities in the Department of Agriculture generally fall into the following categories: research, information, education, regulation, and food assistance. The USDA administers its research in nutrition chiefly through the Agricultural Research Service and the Cooperative State Research Service. The Agricultural Research Service administers a basic, applied, and developmental research program in all aspects of agriculture, as well as nutrition. It supports five major research centers at universities, each devoted to a special area of research.

The Cooperative State Research Service funds and coordinates research at state agricultural experiment stations in land-grant colleges and universities.

Three agencies under the Assistant Secretary for Food and Consumer Services are responsible for most of the department's publications in nutrition: the Human Nutrition Information Service, the Food and Nutrition Service, and the Office of the Consumer Advisor.

The Human Nutrition Information Service (HNIS) conducts research on the nutritional adequacy of diets and the food supply and the nutritive value of foods. It also collects and disseminates technical and educational information in the field of nutrition. Its Nutrient Data Research Branch is responsible for maintaining and updating our national nutrient data bank, the most extensive database of food composition information in existence. This information is available to nutrition professionals and the public in the continuous revisions of Agriculture Handbook No. 8, *The Composition of Foods*. The Human Nutrition Information Service also conducts the Nationwide Food Consumption Surveys and publishes the results.

The Food and Nutrition Service administers USDA food assistance programs such as WIC (Supplemental Food Program for Women, Infants and Children), the Commodity Supplemental Food Program (CSF), and the National School Lunch Program. Its Program Aids series is devoted to such subjects as the school lunch program, menu planning guides, and information on various federal nutrition programs.

The Office of the Consumer Advisor coordinates USDA activities on problems and issues of interest to consumers. It advises those making USDA policy on consumer issues and represents the department in consumer-related matters before Congress and agencies in the executive branch. It also interprets USDA services to consumers.

The Extension Service is the educational arm of the USDA. It works with the land-grant universities and county governments in financing, planning, and conducting agricultural extension programs to educate the public about agricultural production, marketing, natural resources, home economics, nutrition, and related subjects. Its nutrition education efforts include such programs as the Expanded Food and Nutrition Program (EFNEP), aimed at low-income people in both rural and urban areas.

The Food Safety and Inspection Service is responsible for the inspection of the meat supply and is discussed in chapter 21.

The Food and Nutrition Information Center within the National Agricultural Library has been praised by nutrition practitioners as a valuable national resource. It collects journal articles, books, and audiovisual materials on human nutrition, nutrition education, food service, food science, food policy, and related areas and loans these to libraries, federal and state agencies, college and university faculty, cooperative extension personnel, daycare and Head Start personnel, and WIC and CFS personnel. It does not loan materials to the general public.

The center does the nutrition, food service, and food science indexing for the AGRICOLA database (*Bibliography of Agriculture*) produced by the National Agricultural Library. For the years 1973-1978 it produced a catalog of its holdings with abstracts called the *FNIC Catalog*. It was updated by eight supplements and was continued by the *Food and Nutrition Bibliography* and later by the *Food and Nutrition Quarterly Index*.

FNIC has also produced useful, brief bibliographies called "Pathfinders" on food and nutrition topics of current interest, available free of charge. These have appeared in separate editions suitable for use by professionals, consumers, or for teaching. Topics include nutrition misinformation, fad weight loss diets, nutrition, vegetarianism, nutrition and diabetes, nutrition and the handicapped, and diet and cancer.

Department of Health and Human Services

There are a number of agencies within this department which are involved in food safety and nutrition research and education. The National Institutes of Health (NIH), whose mission is to improve the health of the nation, administers a biomedical nutrition research program through its individual institutes, such as the National Cancer Institute, the National Heart, Lung, and Blood Institute, and the National Institute of Arthritis, Metabolism and Digestive Diseases. The NIH has issued a wide variety of publications on nutrition and health.

The Center for Health Statistics within the U.S. Public Health Service is responsible for conducting and publishing the results of the National Health and Nutrition Examination Survey (HANES or NHANES), the major survey of nutrition status of the U.S. population.

The Food and Drug Administration (FDA) is responsible for assuring the safety of the food supply, protecting consumers against unsafe drugs and cosmetics, overseeing the fortification of staple foods, regulating food and nutrition labeling, and many other functions. Its Center for Food Safety and Applied Nutrition produces standards for the composition, safety, and quality of foods and food additives. The FDA has also developed a nutrition program to support its regulatory activities. For instance, it has been concerned with the establishment of nutrient requirement levels under different environmental conditions and with toxic levels of nutrients.

Congress

The day-to-day functioning of the legislative bodies results in a large amount of information on food and nutrition. The Senate and the House both have a committee on agriculture responsible for overseeing federal expenditures on agriculture, food, and nutrition and for legislation.

These committees generate a large number of transcripts of hearings and committee prints. During the years from 1972 to 1977 the U.S. Senate Select Committee on Nutrition and Human Needs conducted a wide-ranging investigation of the American diet and health. It made considerable progress toward developing a national nutrition policy, and issued the *Dietary Goals for Americans*. This document, issued in a revised edition because the original caused so much controversy among food industry and agricultural groups, was nonetheless a major impetus toward dietary change.

The General Accounting Office

This agency was established in 1921 as an independent agency of the legislative branch to provide an audit of government agencies. It assists the Congress and its committees in overseeing the activities of agencies within the executive branch. It provides assistance to the Congressional Budget Office and carries out legal, accounting, and other functions with respect to federal programs and operations, and makes recommendations for more efficient and effective operation of the government. In carrying out these functions, it issues so many reports related to food and nutrition that it has had to publish a continuing bibliography to make them accessible.

INTERNATIONAL

The most important international body producing food and nutrition information is the Food and Agriculture Organization (FAO) of the United Nations. The FAO came into being in 1945. Its purpose, as set forth in the preamble to its constitution, is "raising levels of nutrition and standards of living of peoples under their respective jurisdictions, securing improvements in the efficiency of food production and distribution of all food and agricultural products, bettering the conditions of rural populations and thus contributing toward an expanded world economy."

To achieve its nutrition-related goals, the FAO has issued a large number of publications. Currently, much nutrition and food safety material is published in the Food and Nutrition Papers series. This series contains many reference materials such as a food composition table, bibliographies and reviews of food consumption surveys, and specifications for food chemicals. Together with the World Health Organization, FAO has issued an international dietary standard.

The World Health Organization (WHO), another independent agency of the United Nations, has as its stated goal "health for all by the year 2000." Among its many concerns are a proper food supply and proper nutrition. It has a relatively modest output of materials on nutrition and food safety. Many of them have been issued jointly with the FAO.

In recent years the United Nations University has begun publishing a substantial number of monographs, some dealing with various aspects of the world food problem. Its periodical, *Food and Nutrition Bulletin*, is devoted to international issues in nutrition and food safety.

Described below are the general indexes to the publications of agencies in the executive branch, congressional publications, and international agencies. Materials dealing with food standards, regulations, and inspection are discussed in chapter 21.

INDEXING/ABSTRACTING SERVICES

General

37. **Index to United States Government Periodicals.** Vol. 1- . Chicago: Infordata International, 1970- . quarterly. ISSN 0098-4604.

This author and subject index covers nearly 200 periodicals published by the U.S. government. The intent of the publishers is to provide access to every government periodical that offers substantive articles of lasting research and reference value. The last issue of the year is the annual cumulation.

38.   **Monthly Catalog of United States Government Publications**. No. 672- .
Washington, D.C.: Government Printing Office, 1951- . monthly. ISSN 0362-
6830. GP3.8: .
   The best all-around index to publications of the U.S. government, the
Monthly Catalog has been in existence since 1895 under various titles. It covers
the publications of agencies in the executive branch and congressional publications (but not in depth). Access is by author, title, subject, series/report number,
contract number, stock number, and title keywords. Entries provide detailed
bibliographic description of items, including Superintendent of Documents
numbers.
   Online Equivalent: GPO Monthly Catalog.
   Indexes: Indexes are cumulated annually. Multiyear cumulations of the
indexes are available for 1950-1960, 1961-1966, 1966-1970, and 1971-1976.

Congressional

39.   **Congressional Index**. Vol. 1- . Chicago: Commerce Clearing House,
1937/38- . ISSN 0162-1203.
   Because the *Digest of Public General Bills* is not published fast enough to
cover current material, documents librarians frequently refer to this index for
very recent action on bills. The coverage is essentially the same as in the *Digest*,
but publication is more rapid and information is briefer. *Congressional Index*
also contains such ancillary information as voting records and scheduled
committee meetings and has sections on the status of Senate and House bills.

40.   Congressional Information Service. **CIS/Index to Publications of the
United States Congress**. Vol. 1- . Washington, D.C.: Congressional Information
Service, 1970- . monthly. ISSN 0007-8514.
   This monthly abstracting service covers all congressional publications except
the congressional record and bills. It covers an extensive body of literature totaling more than 800,000 pages per year, including hearings, reports, committee
prints, and congressional papers issued during the previous month. It is divided
into two parts: abstracts and index. The abstracts section is arranged by accession
number and is cumulated annually. The index is cumulated every quarter. It
provides access by subject, personal and corporate names, official and popular
names of bills, names of subcommittees, and affiliation of witnesses. Documents
abstracted are available directly from CIS.
   Online Equivalent: CIS.

41.   United States. Congress. **Congressional Record: Proceedings of the
Debates of the ... Congress**. Washington, D.C.: Government Printing Office,
1873- . daily. ISSN 0363-7239. X/a.
   This is the record of proceedings and debates on the floor of both houses. It
appears daily when Congress is in session and has indexes that appear semi-
monthly. These are cumulated when a final edited version of the *Record* appears.
The index terms are extremely broad, and it may be necessary to search under a
congressperson's name for more specific access.
   Online Equivalent: Congressional Record Abstracts.

42.   United States. General Accounting Office. **Food Bibliography: References to Reports and Other Documents Issued by the U.S. General Accounting Office.** Washington, D.C.: General Accounting Office, 19?- . irregular. GA1.16/6: .

This bibliography of GAO documents directly or indirectly related to food, agriculture, or nutrition contains extensive abstracts. Several cumulated volumes have appeared covering documents from 1977 on.

43.   United States. General Accounting Office. **General Accounting Office Documents: Catalog of Reports, Decisions, Opinions, Testimonies and Speeches.** Vol. 1- . Washington, D.C.: Government Printing Office, 1977- . monthly. ISSN 0193-0419. GA1.16/4: .

A comprehensive record of GAO publications and documents. The following types of publications are indexed: reports—audits of agencies and other organizations, their programs, and activities; staff studies studies which communicate background information on a variety of subjects; decisions—rulings from the Comptroller General on a variety of government matters, including personnel and procurement issues; testimonies—presentations to congressional committees or state and other governmental bodies; speeches; letters—correspondence addressed to congressional committees and federal agencies.

44.   United States. Library of Congress. Congressional Research Service. **Digest of Public General Bills and Resolutions.** Washington, D.C.: Government Printing Office, 1936- . ISSN 0012-2785. LC14.6: .

"Normally published during each session of Congress in five or more cumulative issues with bi-weekly supplementation as may be needed and a final edition at the conclusion of each session. The Digest of Public General Bills and Resolutions has been prepared since the 74th Congress in 1936. Its principal purpose is to furnish, in summary form, the essential features of public bills and resolutions and the changes hitherto made during the legislative process." The *Digest* consists of three parts. Part 1, "Action Taken during the Congress," covers all measures considered on the floor, voted on, receiving conference action, presidential action, and legislative history. Part 2, "Digests of Public General Bills and Resolutions," contains summaries of bills. Part 3, "Indexes to Digested Bills and Resolutions," contains the following indexes: sponsor and cosponsor, identical bills, short title, and subject.

45.   United States. Library of Congress. Congressional Research Service. **Major Legislation of the Congress.** Washington, D.C.: Government Printing Office, 19?- . irregular. ISSN 0277-2183. LC14.18: .

"Designed to provide congressional Washington and district offices with summaries of topical congressional issues and major legislation introduced in response to those issues."

United Nations

46.   **FAO Documentation: Current Bibliography = Documentation de la FAO: Bibliographie Courante = Documentation de la FAO: Bibliografia Corriente.** Rome: Food and Agriculture Organization of the United Nations, 1972- . bimonthly.

This listing of selected publications and documents produced by or for the Food and Agriculture Organization of the United Nations includes indexing of FAO periodicals. Each issue consists of a bibliography arranged in accession number sequence and subject and geographic indexes. Cumulated indexes now appear only in the cumulated microfiche set of the bibliography.

47. Food and Agriculture Organization of the United Nations. Documentation Center. **Food and Nutrition: Annotated Bibliography. Author and Subject Index**. Rome: Food and Agriculture Organization of the United Nations, 1973. 588p.

A useful, selected bibliography of older FAO documents on nutrition and food from 1945 to 1972. An author index and a keyword index are included. Titles of documents and explanatory materials are given in English, French, and Spanish. FAO materials from 1973 on are covered by *FAO Documentation*.

48. World Health Organization. **Publications of the World Health Organization: A Bibliography, 1947-** . Geneva: World Health Organization, 1958- . quinquennial.

Published at five-year intervals, this bibliography represents the only subject listing of WHO publications. It indexes WHO monographs as well as periodicals, but not internal WHO documents. The arrangement is by broad subjects with detailed subject indexes in some issues. It is supplemented by the *WHO Publications Catalogue*.

SELECTED REFERENCES

Downey, James A. *U.S. Official Publications: The International Dimension*. Oxford, New York: Pergamon, 1978. 352p. ISBN 0080218393.

Hernon, Peter, and Charles R. McClure. *Public Access to Government Information: Issues, Trends, and Strategies*. Norwood, N.J.: Ablex Publishing Co., 1984. 457p. ISBN 0893911003.

Hernon, Peter, Charles R. McClure, and Gary R. Purcell. *GPO's Depository Library Program: A Descriptive Analysis*. Norwood, N.J.: Ablex Publishing Co., 1985. 240p. ISBN 0893913138.

Jenkins, Dianne E. "The Food and Nutrition Information Center." *Food and Nutrition* 5 (August 1975): 14-15.

Morehead, Joe. *Introduction to United States Public Documents*. 3rd ed. Littleton, Colo.: Libraries Unlimited, 1983. 309p. ISBN 0872873595.

Nakata, Yuri. *From Press to People: Collecting and Using U.S. Government Publications*. Chicago: American Library Association, 1979. 212p. ISBN 0838902642.

O'Hara, Frederic J. *A Guide to Publications of the Executive Branch*. Ann Arbor, Mich.: Pierian Press, 1979. 287p. ISBN 0876500726.

8
Getting Started on a Research Paper
A Guide for the Student

The difference between people who can efficiently write papers and those who cannot, is usually many years of library experience. This chapter is intended to help narrow the gap for those without this experience. Information on note taking, footnoting, or style of references is not included here; the bibliography lists books on these topics. This chapter is about getting organized to write a paper and using the library to its full advantage. The suggestions are aimed at helping the user reach the point of taking the initial steps as painlessly as possible.

GETTING STARTED EARLY!

Getting an early start on a paper is excellent advice, even if it seems obvious. Unfortunately, not many students take it to heart. Librarians are in a unique position to observe the result: end-of-semester panic. Here are all the reasons why it is good to start early:

1. The earlier a paper is begun, the easier it is for the writer to be in control of the subject, deal with the unexpected (like the flu), and make major changes if required.

2. There will be more time to get important material on interlibrary loan. This can take four to eight weeks.

3. Those who begin early are more likely to find their materials in the library. Because many students procrastinate, they converge on the major journals at roughly the same time, and not surprisingly, many do

not find materials on the shelf. This principle also holds for the photo-copiers. There are likely to be long lines at the machines later in the semester. Starting early helps avoid these frustrations.

4. Librarians are in a position to give more individual attention to students earlier in the semester when they are less busy. This holds both for reference service across the desk and computer searches.

CHOOSING A "DOABLE" TOPIC

Students in search of suitable topics for term papers will find it useful to browse through recent issues of periodicals in the field to get an idea of what is currently under study. Perusing the subjects covered in the course textbook is also a good idea. If narrowed down properly, many of these could be suitable. The instructor can also be approached for suggestions.

Students often have difficulty with papers because they do not know how to select a subject which is "doable" in the amount of time available. They often choose subjects that are either too general or too specific.

Too General

Students who select subjects that are too general sometimes get caught in the morass of an extensive and sometimes contradictory literature and fail to see the forest for the trees. Many researchers have spent a lifetime working and publishing on topics such as the effect of serum cholesterol on heart disease. With only a couple of weeks or months to devote to a paper, a student can't even begin to read enough about the subject to master it. The answer? Picking a narrower subject or focusing on a specific aspect of a broad problem. In the case of cholesterol and heart disease, the topic could be narrowed to specific population groups such as vegetarians or Seventh-day Adventists, postmenopausal women, or even a particular ethnic group. In certain cases, even such "narrowings" might be too broad.

Another example of a broad topic is diet and hypertension. The sodium and hypertension literature alone is enormous. If all aspects of diet are added, it becomes totally unmanageable. Concentrating on a single nutrient which has not been extensively researched, such as calcium and hypertension, results in a more "doable" topic. There are about 20 to 30 recent references on the subject, still a manageable number.

Finding a subject with the appropriate level of specificity is something that is learned by doing. To determine if a subject is "doable" a bit of exploratory literature searching is essential. A good starting point is to go to the chapter on indexing/abstracting services, become familiar with some of the major indexing/abstracting services in the field, and do some "rummaging around in the literature" before making a commitment to a topic. A quick and dirty search through the last two annual cumulations of *Index Medicus* or through *Nutrition Abstracts and Reviews* can provide a rough idea of the amount of literature on the subject. The student can then select a topic based on the course requirements, the amount of time available for doing the paper, and the number of references available.

A good way to narrow a broad topic is to peruse the *Index Medicus* and look for "clusters" of articles on a specific aspect of the topic. Then restrict the search to this narrower aspect.

Too Narrow or Too Soon

At times a topic can be too specific. If there is too little material on a subject, remember that it is impossible to squeeze blood from a turnip. Student papers should be based on published literature, since in most cases students are not actually engaged in original research unless they are working on theses or dissertations. If a topic is insufficiently researched or too current to have much of a literature, don't choose it. There may be one or two articles on the use of ginger to prevent motion sickness, but that is not a sufficient number for a paper.

Another type of topic to avoid is the "hottest" and "latest." Wait until some of these hot topics have cooled a bit to give people a chance to do some research and publish the results. For example, before 1979 there was very little material available on sucrose polyester. Now there are a fair number of articles. It would have been very difficult or impossible to do a paper on the subject in 1979; now it is a reasonable topic to pursue. Watch out for the latest diet fads, also. When a new "health food" product hits the market or a new diet craze sweeps the country, some time elapses before there is a significant amount of scientific literature on the subject. This happened with the so-called starch blockers. Although there was a lot of interest in this topic when the claims for this diet aid first appeared in the media, most of the scientific literature was not available until the fall of 1982.

Availability of Materials

Another important thing to consider is the local availability of materials. Think carefully about which local libraries might hold the journals needed, and spot check a few. A science or medical librarian experienced at a particular library can sometimes "eyeball" a list of references and estimate how many items are likely to be available. The topic selected should mesh with the known strengths of the library being used. For instance, a topic dealing with nutrition in Africa won't be "doable" if local libraries ignore Africa and collect materials relating to Asia and the Pacific Islands. If a library is strong in materials from tropical areas, the paper should be on bananas, not apples.

It is a mistake to choose a topic for which local access to a significant proportion of the materials is limited. It is possible to request materials on interlibrary loan, but it is never smart to rely on obtaining the bulk of the material this way. There could be delays and the paper might not be done on time, not to mention the charges for interlibrary loans, which are often passed on to the user. In summary, these are the most important considerations in selecting a "doable" topic:

1. Do an exploratory literature search (e.g., rummage around in the literature before committing to a topic).

2. Consider the local availability of materials.

3. Avoid broad topics that have been extensively researched, or focus on a narrow aspect of a broad topic.

4. Do not select topics that have been insufficiently researched.

5. Be practical in assessing the time available for the paper.

6. Check with the instructor to determine if a topic is acceptable.

7. Consider carefully before deciding on a topic, but don't change it constantly once a decision has been made.

8. Select controversial topics with caution. When there is controversy surrounding a subject, it is more critical to have a sufficient background to evaluate research designs and statistical methods to determine which studies hold up and which are flawed.

ORGANIZING REFERENCES

Although many people resist this, it is best to organize all references on individual 3-by-5-inch (or larger) cards. This allows sufficient space to note down holding libraries, call numbers, and comments, and makes rearranging easier. It provides a great deal more flexibility than using sheets of paper. Writing references on cards once allows for rearrangement at various stages of the paper, as follows:

1. By journal title, when checking if a library holds the title.

2. Sequentially by call number, when looking for the materials in the library in call number sequence.

3. By specific aspect or subtopic, when making an outline or writing the paper.

4. In the order in which the items are cited when doing footnotes.

5. Alphabetically by author for a bibliography.

When recording references, it is important to make a special effort to record them correctly the first time. Always note the source of the reference. For example, "*Index Medicus* 1985 v. 26 p. 13545" or "*Nutrition Abstracts and Reviews A* 1985 #749." In the event of an error, it is possible to go back and correct it. Otherwise, all or part of the original literature search must be done over again. Also, if it turns out that an item must be requested on interlibrary loan, the library frequently asks for the source of reference, so that it can be identified more easily by the lending institution.

RECORDING REFERENCES

The format of references or citations as recorded in books and periodicals varies enormously from field to field and from publication to publication. Regardless of how they are recorded, it will probably be necessary to alter the citations when writing the paper. Many fields have their own style manuals, sometimes called style sheets. These usually give general recommendations on the style and format for papers. They explain what and how to abbreviate, for instance, and provide standard formats for bibliographic references. The bibliography at the end of this chapter lists some of the most important style manuals. Some instructors simply ask that students follow the format used by a major journal in the field. When unsure of the format to use, the student should make it a practice to ask. The important thing is to use the style consistently.

The information on the facts of publication provided in indexing/abstracting services is usually quite complete. The best policy is to copy it as given, and then make adjustments to comply with the specific guidelines being used.

REVIEWS OF THE LITERATURE

When doing a literature search, it is helpful to keep an eye out for articles or other types of publications which review and discuss the literature on a specific topic. Such articles usually do not present new information. They merely summarize, discuss, or critique existing papers on a subject. They can save a great deal of time in doing a literature search. It generally can be assumed that the literature reviewed is current up to about a year prior to the date of the review, and the searcher can therefore concentrate on locating more recent references. If there is doubt about the period of time covered, the student should scan the dates of the references at the end of the article.

Review articles can usually be identified because they cite an unusually large number of references, frequently over 100. They can be contained in any scientific journal, but are frequently published in special periodicals which contain only review articles. A few are monthly journals, but most are issued annually or irregularly and frequently bear titles beginning with the words "Advances in," "Annual Review of," or "Progress in." These are indexed in the major indexing/abstracting services such as *Nutrition Abstracts and Reviews*, *Food Science and Technology Abstracts*, and *Index Medicus* and its special section, the *Bibliography of Medical Reviews*. A list of review periodicals most relevant to nutrition and food science is given below.

In a sense, recent scientific books on a subject can also serve as reviews of the literature, particularly such excellent books as *Nutrition Review's Present Knowledge of Nutrition*, last revised in 1984.

Review Periodicals in Nutrition
and Food Science

Advances in Lipid Research. Vol. 1- . New York: Academic Press, 1963- . annual. ISSN 0065-2849.

Advances in Food Research. Vol. 1- . New York: Academic Press, 1948- . annual. ISSN 0065-2628.

Advances in Nutritional Research. Vol. 1- . New York, London: Plenum, 1977- . annual. ISSN 0149-9483.

Advances in Protein Chemistry. Vol. 1- . New York: Academic Press, 1944- . annual. ISSN 0065-3233.

Annual Review of Nutrition. Vol. 1- . Palo Alto, Calif.: Annual Reviews, Inc., 1981- . annual. ISSN 0199-9885.

CRC Critical Reviews in Food Science and Nutrition. Vol. 1- . Boca Raton, Fla.: CRC Press, Inc., 1970- . 8/yr. ISSN 0099-0248.

Nutrition and the Brain. Vol. 1- . Edited by R. J. Wurtman and J. J. Wurtman. New York: Raven Press, 1977- . irregular. (Vol. 6, 1986, ISBN 0881671428).

Nutrition Reviews. Vol. 1- . Washington, D.C.: The Nutrition Foundation, 1942- . monthly. ISSN 0029-6643.

Nutrition Update. Vol. 1- . New York: Wiley, 1983- . annual. ISSN 0735-4762.

Progress in Food and Nutrition Science. Vol. 1- . New York: Pergamon, 1975- . quarterly. ISSN 0306-0632.

Vitamins and Hormones: Advances in Research and Applications. Vol. 1- . New York: Academic Press, 1943- . annual. ISSN 0083-6729.

World Review of Nutrition and Dietetics. Vol. 1- . Basel, Switzerland: Karger, 1959- . irregular. ISSN 0084-2230.

HINTS FOR DOING
A LITERATURE SEARCH

1. Use the most appropriate indexing/abstracting service for the topic.

2. Consider a computer search, particularly if the topic has two or more facets. For example, the use of fish oils to lower cholesterol. Try to do a little manual searching beforehand to get a feel for the type and quantity of literature available and to refine the search request.

3. Follow up any review articles first, and then decide if the search should be taken further.

4. Keep a log of what years have been searched, and under what subjects, keywords, or authors.

5. *Record each reference accurately on a card. Record all of the facts of publication exactly as they appear in the indexing/abstracting service or bibliography. Be sure to include information on where the citation was found.*

6. When there are many references in a periodical index such as *Index Medicus*, photocopy the page instead of copying by hand. Then cut the references apart and tape them to the cards. Again, be sure to list the source of the reference.

READING

What to Read

Sometimes students feel a compulsion to read everything ever written on a subject. Don't! Learn to discriminate and to be selective. Learn to pick up the thread of the research from study to study. Concentrate on studies in the primary source journals and also read reviews, but remember, unless the original papers are consulted, this is someone else's interpretation of the research. They may be wrong or have an ax to grind.

How to Read

Even primary source journals publish studies with serious flaws. Certain questions should be considered: Was the research design appropriate? Did it really measure what it was supposed to measure or test what it was supposed to test?

Another consideration is how the sampling was done. If the sample consisted of a specific socioeconomic group, what kind of bias could this have introduced into the study? Is the proper statistical test used? Are the statistical assumptions met? Is there a control group? Should there be? Were baseline measurements properly taken? Was a placebo effect possible?

And what about the researcher's interpretation of his or her work? Does it seem justified? Are there alternative explanations for the findings? If so, what are they? How far can the results of the study be generalized?

Finally, has this research been successfully replicated by others? If the results are inconsistent with what is already known, what is the likely explanation? If the brick does not fit into the edifice, it is more likely that something is wrong with the brick than with the foundation.

OUTLINING

Much has been written about the necessity for outlining; it does not need to be repeated here. Suffice it to say that an outline helps in getting organized. Some people resist outlining just because they can never remember where the capital or lowercase letters go. Remember, the important point is to get one's thoughts in order, not the roman numerals.

AT THE END

Now is the time to sift through all of the material gathered in the literature search and select what is most pertinent for the paper. Students who have followed the tips in this chapter, have started early, located a "doable" topic, done a literature search, and read some reviews and enough of the literature to work up an outline, are now ready to take notes and put the paper together.

SELECTED REFERENCES

American Chemical Society. *Handbook for Authors of Papers in American Chemical Society Publications.* Washington, D.C.: American Chemical Society, 1979. 122p. ISBN 084120425X.

Association of Official Analytical Chemists. *The AOAC Style Manual.* 2nd ed. Washington, D.C.: Association of Official Analytical Chemists, 1975. 35p.

Banes, Joan. *The Medical and Scientific Authors' Guide: An International Reference Guide for Authors to More Than 500 Medical and Scientific Journals.* New York: Le Jacq Publishing, Inc., 1984. 1082p. ISBN 0937716200.

Barclay, William R., M. Therese Southgate, and Robert W. Mayo. *Manual for Authors and Editors: Editorial Style and Manuscript Preparation.* 7th ed. Compiled for the American Medical Association. Los Altos, Calif.: Lange Medical Publications, 1981. 184p. ISBN 0870412434.

Barrass, Robert. *Scientists Must Write: A Guide to Better Writing for Scientists, Engineers and Students.* London: Chapman and Hall; distr., New York: Wiley, 1978. 176p. ISBN 047099388X.

Booth, Vernon H. *Writing a Scientific Paper and Speaking at Scientific Meetings.* 5th ed. London: Biochemical Society, 1981. 48p.

Campbell, William G. *Form and Style in Thesis Writing.* 3rd ed. New York: Houghton Mifflin, 1969. 138p.

CBE Style Committee. *CBE Style Manual: A Guide for Authors, Editors and Publishers in the Biological Sciences.* 5th rev. and expanded ed. Bethesda, Md.: Council of Biology Editors, Inc., 1983. 324p. ISBN 0914340042.

Council of Biology Editors. *Scientific Writing for Graduate Students: A Manual on Teaching Scientific Writing.* Edited by F. Peter Woodford. New York: Rockefeller University Press, 1968. 190p.

Day, Robert A. *How to Write and Publish a Scientific Paper.* 2nd ed. Philadelphia, Pa.: ISI Press, 1983. 181p. ISBN 0894950215.

Garn, Stanley M. *Writing the Biomedical Research Paper.* Springfield, Ill.: Charles C. Thomas, 1970. 65p.

Huth, Edward J. *How to Write and Publish in the Medical Sciences.* Philadelphia, Pa.: ISI Press, 1982. 203p. ISBN 0894950185.

Kass, Edward H. "Reviewing Reviews." In *Coping with the Biomedical Literature: A Primer for the Scientist and Clinician,* Kenneth S. Warren, ed., 79-91. New York: Praeger, 1981. ISBN 0030570360.

Katz, Michael J. *Elements of a Scientific Paper.* New Haven, Conn.: Yale University Press, 1985. 130p. ISBN 0300034911.

Longyear, Marie, ed. *The McGraw-Hill Style Manual: A Concise Guide for Writers and Editors.* New York: McGraw-Hill, 1983. 333p. ISBN 0070386765.

Mauch, James E., and Jack W. Birch. *Guide to the Successful Thesis and Dissertation: Conception to Publication: A Handbook for Students and Faculty.* New York: Marcel Dekker, 1983. 352p. ISBN 0824718003.

Morris, Jackson E. *Principles of Scientific and Technical Writing.* New York: McGraw-Hill, 1966. 257p.

Olsen, Leslie A., and Thomas N. Huckin. *Principles of Communication for Science and Technology.* New York: McGraw-Hill, 1983. 414p. ISBN 007047821X.

Peterson, Martin S. *Scientific Thinking and Scientific Writing.* New York: Reinhold Publishing Corp., 1961. 215p.

Sandman, Peter M., Carl S. Klompers, and Betsy G. Yarrison. *Scientific and Technical Writing.* New York: Holt, Rinehart and Winston, 1985. 451p. ISBN 0030410568.

Shields, Nancy E., and Mary E. Uhle. *Where Credit Is Due: A Guide to Proper Citing of Sources—Print and Nonprint.* Metuchen, N.J.: Scarecrow Press, 1985. 252p. ISBN 0810817888.

Turabian, Kate L. *A Manual for Writers of Term Papers, Theses and Dissertations.* 4th ed. Chicago: University of Chicago Press, 1973. 216p. ISBN 0226816206.

Turabian, Kate L. *Student's Guide for Writing College Papers.* 3rd ed. Chicago: University of Chicago Press, 1976. 256p. ISBN 0226816222.

University of Chicago Press. *The Chicago Manual of Style for Authors, Editors, and Copywriters*. 13th ed. Chicago: University of Chicago Press, 1982. 738p. ISBN 0226103900.

Van Leunen, Mary-Claire. *A Handbook for Scholars*. New York: Alfred A. Knopf, 1978. 354p. ISBN 0394409043.

9
Keeping Current

An earlier chapter has outlined strategies for locating research on a specific subject. This chapter deals with strategies for keeping abreast of new research and developments in the field.

Considering how broadly scattered the food and nutrition literature is and how much of it appears in journals from other disciplines, it requires extra organization and effort to avoid missing important new literature. Because scientific journals are the major vehicle for publishing new research, any strategy for keeping up-to-date must necessarily center on reading major journals in the field and determining which of those not regularly read have articles of interest.

The major strategies for keeping up with the literature are outlined below. They involve the physical browsing of journals in the library, browsing through a current awareness service, monthly online searches of the latest additions to important databases in the field, and other methods.

BROWSING

Libraries recognize the importance of browsing, and usually display the most recently received issues of journals in a prominent place. A good strategy is to find out where the library displays issues of current periodicals in the field, how they are arranged, and how long each issue remains on display. Not all institutions have the space to display each issue of a journal until the next issue arrives. In some libraries issues are displayed for short periods of time on a rotating basis.

Although random browsing occasionally leads to serendipitous finds, working out some type of system is better. Set aside a specific time each week for browsing. Keep a log book of vital information. List those journals to be perused, with classification numbers where pertinent, and note down which issues have been examined. This is especially important if one's routine is interrupted by travel, vacations, and unforeseen events, as it enables one to track down individual issues of journals which may have been removed from the current periodical display shelves during an absence. Finally, it is best not to restrict the list of browsing journals too severely; some important articles may be missed.

USING A CURRENT AWARENESS SERVICE

Current awareness services are a somewhat new phenomenon. Subscribing to one allows one to browse through current periodicals from a distance. Many academic departments and research laboratories have their own subscriptions to such services. However, they are sometimes too costly for individuals and many people make use of those found in the library.

The most common services reproduce tables of contents of current periodicals. Others are organized by subject. The best-known current awareness services are published by the Institute for Scientific Information, the producers of *Science Citation Index* and *Social Sciences Citation Index*. The titles of all of ISI's current awareness services begin with the words "Current Contents" and reproduce tables of contents from recently published journals. The institute now produces such table of contents services for the life sciences, clinical practice, agriculture, biology and environmental sciences, and other fields.

As a general rule, the major journals in medicine are grouped with the life sciences, and most, but not all, major nutrition and food journals are grouped in the agriculture, biology, and environmental sciences series. Described below are the major current awareness services for food and nutrition.

49. **BIOSIS/CAS Selects**. Philadelphia, Pa.: BioSciences Information Service (BioSciences Information Service, Customer Services, Dept. A49186A, 2100 Arch Street, Philadelphia, PA 19103-1399).

A joint effort of BIOSIS and Chemical Abstracts Service, *BIOSIS/CAS Selects* is a series of biweekly current literature listing services which have been customized for specific user groups. It consists of nearly 30 individual titles, focusing on fairly specific areas of interest. Items are selected from the BIOSIS and Chemical Abstracts databases and provide coverage of about 16,000 journals and other publications. Titles relevant to food and nutrition are *Biochemistry of Fermented Foods*, *Cancer and Nutrition*, *Food and Drug Legislation*, and *Vitamins*. *BIOSIS/CAS Selects* sections contain abstracts or content summaries (indexing terminology) and cover research papers appearing in journals, reviews, meeting papers or abstracts, and books.

50. **Breast Feeding Abstracts: A Newsletter for Health Professionals**. Vol. 1- . Franklin Park, Ill.: La Leche League International, 1981- . quarterly.

This newsletter is intended to help health professionals keep up-to-date on new developments and literature. It contains brief articles, reviews, abstracts of the literature, and an annual bibliography of breast feeding literature (without abstracts) of approximately 250 items, published as a supplement. When measured against the MEDLINE database, which contains roughly 750 items for 1984 through mid-1986, this annual bibliography is extensive. However, the abstracts appearing in each issue are a highly select group of items. An annual index appears in the final issue of each volume.

51. **Core Journals in Parenteral and Enteral Nutrition**. Vol. 1- . Amsterdam, New York: Excerpta Medica, 1986- . 11/yr. ISSN 0168-972X.

One of 11 current awareness services covering various field in clinical practice, this publication provides abstracts of new journal literature on all aspects of parenteral and enteral nutrition. Covers material on nutritional therapy in cancer, gastrointestinal tract disorders, critical care, pediatrics, complications, solutions, instrumentation, patient monitoring, and nutritional and metabolic status. Articles are selected from 1,000 journal titles monitored for the Excerpta Medica database. Each issue has a subject index.

52. **Current Contents. Agriculture, Biology and Environmental Sciences**. Vol. 4- . Philadelphia, Pa.: Institute for Scientific Information, 1973- . weekly. ISSN 0090-0508.

Former title: *Current Contents. Agricultural, Food, and Veterinary Sciences*. One of a series of current awareness services published by the Institute for Scientific Information, *Current Contents. Agriculture, Biology and Environmental Sciences* contains the tables of contents of 1,010 journals. It regularly covers approximately 75 food science and nutrition journals. Major English-language publications predominate, but selected foreign-language journals are also included. The *American Journal of Clinical Nutrition* is conspicuously absent, but is included in *Current Contents. Life Sciences*. The arrangement is by broad subject fields. A few journals are included in more than one section of *Current Contents* and are so designated in the table of contents.

Each issue includes a title word and an author index, an author address directory, and a publishers' address directory. Features in the front of each issue include the ever-fascinating essays of Eugene Garfield; changes in journal coverage; a section entitled "ISI Press Digest," containing summaries of interesting articles from the popular press; a list of weekly citation classics; and an essay by the writer of that week's citation classic. Journal articles included may be ordered through the "Genuine Article," ISI's document delivery service.

53. **Current Contents. Life Sciences**. Vol. 10- . Philadelphia, Pa.: Institute for Scientific Information, 1967- . weekly. ISSN 0011-3409.

One of a series of current awareness services publishing tables of contents of journals, *Current Contents. Life Sciences* covers approximately 1,160 journals in chemistry, biochemistry, biophysics, molecular biology, genetics, microbiology, cell biology, pharmacology, immunology, physiology, experimental biology and medicine, clinical medicine, neurosciences and behavior, and plant and animal science. Food and nutrition journals generally appear in the biochemistry section, but occasionally are listed under other subjects.

This service covers a large number of journals in biomedicine which have occasional articles related to food and nutrition, for example *Atherosclerosis, New England Journal of Medicine*, and *Diabetes*. It covers only a handful of nutrition journals, among which are *American Journal of Clinical Nutrition, Nutrition Research, Nutrition Reviews, Journal of Agricultural and Food Chemistry, Annals of Nutrition and Metabolism, Food and Chemical Toxicology, Journal of Nutrition Science and Vitaminology*, and *International Journal for Vitamin and Nutrition Research*.

Current Contents. Life Sciences has the same features as *Current Contents. Agriculture, Biology and Environmental Sciences*. There are title word and author indexes to individual articles, author and publisher address directories, essays by Eugene Garfield, a list of citation classics, the "ISI Press Digest," and the essay by the author of the citation classic.

54. **Foods Adlibra Alerting Bulletin**. Vol. 1- . Minneapolis, Minn.: Foods Adlibra Publications, 1974?- . semi-monthly. ISSN 0146-9304.

A current literature alerting service geared to the needs of the food industry, this periodical corresponds to the General Foods database by the same name, although there are a few more citations in the database than in the printed version. The number issued on the first of each month covers a different group of subjects from the one issued on the fifteenth. In addition to the usual array of food science and technology topics, *Foods Adlibra Alerting Bulletin* covers new products, company news, marketing, retailing, government information relevant to the industry, nutritional information, and new patents. The arrangement is by broad subject categories with subdivisions where appropriate. About 500 periodicals are scanned on a regular basis. These include business periodicals, industry trade magazines, nutrition and food science journals, popular magazines, food service periodicals, and the *Federal Register*. No indexes are produced.

55. **Nutrition Research Newsletter: A Monthly Update for Food, Nutrition, and Health Professionals**. Vol. 1- . Palisades, N.Y.: Lydia Associates, 1982- . monthly. ISSN 0736-0037.

A current awareness service in a newsletter format, *Nutrition Research Newsletter* provides summaries of research appearing in approximately 300 journals. Monitored are major journals from the United States and English-language journals from other countries. Entries usually range from two to five paragraphs in length and tend to be focused on subjects with a great deal of general appeal.

CURRENT AWARENESS SECTIONS IN JOURNALS

Many journals have special sections with abstracts of the current literature as a service to their users. The *Journal of the American Dietetic Association*, for example, has an extensive section entitled, "New in Print/Media/Software" featuring tables of contents of journal issues and summaries of key journal articles. *Cereal Science Today* also has a section of abstracts devoted to new literature. *Food Technology* has a special section summarizing new patents. The time lag between publication of the article and its appearance in such a column or section is sometimes greater than with publications such as *Current Contents*.

SDI

SDI stands for selective dissemination of information and usually refers to regular online searching of databases according to an individualized user interest profile. The user sets up a profile with the help of a librarian trained in computer searching and every month the latest references added to specified databases are searched for material fitting that profile. A printout of the references is sent to the user. As with all online searches there is usually a fee. Many of the databases described in this book can be searched for SDIs. SDIs are often requested by people who have had retrospective searches done on a subject, but have a continuing interest in keeping up with a field.

BITS
(BIOSIS INFORMATION TRANSFER SYSTEM)

In addition to making their databases available through database vendors such as DIALOG Information Services, Inc., some database producers are offering computer search services directly to the user. BioSciences Information Service (BIOSIS), has taken this one step further. Recognizing that we are well into the microcomputer revolution, BIOSIS has arranged to transfer citations from its database directly to the user's microcomputer, through a system called BITS. BITS works as follows: The user fills out a detailed profile, pays a fee based on the estimated number of citations (with or without abstracts) and purchases Biosuperfile, a program which enables him or her to maintain and search a database of bibliographic citations on a personal computer. Each month he or she receives a diskette with the latest citations in the BIOSIS database in the specified profile area. The user performs the routine operation of updating a master index on the program disk, and the file is searchable in-house.

BOOKS

No one would claim that books provide access to up-to-the-minute information. But for keeping up generally, or in peripheral areas, and for delving into new ones, recently published books are very important. Libraries generally have browsing shelves where users can peruse new books.

Many periodicals also have special book review sections and some also list new books received for review. In some fields, such as nutrition education, food technology, and dietetics, virtually the only way to keep abreast of new books, audiovisual materials, diet manuals, materials from food companies, and other publications from societies or nonstandard publishers, is to keep up with these sections in the *Journal of the American Dietetic Association*, *Food Technology*, and the *Journal of Nutrition Education*.

Unfortunately, by the time many materials are reviewed, they may be a year old or even older. For commercially published items, one way to circumvent this time lag is to get on the mailing lists of as many publishers as possible and regulary receive announcements of new titles.

In many institutions users play an active role in developing library collections by requesting that the library purchase new books of interest. Reading reviews and new book announcements is prerequisite to this type of involvement. New books don't just magically appear on library shelves — someone has to select and order them. Librarians try to anticipate user needs working within certain budgetary constraints, but to ensure that needed materials are available, a patron should become actively involved in suggesting materials for purchase.

CURRENT RESEARCH

It is not easy to find out about current research projects before the results are published. The U.S. Department of Agriculture produces a database called USDA/CRIS (Current Research Information System) which is available through commercial vendors. This database describes current research projects conducted by USDA agencies, state agricultural experiment stations, state schools of forestry, and other cooperating institutions. It covers a broad range of subjects related to agriculture including home economics, food and nutrition, consumer health and safety, economics and marketing, etc. It is updated monthly and covers projects active during the last two years.

Research sponsored by the Department of Health and Human Services is published in its *Research Awards Index*, issued annually. It lists grants by detailed subject and by principal investigator, and its broad subject scope reflects the interests of the various agencies within that department.

SELECTED REFERENCES

Garfield, Eugene. "Current Contents: Its Impact on Scientific Communication." *Interdisciplinary Science Reviews* 4 (1979): 318-23.

Garfield, Eugene. "How Do We Select Journals for Current Contents." In *Essays of an Information Scientist*, vol. 4, 309-12. Philadelphia, Pa.: ISI Press, 1981.

Kastl, F. " 'Current Contents' Type Journals and Their Utilization in the Field of Food Science and Technology." *Quarterly Bulletin of the International Association of Agricultural Librarians and Documentalists* 18 (1973): 212-19.

Lever, R. "Current Literature Services." In *Medical Librarianship*, Michael Carmel, ed., 203-20. London: Library Association, 1981.

Rowley, J. E. "Bibliographic Current Awareness Services: A Review." *Aslib Proceedings* 37 (1985): 345-53.

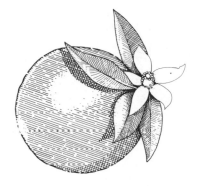

Part III

NUTRITION

10
General Reference Sources

This chapter describes indexing/abstracting services focusing on nutrition. It also lists and describes individual, noncontinuing bibliographies, databases, and other reference materials.

LOCATING RESEARCH—
INDEXING/ABSTRACTING SERVICES

The major organizations providing information services in nutrition are CAB International (formerly Commonwealth Agricultural Bureaux), the Food and Nutrition Information Center at the National Agricultural Library, and the National Library of Medicine.

CAB International is an international nonprofit organization based in the United Kingdom but controlled by member countries. It consists of four research institutes and ten bureaus, each dealing with a specialized aspect of agriculture. Its main objective is to provide information services to agricultural scientists. Although it is best known for over 50 agricultural abstracting services, CAB International has also published over 3,000 annotated bibliographies on specialized topics. It makes its databases available for online searching, and provides copies of abstracted documents through its document delivery services.

CAB International's Commonwealth Bureau of Nutrition is responsible for collecting, indexing, abstracting, and disseminating information on human and animal nutrition. It produces *Nutrition Abstracts and Reviews*, the only major abstracting service specifically devoted to the nutrition literature. This now appears in two sections, one for experimental and human nutrition and one for livestock feeds and feeding.

The Food and Nutrition Information Center at the National Agricultural Library provides indexing of nutrition, food science and technology, nutrition education, and food service material for the *Bibliography of Agriculture*. Its activities are described in chapter 7.

The literature search services provided by the National Library of Medicine's Medical Literature Analysis and Retrieval System (MEDLARS) are vital to nutritionists and dietitians, as is its *Index Medicus*, the major periodical index to journals in the health sciences. These services are discussed in chapters 4 and 5.

Nutrition Indexing/Abstracting Services

56. **Food and Nutrition Quarterly Index**. Vol. 1- . Phoenix, Ariz.: Oryx Press, 1985- . quarterly. ISSN 0887-0535.

This abstracting service succeeds the *Food and Nutrition Bibliography*, which was issued from 1980-1984 and covered the literature from 1978-1980, and was essentially a continuation of the *FNIC Catalog* and its supplements. Like its predecessor, it is based on indexing done by the Food and Nutrition Information Center (FNIC) for the AGRICOLA database. It covers material in about 80 periodicals, as well as books and audiovisual media on human nutrition; nutrition education and extension work; food service management; administrative, legislative, and economic aspects of food and nutrition; food science and technology; food products; home economics; and selected material in peripheral disciplines.

Online Equivalent: AGRICOLA.

Arrangement: Numbered abstracts are arranged by broad subjects.

Indexes: There are personal and corporate author indexes, a title index, a subject index, and an intellectual level index.

Comments: Useful for those working in the areas of applied nutrition and food service, but less useful for researchers. Coverage of the journal literature is highly selective and includes some newsletters and popular magazines. Users of this publication should be aware that there is a considerable gap in coverage between the last volume of its predecessor (volume 11, covering 1980) and the first issue of the new title. Although the *Food and Nutrition Quarterly Index* and the *Food and Nutrition Bibliography* are based on indexing done for the *Bibliography of Agriculture*, they are both quite different from this publication. They provide better subject access by means of an excellent indexing terminology, the *Food and Nutrition Information Center Controlled Vocabulary*. They include abstracts omitted from the *Bibliography of Agriculture*, and they also provide access to material not found there, such as audiovisual materials and books.

57. **Nutrition Abstracts and Reviews**. Vol. 1- . Farnham Royal, England: CAB International, 1931- . monthly. ISSN 0029-6619. (See figure 7.)

Since 1977 this publication has appeared in two sections: *Series A: Human and Experimental* (ISSN 0309-1295) and *Series B: Livestock Feeds and Feeding* (ISSN 0309-135X). *Nutrition Abstracts and Reviews* is one of a series of specialized indexing/abstracting services produced by the CAB International. *NAR* is the most comprehensive indexing/abstracting service in the field of nutrition, providing access to about 8,000 items per year. It indexes and summarizes journals, many in foreign languages, conference publications, reports, selected government publications, and selected books. It does not provide extensive coverage of U.S. government publications or Asian materials.

Online Equivalent: CAB Abstracts.

Arrangement: Continuously numbered abstracts are grouped according to the following categories, each of which is in turn subdivided into more detailed subjects: technique, foods, physiology and biochemistry (divided into literature on various nutrients and physiological processes) human health and nutrition, disease and therapeutic nutrition, reports, conferences, and books. At various times in its history *NAR* has included major review articles on topics of interest, although this practice has been discontinued.

Indexes: Each issue has a subject and an author index which are cumulated annually.

CAB Thesaurus: The indexing vocabulary used in *NAR* has been a problem for American users, who are not used to British terminology. As of January 1984 this situation has been eased by *NAR*'s use of the *CAB Thesaurus*, a listing of index terms used in all CAB abstracting services. Long-time users of *NAR* will notice some major changes in the indexing vocabulary, though the terminology will still seem remote and artificial to many.

List of Periodicals Indexed: Usually periodical titles cited in *NAR* are not abbreviated. Therefore, users have few periodical identification problems. *NAR* has published occasional lists of periodicals scanned, sometimes with the cumulated index or with the January issue. A new *CAB Serials Checklist* for all of the CAB abstracting services was published in 1984, with periodicals coded for the title of the specific CAB service which indexes them.

Comments: One interesting feature of *NAR* is its indexing by country. If a user wished to find out about nutrition in Thailand, he or she could look under "Thailand." When relevant, subject terms in the index are identified by country also (e.g., *Obesity, cardiovascular diseases, risks, USA*). This is a great help in eliminating unwanted citations immediately.

Nutrition Abstracts and Reviews Series A Human and Experimental

Subject Index

Food and Agriculture Organization
fisheries, roles, nutrition, reviews 4786
food additives, reference source 14
food aid, requirements, estimation 4426
reports
  agriculture, food supplies, develop-
    ing countries 5055
  contaminants 4167
  food additives 4167
  food hygiene, health 3777
  statistics, techniques 256
Food aversions (*see* Food preferences)
Food beliefs
  adolescents, athletes, USA 3090, 7062
  Belgium 4451
  beverages 2812
  breast feeding, Fiji 283
  ethnic groups, South Africa 4428
  food supplements, Australia 7716
  ice cream 2812
  infant feeding
    Europe 3821
    Fiji 283

Subject Entry with additional descriptors (note geographic name)

Subject Term

Abstract Number

Author Index

Perkins, E. G. 5312
Perkins, M. J. 6119
Perkkiö, M. 2598, 7150
Perkkiö, M. V. 6944
Perl, I. M. 4725
Perman, J. A. 5216, 6807, 7285
Pernet, A. 3591
Perrenoud, J. P. 7712
Perring, M. A. 3478
Perron, M. 7062
Perrone, R. D. 781
Perry, S. V. 7457
Persaud, C. 7571
Persaud, J. 453
Pershad, D. 6991, 7060
Persson, B. 359, 1181, 4561, 4565, 4604
Persson, H. 5117
Persson, L. 7229
Persson, L. Å. 1108, 1725, 2460, 3826
Pertschuk, M. J. 1299

Author Entry

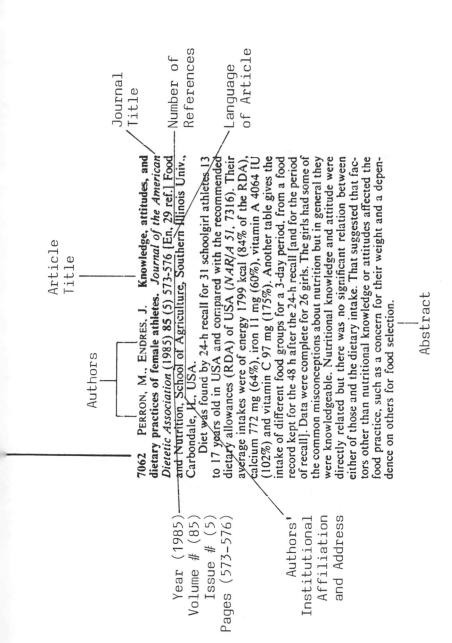

Article Title

Journal Title

Number of References

Language of Article

Authors

Year (1985)
Volume # (85)
Issue # (5)
Pages (573-576)

Authors' Institutional Affiliation and Address

Abstract

7062 PERRON, M., ENDRES, J. **Knowledge, attitudes, and dietary practices of female athletes.** *Journal of the American Dietetic Association* (1985) **85** (5) 573-576 [En, 29 ref.] Food and Nutrition, School of Agriculture, Southern Illinois Univ., Carbondale, IL, USA.

Diet was found by 24-h recall for 31 schoolgirl athletes 13 to 17 years old in USA and compared with the recommended dietary allowances (RDA) of USA (*NAR/A 51*, 7316). Their average intakes were of energy 1799 kcal (84% of the RDA), calcium 772 mg (64%), iron 11 mg (60%), vitamin A 4064 IU (102%) and vitamin C 97 mg (175%). Another table gives the intake of different food groups for a 3-day period, from a food record kept for the 48 h after the 24-h recall [and for the period of recall]. Data were complete for 26 girls. The girls had some of the common misconceptions about nutrition but in general they were knowledgeable. Nutritional knowledge and attitude were directly related but there was no significant relation between either of those and the dietary intake. That suggested that factors other than nutritional knowledge or attitudes affected the food practice, such as a concern for their weight and a dependence on others for food selection.

Fig. 7. Illustration page from *Nutrition Abstracts and Reviews*. Reproduced by permission of Commonwealth Agricultural Bureaux International.

ONLINE DATABASES

58. **CAB Abstracts**
CAB Abstracts is one of the most comprehensive databases in agriculture and related fields. It consists of the specialized abstracting services produced by CAB International. These exist in all fields of agriculture ranging from animal breeding to weeds. *Dairy Science Abstracts* and *Nutrition Abstracts and Reviews* are most relevant to food science and nutrition. This database covers approximately 13,000 periodicals and other types of publications, such as conference proceedings, reports, and selected books in 50 languages. Each year about 150,000 abstracts are added to the database. CAB references can be retrieved by subject headings found in the *CAB Thesaurus*. They can also be retrieved by author, type of publication, journal title, language, publisher, publication date, subject code, and chapter headings. Searches can be limited to specific abstracting services, such as *Nutrition Abstracts and Reviews*.

BIBLIOGRAPHIES AND GUIDES

59. Ashworth, Ann. **Feeding of Infants and Young Children: An Annotated Bibliography**. London: Bureau of Hygiene and Tropical Diseases, 1985. 91p. (Tropical Diseases Bulletin, Vol. 82, Supplement).
This bibliography of over 400 annotated references on infant feeding emphasizes material on the developing countries but is not strictly limited to tropical areas. An index is included.

60. Blanchard, J. Richard, and Lois Farrell, eds. **Guide to Sources for Agricultural and Biological Research**. Berkeley, Calif.: University of California Press, 1981. 735p. ISBN 0520032268.
This excellent guide to reference sources in agriculture contains a lengthy chapter on nutrition and food science reference sources (about 40 pages).

61. Crowhurst, Christine Marie, and Bonnie Lee Kumer. **Infant Feeding: An Annotated Bibliography**. Toronto: Nutrition Information Service, Ryerson Polytechnical Institute Library, 1982. 154p. ISBN 0919351069.
Contains over 700 references with abstracts on breast feeding, infant formulas, comparisons between these feeding methods, solid foods, infant formula use in developing countries, preterm and low birthweight infants, clinical concerns, and recipes. The bulk of the references was published after 1976. Audiovisual materials are included. There is no index.

62. Furse, Alison, and Elyse Levine. **Food, Nutrition, and the Disabled: An Annotated Bibliography**. Toronto: Nutrition Information Service, Ryerson Polytechnical Institute Library, 1981. 82p. ISBN 091935100X.
This bibliography covers primarily books, although some journal literature is included. It also includes a list of organizations and equipment suppliers.

63. Henderson, Jane O., et al. **Bibliography of Infant Foods and Nutrition, 1938-1977**. Melbourne, Australia: Commonwealth Scientific and Industrial Research Organization; distr., Forest Grove, Oreg.: ISBS, 1978. 322p. ISBN 0643003169.

This work contains 2,259 references gleaned in part from searches of *Dairy Science Abstracts*, *Food Science and Technology Abstracts*, *Nutrition Abstracts and Reviews*, and the AGRICOLA database. It is organized by broad subject categories, with author and subject indexes.

64.   Jelliffe, Derrick Brian, et al. **Breast Feeding and Weaning Foods: An Annotated Bibliography of Recent Publications**. Ann Arbor, Mich.: Nutrition Planning Information Service, 1974? 30 leaves.

This brief bibliography provides access to citations on breast feeding practices in developing countries. It includes some references dating from the 1940s and 1950s.

65.   Jelliffe, E. F. Patrice. **Protein-Calorie Malnutrition in Early Childhood: Two Decades of Malnutrition: A Bibliography**. Slough, England: Commonwealth Agricultural Bureaux, 1975. 118p. ISBN 0851983559.

This classified bibliography contains 3,371 references.

66.   Metress, Seamus P., and Cary S. Kart. **Nutrition and Aging: A Bibliographic Survey**. Monticello, Ill.: Vance Bibliographies, 1979. 96p. (Public Administration Series: Bibliography No. P-309).

Included are approximately 1,400 references, chiefly to journal literature, some dating back into the 1950s. Citations without abstracts are arranged according to broad subject categories, for example, vitamins and the elderly. No indexes are provided.

67.   National Research Council. Committee on Nutrition of the Mother and Preschool Child. **A Selected Annotated Bibliography on Breast Feeding, 1970-1977**. Washington, D.C.: National Academy of Sciences, 1978. 58p. ISBN 0309027969.

This work includes over 400 English-language books and articles intended for nurses, nutritionists, physicians, and other health professionals. It is organized by broad topics and has no index.

68.   Read, Merrill S. "Guide to Materials for Use in Teaching Nutrition in Schools of Medicine, Dentistry, and Public Health." **American Journal of Clinical Nutrition** 38 (November 1983): 775-94.

A revision of The Nutrition Foundation's *Selected Nutrition Reference Texts for Physicians and Medical Students* (1976), this bibliography includes materials evaluated by over 100 reviewers for basic sciences, clinical teaching, or continuing education. Included are reference sources, texts, industry publications, teaching modules and audiovisuals, review series, and other periodicals. The emphasis is on recent clinical nutrition materials published after 1976.

69.   Rodgers, Kay. **Human Diet and Nutrition**. Washington, D.C.: Science Reference Section, Science and Technology Division, Library of Congress, 1981. 18p. (LC Tracer Bullet, No. TR 81-16).

This is a brief but useful guide to locating nutrition information in libraries. Intended for the Library of Congress, it is useful anywhere.

70. St. Clair, Barbara Elaine, and Sandra Ann Wong. **Nutrition and Aging: A Selected Bibliography**. Toronto: Nutrition Information Service, Ryerson Polytechnical Institute Library, 1982. 128p. ISBN 0919351050.

Included are over 750 largely unannotated citations to journal articles, books, and pamphlets dealing with such topics as the physiology of aging, common diseases of the aged, nutritional status and requirements, food habits, and meal planning and preparation. Also included are relevant bibliographies, periodicals, and associations.

71. Smith, Anne, et al. **Obesity: A Bibliography, 1974-1979**. London: Information Retrieval, 1980. 340p. ISBN 0904147177.

This updates the earlier bibliography by Hilary Whelan and Trevor Silverstone, published in 1974, and covers the years 1974-1979. It is arranged by broad subjects and has good topical and author indexes.

72. Society for Nutrition Education. **Nutrition Information Resources for Professionals**. rev. ed. Berkeley, Calif.: Society for Nutrition Education, 1979. 15p.

This brief guide to selected sources of information in nutrition now needs updating, but some of it is still relevant, such as its guidelines for evaluating nutrition materials. It lists basic and more specialized books, selected periodicals, and, briefly, names and addresses of government agencies, trade associations, and professional organizations.

73. Trowell, Hubert C. **Dietary Fibre in Human Nutrition: A Bibliography**. London: J. Libbey for Kellog Company of Great Britain, 1979. 56p.

References dating back to classical times are arranged here by year of publication. Subject and author indexes are included.

74. Ullrich, Helen D. **Health Maintenance through Food and Nutrition: A Guide to Information Sources**. Detroit: Gale Research, 1981. 305p. (Health Affairs Information Guide Series, No. 7). ISBN 0810315009.

This bibliography is intended for the nonspecialist and covers the whole spectrum of nutrition literature, especially as related to health. It consists chiefly of selected references to journal literature, but also includes books and government publications. Author, title, and subject indexes are included.

75. Weg, Ruth B., and Anne M. Bailey. **Nutrition and Aging: A Selected Bibliography**. Los Angeles, Calif.: Ethel Percey Andrus Gerontological Center, University of Southern California, 1977. 51p.

This bibliography includes references from 1969 to 1977.

76. Whelan, Hilary, and Trevor Silverstone. **Obesity: A Bibliography, 1964-1973**. London: Information Retrieval, 1974. 253p. ISBN 0904147010.

A substantial bibliography of mostly journal literature for the years 1964 to 1973. Arranged by broad subjects and indexed in detail by specific topics and authors.

DICTIONARIES

Nutrition Dictionaries

77. Anderson, Kenneth, and Lois Harmon. **The Prentice-Hall Dictionary of Nutrition and Health**. Englewood Cliffs, N.J.: Prentice-Hall, 1985. 257p. ISBN 0136956106.

The emphasis in this dictionary is on health rather than nutrition. It is aimed at the health professional, but is also suitable for the general public. Definitions are clear and substantial, but the total number of terms is small—about 900 to 1,000 entries. It includes an appendix.

78. Ashley, Richard, and Heidi Duggal. **Dictionary of Nutrition**. New York: St. Martin's Press, 1975. 236p.

79. Bender, Arnold E. **Dictionary of Nutrition and Food Technology**. 5th ed. Boston: Butterworths, 1982. 309p. ISBN 040810855X.

This edition defines approximately 3,400 nutrition and food science and technology terms, including 250 new items and 350 revised entries. A bibliography is appended for further reference. Tables in the back consist of U.S., U.K., and FAO recommended dietary allowances.

80. Food and Agriculture Organization of the United Nations. **Food and Nutrition Terminology: Definitions of Selected Terms and Expressions in Current Use (English Only)**. Rome: FAO Terminology and Reference Section, 1974. 54p. (Terminology Bulletin, No. 28).

Provided are English-language definitions of 142 basic terms with equivalents in French and Spanish.

81. Lagua, Rosalinda T., Virginia S. Claudio, and Victoria F. Thiele. **Nutrition and Diet Therapy: Reference Dictionary**. 2nd ed. St. Louis, Mo.: C. V. Mosby Co., 1974. 329p. ISBN 0801628075.

"The previous edition was copyrighted in the Philippines in 1969, and this second one has been redesigned for American and international use. It will probably be of use mainly to dietitians and students of dietetics and nursing. After the dictionary proper there is a series of appendices from A to V dealing with a range of subjects from a comparison of dietary standards, through diagrams of the Embden-Meyerhof pathway" (*Nutrition Abstracts and Reviews A*, 1975, #9471).

82. Mayes, Adrienne. **The Dictionary of Nutritional Health: A Guide to the Relationship between Diet and Health**. Wellingborough, England; distr., New York: Thorsons Publishing Group, 1986. 286p. ISBN 0722511469.

This dictionary includes definitions of roughly 2,400 terms. Included are nutrition science terms, selected biochemical terms, and individual nutrients and foods. Many of the entries for individual foods have data on nutrients. Entries for individual nutrients contain data on recommended allowances or intakes, toxicity, and food sources.

Medical Dictionaries

83. **Dorland's Illustrated Medical Dictionary**. 1st ed.- . Philadelphia, Pa.: W. B. Saunders, 1900- .

(This description is based on the twenty-sixth edition, published in 1981.) This extensive dictionary of medical terminology is generally considered a standard. Pronunciation is included. The alphabetical sequence is letter by letter. All spaces and hyphens between words are ignored. Terms consisting of two or more words are ordinarily defined under the major noun. For example, definitions for *acetic acid*, *citric acid*, and *fatty acid* are all grouped alphabetically under *acid*. The book contains a substantial number of illustrations and plates. The medical etymology section preceding the dictionary has word roots derived from the Latin and Greek.

84. **Stedman's Medical Dictionary**. 24th ed. Baltimore, Md.: Williams and Wilkins, 1982. 1678p. ISBN 0683079158.

Stedman's standard medical dictionary contains approximately 100,000 terms with pronunciations. This edition has over 8,000 new entries and about 25,000 revised entries. Multiple-word entries are grouped under major nouns. For instance, *diabetic acidosis*, *lactic acidosis*, and *metabolic acidosis* are grouped under *acidosis*. However, the subentry index in the appendix helps by referring the user from *diabetic acidosis* to *acidosis*. Also included in the appendix are blood groups, reference values for laboratory tests and evaluations, comparative temperature scales, and common Latin terms used in prescription writing. An extensive root word list precedes the dictionary.

ENCYCLOPEDIAS

85. Considine, Douglas M., and Glenn D. Considine, eds. **Foods and Food Production Encyclopedia**. New York: Van Nostrand Reinhold, 1982. 2305p. ISBN 0442216122.

This well-produced one-volume encyclopedia emphasizes agricultural commodities, and contains articles of varying length. It includes information on history, production, varieties, pests, processing, and dietary and nutritional quality as well as handling, storage, and transportation of food. Longer articles have bibliographies. *See* references are plentiful and there is a detailed index. Appendixes include a table of food additives now in use.

86. Coyle, Patrick L. **The World Encyclopedia of Food**. New York: Facts on File, 1982. 790p. ISBN 0871964171.

Descriptions of some 4,000 foods and beverages from throughout the world, including staples and local specialties are arranged alphabetically. This is an excellent source of brief information on foreign or ethnic foods. It contains numerous illustrations.

87. Ensminger, Audrey H., et al. **Foods and Nutrition Encyclopedia**. Clovis, Calif.: Pegus Press, 1983. 2415p. 2v. ISBN 0941218058.

This excellent encyclopedia covers commodities, nutrients, concepts, nutrition disorders, and simple nutritional biochemistry with both brief and extensive entries. The entry under *additives* has extensive tables of food additives now in use. Entries under *agricultural commodities* have material on origin and history, production, propagation and growing, harvesting, processing, selection and preparation, and nutritional value. The entry under *convenience and fast foods* has extensive nutrient tables of foods available at major fast food chains. An extensive food composition table based on USDA data is included. There are illustrations and an index.

88. Lapedes, Daniel N., ed. **McGraw-Hill Encyclopedia of Food, Agriculture and Nutrition**. New York: McGraw-Hill, 1977. 732p. ISBN 0070452636.

"Designed to inform the student, librarian, scientist, teacher, engineer, and lay person about all aspects of agriculture; the cultivation, harvesting, and processing of food crops; food manufacturing; and health and nutrition — from the economic and political to the technological aspects" (*Nutrition Abstracts and Reviews A*, 1978, #9139).

The first part contains articles on the world food problem. The second part has 400 alphabetically arranged and signed articles with occasional bibliographies. An index is included.

89. Tver, David F., and Percy Russell. **Nutrition and Health Encyclopedia**. New York: Van Nostrand Reinhold, 1981. 569p. ISBN 0442248431.

"From abalone to zymogen this volume lists alphabetically terms associated not only with nutrition but with all the related sciences including chemistry, physiology and general medicine. The space allocated varies from one line, e.g., the definition of 'labile', to a page or more for the major vitamins. The text includes chemical structures, useful tables of vitamin sources and composition of foods, and there are some line drawings illustrating, among other things anatomical and histological entries" (*Nutrition Abstracts and Reviews A*, 1982, #2379).

Appendixes include abbreviations, prefixes, atomic weights, weights and measures, conversion tables, weight ranges for heights of men and women, RDAs, mineral and vitamin content of foods, etc.

HANDBOOKS, MANUALS, AND OTHER DATA COMPILATIONS

90. Altman, Philip L., and Dorothy S. Dittmer, eds. **Biology Data Book**. Bethesda, Md.: Federation of American Societies for Experimental Biology, 1972-1974. 3v.

This is the major reference work presenting data in the biological sciences. Two volumes have information of interest to nutritionists: volume 1 includes general data on reproduction, growth, and development; volume 3 has extensive data on nutrition, digestion, excretion, metabolism, respiration, circulation, blood, and other body fluids.

91. Altman, Philip L., and Dorothy S. Dittmer, eds. **Metabolism**. Bethesda, Md.: Federation of American Societies for Experimental Biology, 1968. 737p. (Biological Handbooks).

This revision and updating of *Standard Values in Nutrition and Metabolism*, edited by E. C. Albritton, is an extensive compilation of data related to metabolic functions. It includes food composition and energy values, animal nutrition, plant nutrition, digestion and absorption, nutrient function, deficiency and excess, animal energy exchange, metabolic pathways, plant metabolism, and metabolic end products.

92. Aronson, Virginia, and Barbara Danielson Fitzgerald. **Guidebook for Nutrition Counselors.** North Quincy, Mass.: Christopher Publishing House, 1980. 484p. ISBN 0815803877.

"A practical guide for developing more effective counseling techniques ... intended for dietitians, nutritionists and students involved in a variety of consultative settings (including hospitals, clinics, and physicians', dentists' and private offices)." This guide contains numerous sample forms and handouts (e.g., a food intake record, 24-hour recall record, diet history, activity record, insulin chart). Chapter bibliographies are included; there is no index.

93. Briggs, George M., and Doris Howes Calloway. **Nutrition and Physical Fitness.** 11th ed. New York: Holt, Rinehart and Winston, 1984. 623p. ISBN 0030585872.

This largely rewritten edition of *Bogert's Nutrition and Physical Fitness* (tenth edition, 1979) covers the range of materials commonly found in basic nutrition texts. In addition, there are chapters on the relationship of nutrition to physical fitness and sports, food beliefs and eating patterns, and global malnutrition. The extensive tables in the appendix contain the RDAs, recommended daily nutrient intakes for Canadians, FAO/WHO recommended intakes, a food composition table based primarily on Agriculture Handbook No. 8, height-weight tables, and an extensive bibliography on all of the material covered in the text. An index is included.

94. Cameron, Margaret, and Yngve Hofvander. **Manual on Feeding Infants and Young Children.** 3rd ed. Oxford: Oxford University Press, 1983. 214p. (Oxford Medical Publications). ISBN 0192614037.

Published under the auspices of the FAO/WHO/UNICEF Protein Advisory Group (PAG), this manual is primarily intended for health and nutrition professionals. It focuses on breast feeding and on weaning foods in developing countries. Included are reference values for height and weight.

95. Collins, Douglas. **Illustrated Manual of Fluid and Electrolyte Disorders.** Philadelphia, Pa.: Lippincott, 1976. 180p. ISBN 039750361X.

This manual covers normal fluid and electrolyte metabolism, effects of individual electrolyte alterations, and fluid and electrolyte disorders and their diagnosis. It contains 64 excellent color illustrations.

96. Eagles, Archibald, and Mildred N. Randall. **Handbook of Normal and Therapeutic Nutrition.** New York: Raven Press, 1980. 323p. ISBN 0890043256.

This discussion of basic concepts of normal and therapeutic nutrition is geared to nursing students and others preparing for health science careers. Appendixes have exchange lists, tables of desirable weights, a food composition table, and the RDAs. There is a subject index.

97. Forbes, Gilbert B., and Calvin W. Woodruff, eds. **Pediatric Nutrition Handbook.** 2nd ed. Elk Grove Village, Ill.: Committee on Nutrition, American Academy of Pediatrics, 1985. 421p. ISBN 091076106X.

Thirty-five chapters deal at length with the feeding of normal infants and children, basic nutrition concepts, nutrition in disease, and various dietary modifications, for example, vegetarian diets. Extensive appendixes contain growth charts and other anthropometric data; the RDAs; data on the composition of human milk and infant formulas; laboratory values; and tables listing the calcium, zinc, iron, and sodium content of foods. An index is included.

98.   Garrison, Robert H., and Elizabeth Somer. **The Nutrition Desk Reference.** New Caanan, Conn.: Keats Publishing, 1985. 245p. ISBN 0879833289.

Aimed at health professionals and the general reader, this book covers the basics of nutrition and discusses the following topics: nutrition and cancer, nutrition and cardiovascular disease, dietary recommendations, nutrition and drugs. Controversial topics, such as vitamin supplementation, are represented by authors with differing views. An index, a glossary, and extensive references are included.

99.   Goodhart, Robert S., and Maurice E. Shils, eds. **Modern Nutrition in Health and Disease.** 6th ed. Philadelphia, Pa.: Lea and Febiger, 1980. 1370p. ISBN 0812106458.

The most extensive reference text in nutrition, in a greatly revised, updated edition with 40 chapters by over 80 contributors, this book covers every conceivable topic related to normal and clinical nutrition. The appendix has such information as desirable heights and weights; lipids and polyunsaturates in selected foods; the major exchange lists; protein, sodium, potassium, phosphorus, and zinc contents of major foods; and data on special diets and formula diets. The index is excellent.

100.   Gussler, Judith D., Marlene A. Woo-Lun, and Nancy M. Smith, eds. **The International Breast Feeding Compendium.** 3rd ed. Columbus, Ohio: Ross Laboratories, 1984. (Volume 1, **Eastern Hemisphere**; volume 2, **Western Hemisphere**).

"The purpose of this document is to summarize and present much of the available data on the prevalence and duration of and trends in breast-feeding worldwide." Information is by country within a regional arrangement. A detailed alphabetical country index provides information about the types of data and year of study. (See entry 116 for information on the update to this work.)

101.   Hamilton, Eva May Nunnelley, Eleanor Noss Whitney, and Frances Sienkiewics Sizer. **Nutrition, Concepts and Controversies.** 3rd ed. St. Paul, Minn.: West Publishing Co., 1985. 475, 133p. ISBN 0314852433.

An excellent basic book for the beginning student or layperson, this offers the "straight scoop" on many nutrition controversies and can serve as a useful nutrition education tool. Excellent graphs, line drawings, and color photographs do much to create interest and make the text more understandable. Chapters cover nutrition basics as well as nutrition surveys; energy balance; composition and safety of foods; maternal, child, and adolescent nutrition; and nutrition problems of the elderly. Controversial topics are discussed in the brown pages at the end of each chapter. Among the many subjects treated are natural foods, diet and heart disease, and sugar in the diet and hyperactivity. A section entitled "Controversy Notes and Selected References" lists extensive literature on these topics. Extensive appendixes include a general table of food composition based on Home and Garden Bulletin, No. 72 with added material about vegetarian foods and tables on the following: dietary fiber, sodium, potassium, fats, cholesterol, fatty acids, sugar in foods, and nutrients in fast foods. Also included in the appendixes are the RDAs, recommended nutrient intakes for Canadians, a comparison of vitamin and mineral supplements, and food exchanges. It contains bibliographies and a good index.

102. Helsing, Elisabet, and Felicity Savage King. **Breast-Feeding in Practice: A Manual for Health Workers**. Oxford: Oxford University Press, 1982. 271p. ISBN 0192612980 (pbk).

This manual is intended as a practical manual for health workers who may lack the necessary information to handle problems, answer questions, and provide guidance to nursing mothers. An appendix is included.

103. Hsu, Jens M., and Robert L. Davis. **Handbook of Geriatric Nutrition: Principles and Applications for Nutrition and Diet in Aging**. Park Ridge, N.J.: Noyes Publications, 1981. 372p. ISBN 0815508808.

This book contains 19 chapters on the status of various nutrients in the aged, psychological and sociological aspects of nutrition, food facts, fads and fallacies related to aging, etc., and has bibliographies and an index.

104. International Commission on Radiological Protection. Task Group on Reference Man. **Report of the Task Group on Reference Man**. Oxford, New York: Pergamon, 1975. 480p. (ICRP Publication, No. 23). ISBN 0080170242.

Presents basic biological data for a reference individual developed for the estimation of radiation doses, but useful for any purpose, such as finding out the composition of adipose tissue or calcium content of the human body. Contains general anatomical values and data on the integumentary system, the skeleton, cartilage, connective tissue and teeth, the hematopoietic system, the lymphatic system, the spleen and thymus, the skeletal muscle system, the cardiovascular system, the digestive system, the respiratory system, the urogenital system, the endocrine system, the central nervous system, special sense organs, and pregnancy. It also includes data on the gross and elemental content of the human body.

105. Kirschman, John D., and Lavin J. Dunne. **Nutrition Almanac**. 2nd rev. ed. New York: McGraw-Hill, 1984. 313p. ISBN 0070349053; 0070349061 (pbk).

This is a compendium of nutrition information aimed at the layperson, some of it of uncertain reliability. There are six chapters, one on herbs and herbal preparations, a food composition table, a bibliography, and an index. "Although much of the information in this book is factual, some of it is questionable and problematic" (*Journal of Nutrition Education* 17 [December 1985]: 206).

106. Kutsky, Roman J. **Handbook of Vitamins, Minerals and Hormones**. 2nd ed. New York: Van Nostrand Reinhold, 1981. 492p. ISBN 0442245572.

The first edition was published in 1973 under the title *Handbook of Vitamins and Hormones*. This work provides useful information on 28 vitamins and minerals and 29 hormones. The data are presented in outline format and include information on dietary and medicinal forms, history of biological significance, physiological forms, synergistic agents, antagonistic agents, physiological functions, body content, concentration in organs, deficiencies, excess, essentiality, commercial uses, medicinal applications, hazards and toxicity, distribution and sources, metabolic role, relationship to other vitamins, hormones and minerals, etc. There are summary tables and an index.

107.   Lentner, Cornelius, ed. **Geigy Scientific Tables**. 8th ed. West Caldwell, N.J.: Ciba-Geigy Corp., 1981- . ISBN 0914168509 (vol. 1); 0914168517 (vol. 2); 0914168525 (vol. 3).

Volume 1 contains units of measurement, data on body fluids, body composition, and nutrition. Volume 2 has an introduction to statistics, statistical tables, and mathematical formulae. Volume 3 covers physical chemistry, blood, and somatometric data.

These volumes are useful for such things as body composition, vitamin levels in blood, composition of breast milk, body mass and height, development of teeth, growth, etc.

108.   MacDonald, Donna, Roxanne Buckle, and Rosemary Berardi. **Nutrition and Fitness Manual: Summary of Research and Resources**. Toronto: Nutrition Information Service, Ryerson Polytechnical Institute Library, 1983. 110p. ISBN 0919351107.

Intended for use by fitness instructors, coaches, nutritionists, and other program leaders, this manual covers topics ranging from general nutrition to dietary regimes used by professional athletes. It contains a bibliography of popular and professional references.

109.   Machlin, Lawrence J., ed. **Handbook of Vitamins: Nutritional, Biochemical, and Clinical Aspects**. New York: Marcel Dekker, 1984. 614p. (Food Science and Technology). ISBN 082477051X.

This volume covers history, chemistry, biological assays, analytical procedures, metabolism, biochemical function, deficiency signs, methods of nutritional assessment, nutritional requirements, factors influencing vitamin status, efficacy of pharmacological doses, and hazards of high doses. It also provides some information on substances without vitamin status (e.g., laetrile, pangamic acid, orotic acid). An index is included.

110.   Paige, David M., ed. **Manual of Clinical Nutrition**. Pleasantville, N.J.: Nutrition Publications, 1983. 1003p. ISBN 0316035092.

This manual is updated by a periodical, *Clinical Nutrition*. Major sections on principles of nutrition, nutrition in the normal life cycle, evaluating nutritional status, systemic disorders and nutrition, nutritional management of specific disease states, nutritional deficiencies and abnormalities, nutritional management and counseling are divided into chapters written by specialists. Appendixes include U.S. dietary standards, selected reference diets, food tables, growth standards, analyses of popular diets, and data on U.S. dietary intake. It includes an index. "Invaluable as a day-to-day reference text as well as serving as a quick short course for nutrition in medical practice" (*American Journal of Clinical Nutrition* 39 [1984]: 984-85).

111.   Parkinson, Susan, and Julian Lambert. **The New Hand Book of South Pacific Nutrition**. 3rd ed. Suva, Fiji: Fiji National Food and Nutrition Committee, 1982. 92p.

(The cover title is *The New South Pacific Handbook of Nutrition*.)

"A practical reference for people applying the principles of good nutrition through education, medicine or agricultural programmes in the South Pacific." It contains a food value chart showing whether local foods are good, medium, or poor sources of major nutrients. There is no index.

112. Raab, Constance, and Jean Tillotson, eds. **Heart to Heart: A Manual on Nutrition Counseling for the Reduction of Cardiovascular Disease Risks**. Bethesda, Md.: National Institutes of Health, 1983. 121p. (DHHS Publication. Vol. (NIH) 83-1528). HE20.3008N95.

This manual for nutritionists, dietitians, and other health professionals involved in counseling patients with cardiovascular disease or at risk includes information on nutrition assessment and monitoring techniques, practical nutrition counseling guidelines and skills, nutrition counseling in groups, sources for patient education materials, a checklist for assessing patient education materials, and professional associations and voluntary health groups.

113. Rechcigl, Miloslav, Jr., ed. **CRC Handbook of Nutritional Supplements**. Boca Raton, Fla.: CRC Press, Inc., 1983. 2v. ISBN 0849339693 (vol. 1); 0849339707 (vol. 2).

Volume 1 is entitled *Human Use*; volume 2, *Agricultural Use*. This handbook does not cover vitamin supplements, but a variety of dietary supplements ranging from single nutrients to formulated foods, synthetically produced foods, and enrichment and fortification of foods, as well as foods for special uses such as parenteral nutrition. Volume 1 is a potentially useful source of information for those interested in the practical aspects of preventing malnutrition.

114. Rechcigl, Miloslav, Jr., ed. **CRC Handbook of Nutritional Requirements in a Functional Context**. Boca Raton, Fla.: CRC Press, Inc., 1981. 2v. ISBN 0849339561 (vol. 1); 0849339588 (vol. 2).

Included is information on nutritional requirements related to physiological stress in animals and man. Volume 1 is *Development and Conditions of Physiologic Stress*; volume 2, *Hematopoiesis, Metabolic Function, and Resistance to Physical Stress*.

115. Rechcigl, Miloslav, Jr., ed. **CRC Handbook Series in Nutrition and Food**. Cleveland, Ohio: CRC Press, Inc., 1977- .

This series was projected as a set of 19 or more volumes on nutrition. It was to cover a wide range of topics from culture media to human nutrition, but its structure was altered and unfortunately, many volumes pertaining to human nutrition were never published.

Of interest to nutritionists and dietitians are Section E: *Nutritional Disorders*, volume I, *Effect of Nutrient Excesses and Toxicities in Animals and Man*, 1978 (518p.); and Section E: *Nutritional Disorders*, volume III, *Effect of Nutrient Deficiencies in Man*, 1978 (388p.).

116. Ryan, Alan S., and Judith D. Gussler, eds. **International Breast-Feeding Compendium: Updated Appendix to Volumes 1 and 2, Third Edition, 1984**. Columbus, Ohio: Ross Laboratories, 1986. 1v. (various paging).

"The purpose of this document is to update the material presented in the 1984 edition of the International Breast-Feeding Compendium. This appendix summarizes much of the latest available data on the prevalence and duration of and trends in breast-feeding worldwide."

117.   Van-Lane, Deirdre, and Donna MacDonald. **A Manual on Food and Nutrition for the Disabled**. Toronto: Nutrition Information Service, Ryerson Polytechnical Institute Library, 1981. 73p.

This manual covers basic nutrition principles, nutrition in disabling conditions, homemaking and feeding problems, including information on feeding aids. It includes an extensive annotated bibliography.

118.   Watkin, Donald M. **Handbook of Nutrition, Health and Aging**. Park Ridge, N.J.: Noyes Publications, 1983. 326p. ISBN 0815509294.

This includes general information about nutrition and aging, specific nutrients and their relation to aging, and federally sponsored programs for the aged. It contains a bibliography and an index.

119.   Watson, Ronald R., ed. **CRC Handbook of Nutrition in the Aged**. Boca Raton, Fla.: CRC Press, Inc., 1985. 355p. ISBN 0849329337.

Individually authored chapters provide information on the general nutritional problems of the elderly and the effect of aging on specific nutrients. Contains tables, references, and an index.

120.   Weinsier, R. L., and C. E. Butterworth, Jr. **Handbook of Clinical Nutrition: Clinician's Manual for the Diagnosis and Management of Nutritional Problems**. St. Louis, Mo.: C. V. Mosby Co., 1981. 231p. ISBN 0801654068.

"This pocket-sized handbook contains a remarkable amount of practical information on different aspects of human nutrition. There are five main sections dealing with nutritional assessment, nutritional support with details on formula diets for tube ... and parenteral feeding. Short but concise chapters consider nutrition in burns, cancer, hepatic failure, malabsorption, renal failure, obesity, diabetes, hyperlipaemia and vegetarian diets. Later sections discuss nutrition in growth and pregnancy and drug-nutrient interaction. A short appendix supplies miscellaneous information" (*Nutrition Abstracts and Reviews*, 1982, #2366).

121.   Whitney, Eleanor Noss, and Corrine Balog Cataldo. **Understanding Normal and Clinical Nutrition**. St. Paul, Minn.: West Publishing Co., 1983. 1065p. ISBN 0314696857.

"A two-semester edition of the original *Understanding Nutrition* by E. N. Whitney and E. M. N. Hamilton." In addition to the material on general nutrition principles and normal nutrition, this book provides extensive information on therapeutic nutrition. It is thoroughly readable, with numerous illustrations and a great deal of practical, factual information on nutrition problems and controversies interspersed throughout the text on blue pages (e.g., alcohol and nutrition, surgery for morbid obesity, sugar, protein calorie malnutrition). References are provided for further reading. Appendixes include a list of popular nutrition books which are *not* recommended, basic chemistry concepts, patient/client education materials, aids to calculation, assessment standards and tools (including growth charts), sugar content of foods, a food composition table, information on dietary fiber in selected foods, exchange lists, table of nutrient values in fast foods, dietary standards such as the RDAs, WHO recommendations, and Canadian standards, and a comparison of major vitamin and mineral supplements. A detailed index is appended.

122.   Whitney, Eleanor Noss, and Eva May Nunnelley Hamilton. **Understanding Nutrition**. 3rd ed. St. Paul, Minn.: West Publishing Co., 1984. 573, 215p. ISBN 0314778624.

Style, format, and type of information included here are basically that of previous editions. The material is well presented and highly readable. Highlighted sections explore interesting topics (e.g., "Alcohol and the B Vitamins"). A good reference source for basic nutrition information, the book has two new chapters—"Introduction to Nutrition" and "Nutrition Status, Food Choices, and Diet Planning." Unfortunately, many of the supporting references in the previous editions have been deleted to save space. Extensive appendixes are a gold mine (e.g., history of discoveries in biochemistry and nutrition, summary of basic chemistry concepts, biochemical structures, recommended nutrition references, exchange system, tables of food composition, etc.).

123.   Williams, Sue Rodwell. **A Handbook of Commonsense Nutrition**. St. Louis, Mo.: C. V. Mosby Co., 1983. ISBN 0801655862.

This is an adaptation of Mowry's *Basic Nutrition and Diet Therapy*, sixth edition (1980). It is geared to the nonnutritionist, and seeks to provide "a source of clearly stated nutrition information." It contains a glossary of specialized terms.

124.   World Health Organization. Regional Office for the Western Pacific. **The Health Aspects of Food and Nutrition. A Manual for Developing Countries in the Western Pacific Region of the World Health Organization**. 3rd ed. Manila, Philippines: Regional Office for the Western Pacific, 1979. 380p.

"This is the third edition of a manual first published in 1969 ... and contains sections on foods and nutrition with nutrient requirements and recommended intakes appropriate to the region, nutritional disorders, nutritional surveillance, intervention programmes and a series of appendices embodying reference data" (*Nutrition Abstracts and Reviews A*, 1981, #9255).

DIRECTORIES

Bibliographies and Guides to Directories

125.   **Directory of Directories**. 1st ed.- . Detroit: Gale Research, 1980- . biennial. ISSN 0275-5580.

This lists and describes directories available in a variety of subject areas— health and medicine, science and engineering, humanities, social sciences, business, banking, etc. The yellow pages in the back are title and subject indexes.

126.   Gray, Constance Staten. **U.S. Government Directories, 1970-1981: A Selected Annotated Bibliography**. Littleton, Colo.: Libraries Unlimited, 1984. 260p. ISBN 0872874141.

This bibliography of 575 directories received as Government Printing Office depository items defines directories as "alphabetical or classified lists of organizations, individuals, business places, laws, programs and so forth." Title and subject indexes are included; appendixes include a list of regional federal depository libraries, the GPO Sales Publications Reference File, U.S. government book stores, and departments and agencies.

127. **International Bibliography of Special Directories: Internationale Bibliographie der Fachadressbücher.** 7th ed.- . Munich, New York: K. G. Saur, 1983- . (Handbuch der Internationalen Documentation und Information, Vol. 5). ISSN 0724-4126.
   Printed in English and in German, this continues *International Bibliography of Directories*.

National and International

128. **American Men and Women of Science: Physical and Biological Sciences.** 10th ed.- . New York: R. R. Bowker, 1960- . irregular. ISSN 0192-8570.
   The sixteenth edition (1986) contains biographies of 127,000 living scientists in all disciplines. For a time, this was issued in two sections: *Physical and Biological Sciences*, and *Social and Behavioral Sciences*. Because of limited acceptance the latter section was last issued in 1978.

129. Baldwin, Carol, ed. **Nutrition Professional Directory.** Emmaus, Pa.: Rodale, 1978. 41p.
   This geographic listing of nutritionally oriented physicians docs not list dietitians and nutritionists. It needs updating.

130. **Current Contents Address Directory. Science & Technology.** Philadelphia, Pa.: Institute for Scientific Information, 1985- . annual. ISSN 0882-2360. (1st ed., 1984).
   The author section of this directory is useful for locating the addresses of over one million authors covered by *Current Contents*, *Science Citation Index*, and other publications of ISI. Entries under names contain abbreviated citations to an author's publications as an aid in identifying an author's specialty. The organization section is an alphabetical list of organizations with names of researchers who published during the year covered. The geographic section lists authors by countries and cities. Within a city the arrangement is by organization. The organization and geographic sections can be used to locate addresses of academic and research institutions and to find names of researchers in a specific area.

131. **Encyclopedia of Associations.** 1st ed.- . Detroit: Gale Research, 1961- . annual. ISSN 0071-0202.
   This is the major source of information on American organizations. This directory now lists over 18,000 professional, trade, and other organizations. Volumes 1 and 2 list organizations and contain geographic, keyword, name, and executive indexes. Volume 3 lists new associations and projects and volume 4 is a separate listing of international associations with an index. Entries contain the

following information: name, address, telephone number, name of president or chief officer, date of founding, number of members, purpose and activities, publications, and conventions or conferences.

132. Frank, Robyn C., ed. **Directory of Food and Nutrition Information Services and Resources**. Phoenix, Ariz.: Oryx Press, 1984. 287p. ISBN 0897740785.

"Provides directory and bibliographic information for the food and nutrition sciences. It lists organizations, databases, software, journals and newsletters, abstraets and indexes, producers of books, audiovisuals and microcomputer software, key reference materials, and regional, state, and area agencies and organizations. There are subject, geographic, and organization indexes. Nutrient tables and a listing of American Dietetic Association approved training programs complete this thorough, well-organized directory" (*Choice* 22 [March 1985]: 962).

133. Kruzas, Anthony Thomas, Kay Gill, and Karen Backus, eds. **Medical and Health Information Directory: A Guide to Associations, Agencies, Companies, Institutions, Research Centers, Hospitals, Clinics, Treatment Centers, Educational Programs, Publications, Audiovisuals, Data Banks, Libraries, Information Services in Clinical Medicine, Basic Bio-Medical Sciences, and the Technological and Socio-Economic Aspects of Health Care**. 3rd ed. Detroit: Gale Research, 1985- . ISBN 0810302683.

When this greatly expanded third edition is complete it will consist of three volumes and will be one of the most extensive directories in the field. Volume 1 provides brief descriptive entries for national and international organizations, lists state and regional organizations and local affiliates of national organizations, federal and state agencies, foundations, HMOs, pharmaceutical and health insurance companies, publishers, research centers and institutes, and medical and allied health schools. Volume 2 lists medical journals, newsletters, annuals and review series, indexing and abstracting publications, directories, computerized information services, audiovisual producers and services, libraries and information centers. Most of the sections in volume 1 have separate indexes. Volume 2 has a master index in the back.

134. **The National Faculty Directory**. Detroit: Gale Research, 1983- . annual. ISSN 0077-4472.

"Names, departmental affiliations, and institutional addresses of about 592,800 members of teaching faculties at approximately 3,030 American colleges and universities."

135. **Research Centers Directory**. 1st ed.- . Detroit: Gale Research, 1960- annual. ISSN 0080-1518.

"A guide to approximately 7,500 university-related and other non-profit organizations ... carrying on a continuing research program."

136. Sakura, JoAnne, Nancy Plaatjes, and Kathleen Gordon, eds. **A Directory of Canadian Organizations Involved in Food and Nutrition**. Toronto: Nutrition Information Service, Ryerson Polytechnical Institute Library, 1982. 306p. ISBN 0919351018.

Included are about 300 entries covering consumer health and development agencies; consultants and private practitioners; education and research institutions; food, drug, and health industry groups; government agencies; hospitals and health care facilities; private publishers; and professional associations.

137. Scarpa, Ioannis S., Helen Chilton Kiefer, and Rita Tatum, eds. **Sourcebook on Food and Nutrition**. 3rd ed. Chicago: Marquis Academic Media, 1982. 549p. ISBN 0837945038.

"A compendium of dietary information on current topics ... designed primarily as a reference tool for librarians, dieticians, researchers, biochemists, students, physicians." Major sections deal with dietary directions in the 1980s, nutrition from conception through adolescence, adulthood into old age and resources for further information. This last section includes extensive listings of food, agriculture, and nutrition libraries, relevant organizations, colleges and universities with food and nutrition curricula, nutrition organizations providing grants, food and nutrition periodicals, and publishers. Contains a food composition table (USDA Home and Garden Bulletin, No. 72). There is an index.

138. Union of International Associations. **Yearbook of International Organizations**. 11th ed.- . Munich, New York: K. G. Saur, 1966- . ISSN 0084-3814.

(This description is based on the twenty-second edition, 1985/86.)

Volume 1, *Descriptions and Index*, provides essential information on over 18,000 international organizations. Volume 2 is *International Organization Participants, Country Directory of Secretariats and Memberships*. Volume 3 is *Global Action Networks; Classified Directory by Subject and Region*.

139. United States. Department of Agriculture. Food and Nutrition Service. **Directory of Cooperating Agencies**. Washington, D.C.: Food and Nutrition Service, 1981?- . irregular. A98.2:D62/2.

State education and health and human service agencies working with USDA on food assistance programs are listed here with contact persons, addresses, and telephone numbers.

140. United States. Department of Agriculture. Office of Operations. **Telephone Directory—United States Department of Agriculture**. Washington, D.C.: Government Printing Office, 1974- . irregular. A1.89.

The white pages list individuals, the blue pages are the organizational listing.

141. United States. Department of Agriculture. Policy and Coordination Council. Committee of Research and Education. **Directory, Human Nutrition Activities: Food and Fitness**. Washington, D.C.: Department of Agriculture, 1984. 21p. A1.2:D83/5.

This is a directory of data gathering, research, service, and other nutrition activities within the USDA.

142. United States. Department of Agriculture. Science and Education Administration, Cooperative Research. **Directory of Professional Workers in State Agricultural Experiment Stations and Other Cooperating State Institutions**. Washington, D.C.: Government Printing Office, 1981- . irregular. A1.76:305.

This includes nutrition and food science personnel.

143.   United States. Department of Health and Human Services. **Telephone Directory**. Washington, D.C.: Government Printing Office, 1980- . HE1.28.

The white pages list individuals; the yellow pages are the organizational section.

144.   Verrel, Barbara, and Helmut Opitz, eds. **World Guide to Scientific Associations and Learned Societies: Internationales Verzeichnis Wissenschaftlicher Verbände und Gesellschaften**. 4th ed. Munich, New York: K. G. Saur, 1984. 947p. ISBN 3598205228.

A revised edition of *World Guide to Scientific Associations*, this directory is a country-by-country list of scientific and technical associations. It provides chief officers, address, and number of members. Organization names are also listed by broad subject categories.

State and Local

145.   Broering, Naomi C., Helen C. Bagdoyan, and Linda S. Blackburn, eds. **Directory of Food and Nutrition Programs in the District of Columbia, Maryland and Virginia**. Washington, D.C.: Food and Nutrition Information Center, U.S. Department of Agriculture, 1980. 86 leaves. A106.102:D62. (available from EDRS, ED 204 435).

Prepared under a grant from the Food and Nutrition Information Center at USDA, this directory describes nutrition programs and resources in the District of Columbia, Maryland, and Virginia. It includes information on programs of federal and state agencies, health-related organizations, special interest groups, businesses, and professional organizations. Entries include name of organization, purpose, clientele, research, availability of service, and publications. Also included is a list of libraries, information services, and databases that provide information on food and nutrition. Title and subject indexes refer to entry numbers.

146.   The Greater New York Dietetic Association. **Directory of Nutrition: Resources and Consultation Services for New York City**. New York: Nutrition Information Center, 1982. 33p. (Greater New York Dietetic Association, P.O. Box 416, Lenox Hill Station, New York, NY 10021. $4.00).

An updated version of the 1979 *Directory of Nutrition Sources, Counseling and Resource Information* issued by the association, this directory lists a range of nutrition and nutrition information services available from qualified professionals. It lists nutritionists and dietitians in private practice, with a specialty and geographic index; counseling services, such as weight control programs, hospital outpatient services, and specialty clinics and private organizations; government nutrition programs; and resources for nutrition information.

147.   Illinois State Council on Nutrition. **Nutrition Services in Illinois. Feeding Programs and Nutrition Education**. 2nd ed. Springfield, Ill.: Illinois State Council on Nutrition, 1984. 88p. (available from EDRS, ED 244 911).

"This publication lists information about Illinois state agencies and organizations that participate in feeding programs and/or have nutrition programs and nutrition services available to the public. This nutrition services sourcebook also lists where one can go for help and available information and services."

148. Iowa Dietetic Association. **Directory of Iowa Food and Nutrition Services.** Iowa: Prepared by the Iowa Dietetic Association in cooperation with the Iowa Corn Promotion Board, 1981- . looseleaf.

149. Nebraska Nutrition Council. **Directory of Food and Nutrition Services.** Lincoln, Nebr.: Nebraska Nutrition Council, 1975? 53p.

150. New Jersey. State Department of Health. Office of Local Health and Regional Operations. Nutrition Consultation Services. **Directory of New Jersey's Resources for Food and Nutrition.** Trenton, N.J.: New Jersey Department of Health, 1983- . (New Jersey State Department of Health, CN 364, Trenton, NJ 08625. $5.00).

"This directory has been compiled to update health providers with information about current food assistance programs and community resources that can be used to improve the diets of individuals and families served at all levels of the health system."

SELECTED REFERENCES

Frank, Robyn C. "Information Resources for Food and Human Nutrition." *Journal of the American Dietetic Association* 80 (1982): 344-49.

Leitch, Isabella. "The Collection and Dissemination of Information on Nutrition Science with Special Reference to the United Kingdom." *Progress in Food and Nutrition Science* 2 (1976): 59-79.

11
Food Composition Data

Knowledge of the nutrients contained in foods is essential not only for the practical application of nutrition principles, but also for research, nutrition planning, and food policy implementation. This type of information is conveniently collected in food composition tables for easy reference. Frequently such tables are issued by national and international governmental bodies. To be of practical use these tables must actually contain data on foods eaten by most of the population. Unfortunately, few general tables have many of the foods commonly eaten by ethnic minorities. However, there are numerous international and foreign tables which contain these specialty foods.

The data in food composition tables may be derived from a combination of the following sources: analyses done by government agencies and universities; food industry analyses; and information from analyses published in food science, agriculture, and nutrition journals. In the case of the major tables available to professionals in the United States—the various sections of the revised Agriculture Handbook No. 8—the latest information from all of the above sources is critically evaluated before it is added. In this country much of the data that find their way into commercially published food tables are derived from Agriculture Handbook No. 8.

SEARCHING SUGGESTIONS

It is advisable to use the most general tables first. If these are not useful, the various ethnic or foreign tables or tables devoted to specific nutrients, listed below, may help. For tables that are not listed in this guide, consult the following bibliographies and guides to food composition tables.

Bibliographies and Guides
to Food Composition Tables

151. Boston Area Research Dietitians, Special Practice Group, and Massachusetts Dietetic Association. **Nutrient Composition of Foods: Selected References and Tables**. Boston: Boston Area Research Dietitians, 1978. 41 leaves.

This bibliography of food composition sources includes many citations to journals for difficult to locate nutrients, such as vitamin E, copper, iodine, zinc, trace metals, etc.

152. Food and Agriculture Organization of the United Nations. Nutrition Policy and Programmes Service. **Food Composition Tables, Updated Annotated Bibliography**. Rome: Food and Agriculture Organization of the United Nations, 1975. 181p.

This international bibliography covers some 165 food composition tables. Annotations include information on background, portion analyzed, nutrients included, arrangement, etc.

153. International Network of Food Data Systems (INFOODS). **International Directory of Food Composition Tables**. 1st ed. Cambridge, Mass.: INFOODS Secretariat, 1986. 18p. (INFOODS Secretariat, Massachusetts Institute of Technology, Room 20A-226, 77 Massachusetts Avenue, Cambridge, MA 02139).

"This first edition lists only titles, compilers and publishers; later editions will be expanded to include descriptions of contents of these data tables and sources of data. It is the intention of this directory to list food composition data tables that have been compiled for use around the world. No attempt has been made to list the many journal articles which contain valuable food composition data, except in those cases where very limited data are available." The directory is organized by geographic area. The language is noted when it is not English.

154. Robson, John R. K., and Joel W. Elias. **The Nutritional Value of Indigenous Wild Plants**. New York: Whitston Publishing Co., 1978. 232p. ISBN 0878751122.

This does not include information more recent than 1972 or 1973. Indexes of common and scientific plant names are included.

If these sources do not lead to the necessary data, consider a search of the journal literature. The indexing and abstracting services of choice are *Food Science and Technology Abstracts* and *Agrindex*. Although *Biological Abstracts* is a good source of food composition information, computer searching is preferable to manual searching because it allows refinement of the search strategy enabling the user to combine such elements as genus and species of a food plant with terms for specific nutrients or nutrient groups. *Agrindex* is a good source for information of this type. Each issue has an entire section devoted to food composition information. However, cumulative indexes currently are not being published at reasonable intervals. The database is now available for online searching in the United States.

The citations below include many references to the journal literature. These are highly selective because of space limitations. To be included, an article had to deal with nutrients or foods not easily located in commonly available food composition tables, and had to cover a substantial number of foods. Reports in the literature on a single nutrient in a single food or in a small group of foods were automatically excluded.

GENERAL TABLES (NORTH AMERICA)

155. U.S. Department of Agriculture. Consumer and Food Economics Institute. **Composition of Foods: Raw, Processed, Prepared**. (Agriculture Handbook No. 8).

> No. 8-1, *Dairy and Egg Products; Raw, Processed, Prepared*. Washington, D.C.: Government Printing Office, 1976. A1.76:8-1.

> No. 8-2, *Spices and Herbs; Raw, Processed, Prepared*. Washington, D.C.: Government Printing Office, 1977. A1.76:8-2.

> No. 8-3, *Baby Foods; Raw, Processed, Prepared*. Washington, D.C.: Government Printing Office, 1978. A1.76:8-3.

> No. 8-4, *Fats and Oils; Raw, Processed, Prepared*. Washington, D.C.: Government Printing Office, 1979. A1.76:8-4.

> No. 8-5, *Poultry Products; Raw, Processed, Prepared*. Washington, D.C.: Government Printing Office, 1979. A1.76:8-5.

> No. 8-6, *Soups, Sauces, and Gravies; Raw, Processed, Prepared*. Washington, D.C.: Government Printing Office, 1980. A1.76: 8-6.

> No. 8-7, *Sausages and Luncheon Meats; Raw, Processed, Prepared*. Washington, D.C.: Government Printing Office, 1980. A1.76: 8-7.

> No. 8-8, *Breakfast Cereals; Raw, Processed, Prepared*. Washington, D.C.: Government Printing Office, 1982. A1.76:8-8.

> No. 8-9, *Fruits and Fruit Juices; Raw, Processed, Prepared*. Washington, D.C.: Government Printing Office, 1983. A1.76:8-9.

> No. 8-10, *Pork and Pork Products; Raw, Processed, Prepared*. Washington, D.C.: Government Printing Office, 1983. A1.76:8-10.

> No. 8-11, *Vegetables and Vegetable Products; Raw, Processed, Prepared*. Washington, D.C.: Government Printing Office, 1984. A1.76:8-11.

> No. 8-12, *Nut and Seed Products; Raw, Processed, Prepared*. Washington, D.C.: Government Printing Office, 1984. A1.76:8-12.

> No. 8-14, *Beverages; Raw, Processed, Prepared*. Washington, D.C.: Government Printing Office, 1986. A1.76:8-14.

When completed, this handbook is expected to contain data on over 4,000 foods, and will be the largest and most comprehensive compilation of its type. It is a revision of the 1963 edition (K. Watt, *Composition of Foods*), which contained 2,483 foods. Published in sections according to food groups, it is expected to be complete in 1988. Individual components on which data are included are:

food energy, fat, protein, carbohydrates, water, fiber, ash, calcium, iron, magnesium, phosphorus, potassium, sodium, and zinc, ascorbic acid, thiamin, riboflavin, niacin, pantothenic acid, vitamin B-6, folacin, vitamin B-12, vitamin A, saturated, monounsaturated and polyunsaturated fatty acids, cholesterol and phytosterols, and 18 amino acids. Surprisingly, vitamin E or tocopherol values are omitted in most sections—even with foods that are expected to be good sources of this nutrient. Data in the tables are provided on 100-gram quantities, edible portion only, although equivalents to common household measures are given at the top of the page. For most items, data are also provided for one pound as purchased. Values are provided as mean values with standard error and number of samples.

156. Adams, Catherine F. **Nutritive Value of American Foods in Common Units**. Washington, D.C.: Government Printing Office, 1975. 291p. (Agriculture Handbook No. 456). A1.76:456.

"Basic reference data on nutrients in frequently used household measures and market units of food.... This handbook includes data on approximately 1500 foods.... The nutritive values on which data are provided include water, food energy, protein, fat, carbohydrate, five mineral elements (calcium, phosphorus, iron, sodium, and potassium), five vitamins (vitamin A, thiamin, riboflavin, niacin, and ascorbic acid), total saturated fatty acids and two unsaturated fatty acids."

157. Adams, Catherine F. **Nutritive Value of Foods**. Washington, D.C.: Government Printing Office, 1981. 34p. (Home and Garden Bulletin, No. 72). A1.77:72.

Intended for home use, this food table provides information on caloric values, water, protein, fat (saturated, unsaturated), oleic and linoleic acid, carbohydrates, calcium, phosphorus, iron, potassium, vitamin A, thiamin, riboflavin, niacin, and vitamin C, in common household measures with equivalents in grams.

158. Bowes, Anna de Planter. **Bowes and Church's Food Values of Portions Commonly Used**. 14th ed. Revised by Jean A. T. Pennington and Helen Nichols. Philadelphia, Pa.: Lippincott, 1984. 257p. ISBN 0397544901.

This newly revised edition of one of the major American food composition tables has been greatly expanded. Saturated fatty acids, vitamin B-6, vitamin B-12, vitamin E, pantothenic acid, cholesterol, zinc, copper, and manganese have been added to the main table. Vitamin A is given both in international units and retinol equivalents. A section of supplementary tables provides amino acid values, data on selected alcoholic beverages, sources of protein, fat and carbohydrate in infant formulas, brand name information on polyunsaturated fatty acids and saturated fatty acids in margarines, chromium, cobalt, fluorine, iodine, molybdenum, nickel, selenium, tin, biotin, vitamin D, vitamin E as alpha tocopherol, vitamin K, choline, caffeine, dietary fiber, myo-inositol, nitrite and nitrate, oxalate and phytate in selected foods. Also included in this section are a list of purine-yielding foods, foods high in salicylates, tyramine, and theobromine, and an extensive table of sugars in selected foods. An index is appended.

159.   Canada. Health Services and Promotion Branch. **Nutrient Values of Some Common Foods**. rev. ed. Ottawa, Ont.: Health Services and Promotion Branch, 1979. 35p. ISBN 0662113470.

This is a table of nutrient values of over 600 common foods eaten in Canada. Entirely in metric units, this table provides information on 15 nutrients. Vitamin A values are presented in retinol equivalents and niacin values in niacin equivalents. There are separate tables on total dietary fiber in food and recommended nutrient intakes. A bibliography of sources is included. This table is very similar in scope to *Nutritive Value of Foods* (Home and Garden Bulletin, No. 72).

160.   Dadd, Robert C. **Nutritional Analysis System: A Physician's Manual for Evaluation of Therapeutic Diets, with Special Emphasis on the Rotary Diversified Diet**. Springfield, Ill.: Charles C. Thomas, 1980. 137p. ISBN 0398046816.

Intended to help physicians analyze nutrient values in special diets, this book contains an extensive food value table which translates information on nutrients in 700 unprocessed foods into percentages of the RDA on a per-100-gram basis.

161.   Dreifke, Colleen K., et al., eds. **Infant Formulas and Selected Nutritional Supplements**. Columbus, Ohio: Children's Hospital, Department of Dietetics, 1984. 26p.

This includes information on the composition of more than 100 infant and adult formulas, modular components, and electrolyte solutions.

162.   **The Fast-Food Nutrition Guide: Nutritional Data for Menu Items of Fast Service Restaurants**. Wichita, Kans.: Fortrex Corp., 1983. 96p.

This guide provides information on energy values, protein, carbohydrates, total fat, vitamin A, thiamin, riboflavin, niacin, calcium, iron, sodium, potassium, and cholesterol content of foods served at major fast food chains. It also provides exchange list information for diabetics.

163.   First National Supermarkets. Pick-n-Pay Consumer Center. **Nutri-Scan: A Shopping Guide to Calories, Fat, and Sodium**. Cleveland, Ohio: First National Supermarkets, 1980. 70p.

Aimed at the layperson, this guide to nutrients in common foods graphically presents information on calories, fat, and sodium arranged by major food groups.

164.   Fordham, J. R., et al. "Sprouting of Seeds and Nutrient Composition of Seeds and Sprouts." **Journal of Food Science** 40 (1975): 552-56.

Data are included on water, ash, protein, lipids, ascorbic acid, tocopherol, carotene, thiamin, riboflavin, niacin, iron, magnesium, manganese, phosphorus, and potassium in 18 varieties of sprouted peas and beans.

165.   Franz, Marion J. **Fast Food Facts: Nutritive and Exchange Values for Fast Food Restaurants**. Minneapolis, Minn.: International Diabetes Center, St. Louis Park Medical Center Research Foundation, 1983. 31p.

Information is provided here on calories, carbohydrates, protein, fat, sodium, and exchanges of foods sold in 21 fast food chains.

166.   Gelb, Barbara Levine. **The Dictionary of Food and What's in It for You**. New York: Paddington Press, 1978. 253p. ISBN 0448223651.

A prefatory chapter entitled "Eater's Digest" offers a brief overview of essential nutrients for the layperson. The dictionary that follows provides nutrient information for 180 to 190 foods, along with a brief description of how they are made and their history.

167.   Hansen, Roger Gaurth, Bonita W. Wyse, and Ann W. Sorenson. **Nutritional Quality Index of Foods**. Westport, Conn.: AVI, 1979. 636p. ISBN 0870553208.

"This book explains how nutrient density (expressed as a ratio) can be used to describe nutritional quality. The numerator is the nutrient composition of the food supply or the diet or the meal, or even the individual food. The denominator is human need or allowance for individual nutrients. Both parameters are expressed on a common kilocalorie base. In Part II of the book, individual nutrient profiles are displayed for over 700 foods. Knowing the foods that form a meal, and using the erasable plastic overlay ruler, which is provided with the book, one can examine the balance of nutrients in any combination of foods or diet."

168.   Kylen, Ann M., and Rolland M. McGrady. "Nutrients in Seeds and Sprouts of Alfalfa, Lentils, Mung Beans and Soy Beans." **Journal of Food Science** 40 (1975): 1008-9.

Values for water, food energy, protein, fiber, ash, calcium, zinc, thiamin, riboflavin, niacin, and ascorbic acid are provided.

169.   Lantz, Edith M., Helen W. Gough, and Mae Martha Johnson. **Nutritive Values of Some New Mexico Foods**. Las Cruces, N. Mex.: New Mexico College of Agriculture and Mechanic Arts, 1953. 20p. (Agricultural Experiment Station Bulletin, No. 379).

Data on approximately 40 foods are included, but for a limited number of nutrients.

170.   Leveille, Gilbert A., et al. **Nutrients in Foods**. Cambridge, Mass.: Nutrition Guild, 1984. 291p. ISBN 0938550004.

Included are nutrient composition data on more than 2,700 foods, with a total of 62 factors. The data are from the Michigan State University Nutrient Data Bank, which in turn is based on information from USDA and food industry sources. Many nutrients are presented in more than one unit of measurement, for example, electrolytes are given in both milligrams and milliequivalents, vitamin E values in international units and milligrams of alpha and other tocopherols, vitamin A in international units and retinol equivalents. Also included are both crude and dietary fiber and polyunsaturated to saturated fatty acid ratio. A conversion factor is included that enables the user to convert nutrient values from portion size to 100-gram units. One of the most useful features of the table are data on the percentage of the U.S. RDA of selected nutrients provided by a 100-gram portion of food. The appendix contains information on the caffeine and alcohol content of selected foods.

171.   Pennington, Jean A. Thompson. **Dietary Nutrient Guide**. Westport, Conn.: AVI, 1976. 276p. ISBN 0870551965.

This is a guide to diet analysis and planning based on index nutrients (vitamin B-6, magnesium, pantothenic acid, folacin, vitamin A, iron, and calcium), which if present in adequate amounts will automatically insure the adequacy of other essential nutrients. It includes various tables of nutrients in foods.

172.   Peterkin, Betty B., Jennie Nichols, and Cynthia Cromwell. **Nutrition Labelling: Tools for Its Use**. Washington, D.C.: Government Printing Office, 1975. 57p. (Agriculture Information Bulletin, No. 382). A1.75:382.
Intended to assist the general public in using nutrition labeling information to improve dietary practices, this food table provides information on those nutrients appearing on food labels – calories, protein, vitamin A, vitamin C, thiamin, riboflavin, calcium, and iron. It also provides lists of foods which are considered good sources of these nutrients.

173.   Rechcigl, Miloslav, ed. **Handbook of Nutritive Value of Processed Food**. Boca Raton, Fla.: CRC Press, Inc., 1982. 2v. ISBN 0849339510 (vol. 1).
Although volume 1, *Food for Human Use*, does not contain nutrient tables as such, it has valuable information on the effects of various types of processing techniques on nutrients. Arranged by specific processes, specific foods, and by specific nutrients, many of the data are presented in tabular form.

174.   Truesdell, D. D., E. N. Whitney, and P. B. Acosta. "Nutrients in Vegetarian Foods." **Journal of the American Dietetic Association** 84 (1984): 28-35.
Data on energy, approximate composition, calcium, phosphorus, iron, potassium, zinc, vitamin A, thiamin, riboflavin, niacin, vitamin C, and folacin in approximately 70 foods are included here.

175.   Wilford, Laura, ed. **Nutritive Value of Convenience Foods**. 3rd ed. Hines, Ill.: West Suburban Dietetic Association, 1982. 168p.
This contains information on calories, protein, carbohydrates, fat, cholesterol, sodium, and potassium.

INDIVIDUAL NUTRIENTS

Calories, Carbohydrates, and Fiber

176.   Groves, Phil, Carol Lissance, and Mele Olsen. **The Natural Food Calorie Counter**. Toronto: Bantam Books, 1983. 164p. ISBN 0553237020 (pbk).
This is a very useful book for hard to locate energy values of fresh and prepared "natural" foods. The arrangement is alphabetical by food. Included are brand name comparisons and charts comparing different types of commercial products (e.g., yogurt, breads, crackers, popcorn, etc.).

177.   Kraus, Barbara. **The Barbara Kraus Guide to Fiber in Foods**. New York: New American Library, 1975. 204p.

178.   Kraus, Barbara. **The Barbara Kraus 1983 Carbohydrate Guide to Brand Names**. New York: New American Library, 1983. 147p. ISBN 0451119975 (pbk).

179.   Kraus, Barbara. **The Barbara Kraus 1985 Calorie Guide to Brand Names and Basic Foods**. rev. ed. New York: New American Library, 1985. 147p. ISBN 0451119967 (pbk).

"Excerpted from the *Dictionary of Calories and Carbohydrates....* A smaller and handier version." Gives calorie information for over 8,000 brand names and basic foods.

180.   Kraus, Barbara. **Calories and Carbohydrates**. 6th rev. ed. New York: New American Library, 1985. 353p. ISBN 0452256631 (pbk).

181.   Kraus, Barbara. **The Dictionary of Calories and Carbohydrates**. New York: Grosset and Dunlap, 1973. 388p.

182.   La Gette, Bernard. **La Gette's Calorie Encyclopedia**. New York: Greenwich House, 1984. 431p. ISBN 0517455935.

Caloric values of fresh, commercial, and home prepared foods are arranged by food category—beverages, dairy, breads, etc. Quantities are not given for some items; therefore, it is impossible to tell how large an average portion of sauerbraten one can eat for 570 calories, or the precise amount of sauerkraut totaling 257 calories. Many brand name foods are included. This is aimed at dieters. There is no index.

183.   Lanza, Elaine, and Ritva R. Butrum. "A Critical Review of Food Fiber Analysis and Data." **Journal of the American Dietetic Association** 86 (1986): 732-40.

This article presents a provisional dietary fiber table containing data on approximately 130 foods. Entries are coded as to method of analysis.

184.   LaSota, Marcia. **The Fast Food Restaurant Calorie Guide**. Mankato, Minn.: Gabriel Books, 1979. 137p.

185.   Merrill, A. L., and B. K. Watt. **Energy Value of Foods**. Washington, D.C.: Government Printing Office, 1973. 105p. (Agriculture Handbook No. 74). A1.76:74.

"This publication has been prepared to provide more background information on food energy data than is given in current textbooks and food tables and to show the basic data drawn upon in deriving the revised calorie factors now used in tables of food composition in this country."

186.   Page, Louise, and Nancy Raper. **Calories and Weight: The USDA Pocket Guide**. Washington, D.C.: Government Printing Office, 1981. 80p. (Agriculture Information Bulletin, No. 364). A.175:364/3.

Aimed at the public, this pamphlet offers advice on weight loss and provides information on the caloric values of commonly eaten foods. It is arranged by major food groups.

187.   Ross, Jane K. "Dietary Fiber Constituents of Selected Fruits and Vegetables." **Journal of the American Dietetic Association** 85 (1985): 1111-16.

Data are included on dietary fiber, neutral detergent fiber, cellulose, hemicellulose, lignin, and pectin content of common fruits and vegetables.

188.   Southgate, D. A. T., and S. A. Bingham. "The Contribution of Different Groups of Foodstuffs to the Intake of Dietary Fibre." **Qualitas Plantarum— Plant Foods for Human Nutrition** 29 (1979): 49-58.

Included are tables of data for dietary fiber content of various fruits, vegetables, and cereal products.

189.   Spear, Tziporah. **Kosher Calories**. New York: Genesis, 1985. 352p.

190.   Spiller, Gene A., ed. **Topics in Dietary Fiber Research**. New York: Plenum, 1978. 223p. ISBN 0306311267.

This is a supplement to *Fiber in Human Nutrition*. The appendix contains data on total dietary fiber, noncellulosic polysaccharides, cellulose, and lignin in about 50 foods. Also included are indigestible residue and cell wall (NDF) fractions.

191.   Wenlock, Robert W., Lorna M. Sivell, and Irene B. Agater. "Dietary Fiber Fractions in Cereal and Cereal-Containing Products in Great Britain." **Journal of the Science of Food and Agriculture** 36 (1985): 113-21.

Data are presented on hexoses, pentoses, uremic acids, cellular lignin, and total dietary fiber in wheat flours, and other cereals and cereal products including bread, rolls, buns, scones, cakes, pastry, breakfast cereals, and other foods.

192.   Zyren, J., E. R. Elkins, J. A. Dudek, and R. E. Hagen. "Fiber Contents of Selected Raw and Processed Vegetables, Fruits and Fruit Juices as Served." **Journal of Food Science** 48 (1983): 600-603.

Data on pectin and neutral detergent fiber (NDF) content in 28 foods are presented.

Fat and Cholesterol

193.   Carpenter, D. L., et al. "Lipid Composition of Selected Vegetable Oils." **Journal of the American Oil Chemists Society** 53 (1976): 713-18.

Data on the composition of 14 vegetable oils are presented.

194.   Feeley, R. M., P. E. Criner, and B. K. Watt. "Cholesterol Content of Foods." **Journal of the American Dietetic Association** 61 (1972): 134-49.

About 200 foods are covered.

195.   Giant Food, Inc. **Special Diet Alert: Low Calorie, Low Fat/Cholesterol, Low Sodium: A Guide to Help You Find Products for Your Special Diet Needs in Cooperation with the Food and Drug Administration**. rev. ed. Washington, D.C.: Giant Food, Inc., 1984. 100p.

Developed as a nutrition education tool by Giant Food, Inc. (a large eastern supermarket chain) in conjunction with the FDA, this table of sodium, fat, cholesterol, and energy values was intended to be used by consumers along with shelf labels. However, it stands by itself as a useful guide for consumers in search of low calorie, low fat, low cholesterol, and low sodium foods and for the dietitians and nutritionists advising them.

196. Kraus, Barbara. **The Dictionary of Sodium, Fats, and Cholesterol.** New York: Putnam, 1983, c1974. 366p. ISBN 0399509453.

Included here are data on many brand name products.

197. United States. Department of Agriculture. Human Nutrition Information Service. **Provisional Table on the Content of Omega-3 Fatty Acids and Other Fat Components of Selected Foods.** Hyattsville, Md.: Nutrient Data Research Branch, U.S. Department of Agriculture, 1986. folded leaflet. (HNIS/PT-103).

"Provides data on the linolenic (18:3), eicosapentaenoic (20:5), and docosahexaenoic (22.6) fatty acid content of approximately 140 items of fish origin and on the linolenic acid content of more than 100 other foods. Also provides data on total fat; total saturated, monounsaturated, and polyunsaturated fatty acids; and cholesterol in all items" (*Journal of the American Dietetic Association* 86 [1986]: 292. The table was also published in this volume, pp. 788-93).

Minerals
(General and Macrominerals, Except Sodium)

198. Dyer, W. J., D. Fraser Hiltz, E. R. Hayes, and V. G. Munro. "Retail Frozen Fishery Products—Proximate and Mineral Composition of the Edible Portion." **Canadian Institute of Food Science and Technology Journal** 10 (1977): 185-90.

Included are data on phosphorus, sodium, potassium, and calcium in approximately 200 retail products.

199. Gormican, A. "Inorganic Elements in Foods Used in Hospital Menus." **Journal of the American Dietetic Association** 56 (1970): 397-403.

Data are presented on phosphorus, potassium, calcium, magnesium, sodium, aluminum, barium, iron, strontium, copper, zinc, manganese, and chromium in 128 foods.

200. Gregor, J. L., S. Marhefka, and A. H. Geissler. "Magnesium Content of Selected Foods." **Journal of Food Science** 43 (1978): 1610-12.

Included are 145 foods.

201. Sidwell, V. D., et al. "Composition of the Edible Portion of Raw (Fresh or Frozen) Crustaceans, Finfish, and Mollusks II: Macroelements: Sodium, Potassium, Chloride, Calcium, Phosphorus, and Magnesium." **Marine Fisheries Review** 39 (1977): 1-11.

Covered are 161 seafoods.

202. Wong, N. P., D. E. LaCroix, and J. A. Alford. "Mineral Content of Dairy Products I: Milk and Milk Products." **Journal of the American Dietetic Association** 72 (1978): 288-91.

Included are calcium, magnesium, sodium, potassium, phosphorus, iron, zinc, copper, and manganese in 16 foods.

203. Wong, N. P., D. E. LaCroix, and J. A. Alford. "Mineral Content of Dairy Products II: Cheeses." **Journal of the American Dietetic Association** 72 (1978): 608-11.

Calcium, magnesium, sodium, potassium, zinc, copper, iron, phosphorus, and manganese in 21 types of cheese are covered.

Protein and Amino Acids

204.   Food and Agriculture Organization of the United Nations. Food Policy and Food Science Service. **Amino-Acid Content of Foods and Biological Data on Proteins**. Rome: Food and Agriculture Organization of the United Nations, 1970. 285p. (FAO Nutritional Studies, No. 24).

This remains a major work of reference on amino acid and protein quality data. Part I contains tables with 20 amino acid values in foods by food groups. Part II has biological data (e.g., biological value, PER, NPU) of single foods and mixtures of foods. Part III lists sources of data and part IV is a supplement. Plants are identified to genus and species, animals are frequently identified to broader taxa. Title, headings, and text preceding the tables are in English, Spanish, and French.

205.   Harvey, Douglas Graham. **Tables of the Amino Acids in Foods and Feedingstuffs**. 2nd ed. Farnham Royal, England: Commonwealth Agricultural Bureaux, 1970. 105p. (Commonwealth Bureau of Animal Nutrition. Technical Communication, No. 19). ISBN 0851980139.

Data on 18 amino acids in over 1,900 foods including vegetables, cereals, and cereal products, nuts, legumes, and seeds are included. There is a bibliography.

206.   Hunt, Melanie M., ed. **Phenylalanine, Protein and Calorie Content of Selected Foods**. Cincinnati, Ohio: Children's Hospital Research Foundation, 1977. 39p.

"This book is for use with older PKU children who no longer take just formula. Containing over 900 entries, the booklet lists foods in normal serving sizes. Although not complete by any means, it provides information not readily available elsewhere" (*Environmental Nutrition Newsletter* 9 [May 1986]: 4).

207.   International Association for Cereal Chemistry Symposium on Amino Acid Composition and Biological Value of Cereal Proteins, Budapest, 1983. **Proceedings**. Edited by R. Lasztity and M. Hidvegi. Dordrecht, Netherlands, Boston: Reidel, 1985. 662p. ISBN 9027719373.

Many of the papers presented here contain tables of amino acid values of selected grains, as well as data on protein quality.

208.   Kraus, Barbara, **The Barbara Kraus Dictionary of Protein: Over 8,000 Brand Names and Basic Foods with Their Protein (and Caloric) Count**. New York: Harper's Magazine Press, 1975. 344p. ISBN 0061251011.

Provided is information on total protein in over 8,000 foods. Arrangement is by broad food groups. Many of the values are taken from USDA sources and from data submitted by manufacturers.

209.   Sidwell, V. D., et al. "Composition of the Edible Portion of Raw (Frozen or Unfrozen) Crustaceans, Finfish, and Mollusks. I: Protein, Fat, Moisture, Ash, Carbohydrate, Energy Value, Cholesterol." **Marine Fisheries Review** 36 (March 1974): 21-35.
Included are data on 154 foods.

210.   U.S. Department of Agriculture. **Amino Acid Content of Foods**. By M. L. Orr and B. K. Watt. Washington, D.C.: Government Printing Office, 1957. (Home Economics Research Report, No. 4). A1.87:4.
The two tables presented here have data for the 18 most frequently occurring amino acids. "The first, which is the basic table, gives average, maximum and minimum amino acid values in grams per total grams of nitrogen in the edible portion of the food. The second, calculated from the average values in the first, ... may be used directly to estimate amino acid content of the food."

Sodium

211.   Jacobson, Michael, Bonnie F. Liebman, and Greg Mower, comps. **Salt, the Brand Name Guide to Sodium Content**. New York: Workman Publishing, 1983. 300p. ISBN 0894803611 (pbk).
In addition to general information on the risks associated with our typically high sodium diets, this book has a lot of very useful information. It lists low or reduced sodium foods, sodium content of nonprescription drugs, sodium content of municipal water supplies, sodium containing additives, and a section of 160 pages listing the sodium content of fresh foods, and prepared foods by brand name.

212.   Kraus, Barbara. **The Barbara Kraus 1983 Sodium Guide to Brand Names and Basic Foods**. New York: New American Library, 1982. 129p. ISBN 0451122380 (pbk).
Provided is information on the sodium content of approximately 4,000 fresh and processed foods with brand names.

213.   Vaughn, William. **Low Salt Secrets for Your Diet**. New York: Warner Books, 1982. 144p. ISBN 0446372234.
Sodium content of over 2,000 brand name and natural foods is given. There is an index.

Trace Minerals

214.   Deeming, S. B., and C. W. Weber. "Trace Minerals in Commercially Prepared Baby Foods." **Journal of the American Dietetic Association** 75 (1979): 149-51.
Data are provided on iron, copper, zinc, magnesium, strontium, and cadmium.

215. Mahoney, A. W. "Mineral Contents of Selected Cereals and Baked Products." **Cereal Foods World** 27 (1982): 147-50.
Included are data on moisture, ash, zinc, copper, iron, and manganese.

216.   McNeill, D. A., S. A. Perveen, and S. S. Young. "Mineral Analyses of Vegetarian, Health, and Conventional Foods: Magnesium, Zinc, Copper, and Manganese Content." **Journal of the American Dietetic Association** 85 (1985): 569-72.
   Information is provided on 22 health and vegetarian foods.

217.   Sidwell, V. D., et al. "Composition of the Edible Portion of Raw (Fresh or Frozen) Crustaceans, Finfish and Mollusks III: Microelements." **Marine Fisheries Review** 40 (September 1978): 1-20.
   Data on 21 trace elements in 167 foods are included.

218.   Zook, E. G., F. E. Greene, and E. R. Morris. "Nutrient Composition of Selected Wheats and Wheat Products VI: Distribution of Manganese, Copper, Nickel, Zinc, Magnesium, Lead, Tin, Cadmium, Chromium, Selenium as Determined by Atomic Absorption Spectroscopy and Colorimetry." **Cereal Chemistry** 47 (1970): 720-31.

CHROMIUM

219.   Thomas, B., J. A. Roughan, and E. D. Watters. "Cobalt, Chromium and Nickel Content of Some Vegetable Foodstuffs." **Journal of the Science of Food and Agriculture** 25 (1974): 771-76.
   Data on 50 foods are provided.

220.   Zook, E. G., et al. "National Marine Fisheries Service Preliminary Survey of Selected Seafoods for Mercury, Lead, Cadmium, Chromium, and Arsenic Content." **Journal of Agricultural and Food Chemistry** 24 (1976): 47-53.

IRON

221.   Exler, Jacob. **Iron Content of Food**. Washington, D.C.: Government Printing Office, 1982. (Home Economics Research Report, No. 45). A1.87:45.
   "This publication presents newly compiled compositional data on the iron content of 277 foods commonly eaten in this country. Values are given for food groups for which sections of the revised Agriculture Handbook No. 8 have not yet been published." Data will be superseded when all sections of the handbook are completed. It was slightly revised in 1983.

SELENIUM

222.   Lane, H. W., et al. "Selenium Content of Selected Foods." **Journal of the American Dietetic Association** 82 (1983): 24-28.
   Data are presented on selenium content in 62 foods.

223.   Maxon, A. S., and D. L. Palmquist. "Selenium Content of Foods Grown or Sold in Ohio." **Ohio Report of Research and Development** 65 (1980): 13-14.
   Information on about 90 foods is included.

224. Morris, V. C., and O. A. Levander. "Selenium Content of Foods." **Journal of Nutrition** 100 (1970): 1383-88.
Data for nearly 100 foods are included.

225. Olson, E., and I. S. Palmer. "Selenium in Foods Purchased or Produced in South Dakota." **Journal of Food Science** 49 (1984): 446-52.
Data on 222 foods are given.

226. Schroeder, Henry A., et al. "Essential Trace Elements in Man: Selenium." **Journal of Chronic Diseases** 23 (1970): 227-43.
Data on selenium content of about 160 foods, plus concentration in wild animal and human tissue, are provided.

ZINC AND COPPER

227. Allen, K. G. D., L. M. Klevay, and H. L. Springer. "The Zinc and Copper Content of Seeds and Nuts." **Nutrition Reports International** 16 (1977): 227-30.
Data on 19 seeds and nuts are included.

228. Freeland, J. H., and R. J. Cousins. "Zinc Content of Selected Foods." **Journal of the American Dietetic Association** 68 (1976): 526-29.
Zinc values for 174 foods are presented.

229. Freeland-Graves, J. H., M. Lavone Ebangit, and P. W. Bodzy. "Zinc and Copper Content of Foods Used in Vegetarian Diets." **Journal of the American Dietetic Association** 77 (1980): 648-54.
Information on zinc and copper in 74 foods is provided.

230. Haeflein, K. A., and A. I. Rasmussen. "Zinc Content of Selected Foods." **Journal of the American Dietetic Association** 70 (1977): 610-19.
About 50 foods are included.

231. Lawler, Marilyn, and Leslie M. Klevay. "Copper and Zinc in Selected Foods." **Journal of the American Dietetic Association** 84 (1984): 1028-30.
Included is information on 33 foods with brand names.

232. Murphy, E. W., B. W. Willis, and B. K. Watt. "Provisional Tables on the Zinc Content of Food." **Journal of the American Dietetic Association** 66 (1975): 345-55.
Data on about 200 foods are included.

233. Pennington, J. T., and D. H. Calloway. "Copper Content of Foods." **Journal of the American Dietetic Association** 63 (1973): 143-53.
Data on copper in over 400 foods are presented.

Vitamins

FOLIC ACID, BIOTIN, AND CHOLINE

234. Hoppner, K., B. Lampi, and D. E. Perrin. "The Free and Total Folate Activity in Foods Available on the Canadian Market." **Canadian Institute of Food Technology Journal** 5, no. 2 (1972): 60-66.
Included is information on 162 foods.

235. Perloff, B. P., and R. R. Butrum. "Folacin in Selected Foods." **Journal of the American Dietetic Association** 70 (1977): 161-72.
Information on 299 foods is given.

236. Wilson, J., and K. Lorenz. "Biotin and Choline in Foods—Nutritional Importance and Methods of Analysis—A Review." **Food Chemistry** 4 (1979): 115-29.
This article includes a table of choline and biotin contents in foods.

PANTOTHENIC ACID

237. Hoppner, K., and B. Lampi. "Total Pantothenic Acid in Strained Baby Foods." **Nutrition Reports International** 15 (1977): 627-33.
Data for 50 strained baby foods are presented.

238. Walsh, J. H., B. W. Wyse, and R. G. Hansen. "Pantothenic Acid Content of 75 Processed and Cooked Foods." **Journal of the American Dietetic Association** 78 (1981): 140-44.
Content is estimated here by radioimmunological methods.

VITAMINS B-6 AND B-12

239. Augustin, J., et al. "B Vitamin Content of Selected Cereals and Baked Products." **Cereal Foods World** 27 (1982): 159-61.
Thiamin, riboflavin, niacin, vitamin B-6, and pantothenic acid values are provided.

240. Dong, M. H., et al. "Thiamin, Riboflavin, and Vitamin B-6 Contents of Selected Foods as Served." **Journal of the American Dietetic Association** 76 (1980): 156-60.
Data on 81 foods are provided.

241. Hoppner, K., B. Lampi, and D. C. Smith. "An Appraisal of the Daily Intakes of Vitamin B-12, Pantothenic Acid and Biotin from a Composite Canadian Diet." **Canadian Institute of Food Science and Technology Journal** 11 (1978): 71-74.
Over 80 foods are discussed.

242. Orr, Martha Louise. **Pantothenic Acid, Vitamin B-6, and Vitamin B-12 in Foods.** Washington, D.C.: Government Printing Office, 1969. 53p. (Home Economics Research Report). A1.87:36.

This publication "provides values for three important B vitamins — pantothenic acid, vitamin B-6 and vitamin B-12. Data reported from scientific investigations in many laboratories have been summarized."

VITAMIN E AND TOCOPHEROLS

243. Bauernfeind, J. "Tocopherols in Foods." In **Vitamin E; a Comprehensive Treatise**, Lawrence J. Machlin, ed., 99-167. New York: Marcel Dekker, 1980. ISBN 0824768426.

"A review with 208 references on the effects of processing and storage on food tocopherols, dietary uptake of tocopherols and the tocopherol content of a variety of foods" (*Chemical Abstracts*, 93:44014).

244. Dicks, Martha W. **Vitamin E Content of Foods and Feeds for Human and Animal Consumption.** Laramie, Wyo.: University of Wyoming, 1965. 194p. (Agricultural Experiment Station Bulletin, No. 435).

This is an extensive table of tocopheral values with literature references.

245. McLaughlin, P. J., and J. L. Weihrauch. "Vitamin E Content of Foods." **Journal of the American Dietetic Association** 75 (1979): 647-65.

"Representative values of vitamin E contents in foods are presented in 3 tables: meat and animal products; plant and plant products; and miscellaneous foods and foods prepared from a combination of ingredients" (*Food Science and Technology Abstracts*, 1980, 8A560).

246. Slover, H. T. "Tocopherols in Food and Fats." **Lipids** 6 (1971): 291-96.

Tocopherols and tocotrienols in more than 40 oils and seeds are covered.

GEOGRAPHIC AREAS

Africa

247. Ågren, Gunnar, and Rosalind Gibson. **Food Composition Table for Use in Ethiopia.** Stockholm, Sweden: Almqvist and Wiksell, 1969. 31p. (Children's Nutrition Unit. CNU Report, No. 16).

Arranged by major food groups, this table provides data on energy, moisture, nitrogen, protein, fat, carbohydrates, fiber, calcium, phosphorus, iron, beta carotene, thiamin, riboflavin, niacin, tryptophan, and ascorbic acid. Local names of foods are included.

248. Ågren, Gunnar, Anders Eklund, and Sten-Åke Lieden. **Food Composition Table for Use in Ethiopia II: Amino Acid Content and Biological Data on Proteins in Ethiopian Foods: A Research Project Sponsored by the Swedish International Development Authority, SIDA, Stockholm, Sweden and the Ethiopian Nutrition Institute, Addis Ababa, Ethiopia, 1964-1975.** Uppsala, Sweden: Institute of Medical Chemistry, Biomedical Centre, 1975? 72p.

249. Busson, Félix François. **Plantes Alimentaires de l'Ouest Africain; Étude Botanique, Biologique et Chimique, avec la Collaboration Technique de P. Jaeger, P. Lunven et M. Pinta**. Marseille, France: L'Imprimerie Leconte, 1965. 568p.

Nutrient information on foods is interspersed in text throughout this book.

250. United States Nutrition Program. **Food Composition Table for Use in Africa**. Compiled by Woot-tsuen Wu Leung, Félix Busson, and Claude Jardin. Bethesda, Md.: U.S. Department of Health, Education and Welfare in cooperation with the Food Consumption and Planning Branch, FAO, 1968. 306p. FS2.2 Af8.

Data on over 1,600 foods are arranged here in 14 food groups. Values for moisture, food energy, protein, carbohydrates, calcium, phosphorus, iron, vitamin A in the form of both retinol and beta carotene equivalents, tryptophan, ascorbic acid, thiamin, riboflavin, and niacin are given. Appendixes include indexes of scientific names for plants, animals, insects, and fish and shellfish. There is a bibliography.

Asia

251. Chen, M. L., S. C. Chang, and J. Y. Guoo. "Fiber Contents of Some Chinese Vegetables and Their In Vitro Binding Capacity of Bile Acids." **Nutrition Reports International** 26 (1982): 1053-59.

NDF content of legumes, gourds, and leafy and miscellaneous vegetables is given.

252. Chung-Kuo. Hsüeh k'o Hsüeh Yüan. Wei Sheng Yen Chiu So. **Shih Wu Ch'eng Fen Piao**. 3rd ed. Pei-ching, China: Jen Min Wei Sheng Ch'u Pan She, 1981. ca.260p.

This is a table of food values from the People's Republic of China, in Chinese.

253. Dimaunahan, L. B., A. V. Lontoc, and I. Abdon. "Cholesterol Content of Philippine Foods." **Philippine Journal of Nutrition** 29 (1976): 33-44.

Information is given on some 75 foods.

254. Food and Nutrition Research Institute, Philippines. **Food Composition Table Recommended for Use in the Philippines: Nutritional Value of Local Foods, Fresh and Processed**. Manila, Philippines: Food and Nutrition Research Institute, National Science Development Board, 1980. 134p. (FNRI Handbook, No. 1).

255. Gopalan, C., B. V. Ramasastri, and S. C. Balasubramanian. **Nutritive Value of Indian Foods**. Hyderabad, India: National Institute of Nutrition, 1982. 204p.

256. Hanguk. Nongch'on Chinhungch'ong. Nongch'on Yŏngyang Kaesŏn Yŏnsuwŏn. **Sikp'um Punsok P'yo: Food Composition Table**. Suwon, Korea: Rural Nutrition Institute, 1980. ca.149p.

This is a food composition table from Korea, in Korean.

257. Harris, L. E., et al. **Central and Southeast Asia Tables of Feed Composition**. Logan, Utah: International Feedstuffs Institute, Department of Animal, Dairy, and Veterinary Sciences, Utah State University, 1982. 513p. ISBN 0874211182.

This compendium of animal feed composition information is a good source on unusual varieties of grains, unusual greens and starchy foods, berries, etc. (e.g., fresh amaranth leaves, cassava, and different varieties of corn). It includes tables with proximate composition and energy values, cell wall constituents, mineral contents, vitamins, and amino acid content.

258. Kagaku Gijutsucho Shigenchōsakai, ed. **Shokuhin Seibunhyō: Tables of Food Composition**. 4th ed. Tokyo: Daiichi Shuppan, 1983. 279p.

This volume contains data on energy values (kcal and J), fats, carbohydrates, fiber, ash, calcium, phosphorus, iron, sodium, potassium, retinol, carotene, thiamin, niacin, and ascorbic acid of foods used in Japan. The text is in Japanese. Arrangement is by major food groups. Foods are accompanied by names in English, but not all nutrients are so identified.

259. Lakshimiah, N., and B. V. Ramasastri. "Folic Acid Content of Some Indian Foods of Plant Origin." **Journal of Nutrition and Dietetics** 6 (1969): 200-203.

Information on 38 foods is included.

260. Lontoc, A. V., and O. N. Gonzalez. "Vitamin B-12 Content of Some Philippine Foods." **Philippine Journal of Nutrition** 21 (1968): 163-71.

Over 50 foods are included.

261. Oomen, H. A. P. C., and G. J. H. Grubben. **Tropical Leaf Vegetables in Human Nutrition**. Amsterdam, Netherlands: Koninklijk Instituut voor de Tropen, 1977. 133p. (Koninklijk Instituut voor de Tropen. Afdeling Agrarisch Onderzook. Communication No. 69).

This title contains a chapter on nutritional value with tabular information on 35 leafy vegetables.

262. Palad, J. G., et al. "Nutritive Value of Some Foodstuffs Processed in the Philippines." **Philippine Journal of Science** 93 (1964): 355-84.

Data on caloric values, moisture, protein, fat, ash, carbohydrate content, crude fiber, calcium, phosphorus, iron, vitamin A, thiamin, riboflavin, niacin, and ascorbic acid in 218 processed foods are included. Each entry is identified by local and English name.

263. Santa Banerjee, and B. Pal. "Zinc Content of Foodstuffs." **Indian Journal of Nutrition and Dietetics** 16 (1979): 320-25.

"One hundred twenty-two foods available in the Calcutta region" (*Food Science and Technology Abstracts*, 1980, 8A588).

264. Shih P'in Kung Yeh Fa Chan Yen Chiu So. **Tai-wan Shih P'in Cheng Fen Piao: Table of Taiwan Food Composition**. Hsinchu, Taiwan: Rural Research Institute, 1971.

In Chinese and in English, this title includes proximate composition, minerals and vitamins in cereals, seeds and nuts, legumes, vegetables, by-products, and wastes. A second table published by the institute contains amino acid data.

265. Take, A., K. Yano, Y. Suzuki, and K. Noda. "Magnesium, Manganese, Zinc and Copper Contents in Japanese Foodstuffs." **Journal of the Japanese Society of Food and Nutrition [Eiyo to Shokuryo]** 30 (1977): 381-93.
    The article is in Japanese; the tables are in English. About 200 foods are covered.

266. Tee, E. S., T. K. W. Ng, and Y. H. Chong. "Cholesterol Content and Fatty Acid Composition of Some Malaysian Foods." **Medical Journal of Malaysia** 33 (1979): 334-41.
    About 45 foods are included.

267. Tsuji, K., Y. Nakagawa, E. Tsuji, and S. Suzuki. "Cholesterol Content of Foods." **Japanese Journal of Nutrition [Eiyogaku Zazzhi]** 35 (1977): 159-65.
    The article is in Japanese; the tables are in English. About 170 foods are covered.

268. United States. National Institutes of Health. **Food Composition Table for Use in East Asia.** Bethesda, Md.: National Institutes of Health, 1972. 334p. (DHEW Publication, No. NIH 73-465). HE20.3302:F73.
    The most extensive table of its kind accessible to the Western user, this provides information on some 1,600 foods. It is divided into two major parts; *Proximate Composition, Mineral and Vitamin Contents of East Asian Foods*, by Woot-tsuen Wu Leung, R. R. Butrum, and Flora Huang Chang; and *Amino Acid, Fatty Acid, Certain B Vitamin and Trace Mineral Content of Some Asian Foods*, by M. Narayana Rao and N. Polacchi. Values are listed by major food groups. Part I contains data on food energy, moisture, fat, carbohydrate, fiber, ash, calcium, phosphorus, iron, sodium, potassium, retinol and beta carotene equivalents, thiamin, riboflavin, niacin and ascorbic acid. Part II contains data on moisture, protein, 18 amino acids, vitamin B-6, pantothenic acid, vitamin B-12, folic acid, magnesium, manganese, copper, cobalt, molybdenum, selenium, fluorine, iodine, total saturated fatty acids with separate values for palmitic, and stearic acids and total unsaturated fatty acids with separate values for oleic, linoleic, and linolenic acids.

269. Villegas, N. M. "Philippine Food List for Sodium Restricted Diets." **Philippine Journal of Nutrition** 26 (1973): 33-42.

Australia and New Zealand

In addition to the sources cited below, the journal *Food Technology in Australia* is an excellent source of information for nutrient values of Australian foods. It has published numerous tables on various groups of foods (e.g., fast foods, Greek foods, fried foods, etc.). These are too numerous to list here.

270. Maples, J., R. B. H. Wills, and H. Greenfield. "Sodium and Potassium Levels in Australian Processed Foods." **Medical Journal of Australia** 2 (1982): 20-22.
    Covered are 118 foods.

271. Nobile, S., and J. M. Woodhill. "A Survey of the Vitamin Content of Some 2,000 Foods as They Are Consumed by Selected Groups of the Australian Population I: Tables of Vitamin Content Analysed per 100g. Portions. II. Dietary and Biochemical Findings." **Food Technology in Australia** 25 (1973): 80-100.

272. Shirlow, M. "Sodium, Potassium, and Magnesium Content of Some Australian Foods." **Journal of Food and Nutrition** 39 (1982): 136-43.
"Values for sodium, potassium, and magnesium in selected Australian foods are tabulated" (*Nutrition Abstracts and Reviews*, 1983, #3461).

273. Thomas, Sucy, and Margaret Corden. **Metric Tables of Composition of Australian Foods**. rev. 6th ed. Compiled by Sucy Thomas and Margaret Corden, under the direction of the Nutrition Committee of the National Health and Medical Research Council. Canberra, Australia: Australian Government Publishing Service, 1982. 29p. ISBN 0642029385.
This is essentially a revision of Table III of *Tables of Composition of Australian Foods*, 1970. Data are obtained from a variety of sources. Nutrients included are energy, carbohydrates, protein, fat, calcium, phosphorus, iron, sodium and potassium, beta carotene, thiamin, riboflavin, and ascorbic acid.

274. Thomas, Sucy, and Margaret Corden. **Tables of Composition of Australian Foods**. rev. 5th ed. Compiled by Sucy Thomas and Margaret Cordon, under the direction of the Nutrition Committee of the National Health and Medical Research Council. Canberra, Australia: Australian Government Publishing Service, 1970. 60p.

275. Visser, F. R., and J. K. Burrows. **Composition of New Zealand Foods**. Vol. 1- . Wellington, New Zealand: New Zealand Department of Scientific and Industrial Research, 1983- . (Vol. 1, ISBN 047706728X [pbk]).
Volume 1, *Characteristic Fruits and Vegetables*, contains information on only a small number of foods characteristic of New Zealand. Detailed information on the collection and handling of samples is provided.

Europe

276. Hansen, Holger Hovgård. **Bly, Cadmium, Kobber og Zink i Frugt og Groentsager 1977-80 = Lead, Cadmium, Copper and Zinc in Fruit and Vegetables 1977-80**. Søborg, Denmark: Statens Levnedsmiddelinstitut, Centrallaboratoriets Afdeling B, Pesticider og Forureninger, 1983. 54p. (Publikation Nr. 84). ISSN 0106-8423.
This is in Danish and English.

277. Koivistoinen, P., ed. "Mineral Element Composition of Finnish Foods: N, K, Ca, Mg, P, S, Fe, Cu, Mn, Zn, Mo, Co, Ni, Cr, F, Se, Si, Rb, Al, B, Br, Hg, As, Cd, Pb, and Ash." **Acta Agriculturae Scandinavica, Supplement** 22 (1980): 171p.
The entire supplement is devoted to the mineral composition of Finnish foods.

278.   McCance, R. A. **McCance and Widdowson's The Composition of Foods**.
4th ed. Revised and extended by A. Paul and D. A. T. Southgate. London:
H.M.S.O.; distr., Amsterdam, New York: Elsevier/North-Holland Biomedical
Press, 1978. 418p. (MRC Special Report, No. 297). ISBN 0114500363
(H.M.S.O.); 0444800271 (Elsevier).

This is a revised and expanded edition of the standard British food composition table, based on extensive new analyses and values obtained from the literature, organized into four major sections and within each section by food groups.
Values are presented per 100 grams of food, edible portion.

Section 1 covers proximate composition (including dietary fiber), energy
values, 13 vitamins, and 16 minerals. Section 2 covers amino acid composition,
with values for 18 amino acids. Section 3 is on fatty acid composition, with values
for 18 fatty acids. Section 4 is on cholesterol, phytic acid, iodine, and organic
acids. Supplements to this table are described in entries 283 and 287.

279.   Meyland, Inge. **Magnesium-, Natrium-, og Kaliumindholdet i Danske
Levnedsmidler = The Content of Magnesium, Sodium, and Potassium in Danish
Foods**. Søborg, Denmark: Statens Levnedsmiddelinstitut, Centrallaboratoriets
Afdeling A, Naeringsstoffer og Tilsaeninsstoffer, 1983?. 70p. (Publikation Nr.
82). ISSN 0106-8423.

This is in Danish and English.

280.   Nederlands Voedingsraad. "Nederlandse Voedingsmiddelentabel."
Voeding 39 (1978): 366-80.

"31st edition of the Netherlands food table" (*Nutrition Abstracts and
Reviews A*, 1979, #5223). This article is in Dutch.

281.   Ostrowski, Z. L. **Les Aliments: Tables des Valeurs Nutritives**. Paris:
Jacques Lanore, 1978. 125p. ISBN 2862680028.

This volume, which is in French, contains information on energy and
nutrient requirements and explanatory material on the tables and cholesterol
values of 59 foods. The tables proper contain data on approximately 600 foods
arranged by food groups. Values are provided for energy, protein, lipids, carbohydrates, phosphorus, magnesium, calcium, iron, sodium, potassium, ascorbic
acid, thiamin, riboflavin, and vitamins B-6, A, D, and E.

282.   Ostrowski, Z. L. **Les Aliments: Tables des Valeurs Nutritives: Les
Aliments Preparés Industriellement pour l'Enfance**. Paris: Jacques Lanore, 1978.
32p.

Covered are "about 546 baby and infant foods grouped under about 20
brand names" (*Nutrition Abstracts and Reviews A*, 1978, #8558). It is in French.

283.   Paul, A. A., D. A. T. Southgate, and J. Russell. **First Supplement to
McCance and Widdowson's The Composition of Foods: Amino Acids**. London:
H.M.S.O.; distr., Amsterdam, New York: Elsevier/North-Holland Biomedical
Press, 1979. 112p. ISBN 0444802207 (Elsevier).

This supplement presents amino acid and fatty acid values per 100 grams of
food in contrast to the main volume, which presents these data per 100 grams of
nitrogen and fatty acids, respectively.

284. Randoin, Lucie, et al. **Tables de Composition des Aliments**. Paris: Jacques Lanore, 1982. 116p. ISBN 2862680559.
This is in French. Foods are arranged by major groups. Plants and animals are identified to genus and species. Nutrients covered are protein, fats, carbohydrates, energy value, 11 minerals, and 10 vitamins.

285. Schlettwein-Gsell, Daniela, and Sibylle Mommsen-Straub. **Spurenelemente in Lebensmitteln**. Bern, Switzerland: H. Huber, 1973. 188p. (Internationale Zeitschrift für Vitamin- und Ernährungsforschung. Beiheft Nr. 13). ISBN 3456003633.
These tables are in German and English. They provide values on trace elements in food. Covered are zinc, cobalt, chromium, manganese, nickel, copper, magnesium, selenium, boron, molybdenum, vanadium, and aluminum.

286. Souci, S. Walter. **Food Composition and Nutrition Tables: A Comprehensive Work on Modern Nutrition**. 2nd ed. Stuttgart, W. Germany: Wissenschaftliche Verlagsgesellschaft; distr., Philadelphia, Pa.: Heyden and Son, 1983. 417p. ISSN 0721-6912.
This revised edition of one of the major German food tables provides proximate composition and information on 50 individual nutrients in nearly 700 European and exotic foods. Data are based on LINDAS (Lebensmittel-Inhaltstoff-Daten-System, Food Constituent Data System). Table headings are given in English, French, and German. The index and a glossary of food also appear in all three languages.

287. Tan, S. P., R. W. Wenlock, and D. H. Buss. **Immigrant Foods: The Composition of Foods Used by Immigrants in the United Kingdom: Second Supplement to McCance and Widdowson's The Composition of Foods**. London: H.M.S.O.; distr., Amsterdam, New York: Elsevier/North-Holland Biomedical Press, 1985. 74p. ISBN 0112427170.
Compiled to meet the increasing demand for information on the nutritional value of foods used by immigrants in the United Kingdom, this table presents data from direct analysis or from the published literature. Foods are arranged by categories: cereals and cereal products, milk and milk products, eggs, fats and oils, composite dishes, etc. Data presented are for energy value, dietary fiber, water, protein, fat, carbohydrate, seven minerals and nine vitamins. Appendixes consist of standard recipes for composite dishes and systematic names of fish and plant foods. A detailed index of foods is included.

288. United Kingdom. Working Party on the Monitoring of Foodstuffs for Heavy Metals. **Survey of Copper and Zinc in Foods: Fifth Report of the Steering Group on Food Surveillance**. London: H.M.S.O., 1981. 50p. (Food Surveillance Paper, Ministry of Agriculture, Fisheries, and Food, No. 5). ISBN 0112411991.

Hawaii and the Pacific

289. Hawaii. Department of Health. Nutrition Branch. **Count Your Calories and Protein Values**. Honolulu, Hawaii: Department of Health, 1979. 12p.
Compiled from other sources, this publication contains data on 275 foods.

290.   Hertzler, Ann A., and Bluebell R. Standal. **Food Sources and the Nutritional Role of Sodium and Potassium**. Honolulu, Hawaii: Cooperative Extension Service, College of Tropical Agriculture and Human Resources, 1979. 11p. (Circular No. 493).

This circular contains data on some 150 foods.

291.   Jardin, Claude, and Jacques Grosnier. **Un Taro, un Poisson, un Papaye: Manuel d'Education Alimentaire et de Nutrition Appliquée a l'Usage des Éducateurs de l'Océanie Tropicale**. Nouméa, Nouvelle Calédonie: Commission du Pacifique Sud, 1975. 476p.

This is a basic nutrition education manual. Appendixes include a food table of 185 foods with values presented per 100 grams, edible portion. Nutrients covered are protein, moisture, fat, carbohydrates, fiber, calcium, iron, vitamin A, riboflavin, thiamin, vitamin C, and niacin. English names are provided, with descriptions in French.

292.   Jordan, Sandra Kai, and G. Flick. **Hawaiian Calories**. Kailua-Kona, Hawaii: S. Jordan, 1984. 32p.

Caloric values are given for approximately 380 foods commonly eaten in Hawaii per 3½ ounces (100 grams) or typical household measures. Included are ethnic specialities and some mixed dishes. Sources of data are not cited.

293.   Miller, Carey D., and B. Branthoover. **Nutritive Values of Some Hawaiian Foods in Household Units and Common Measures**. Honolulu, Hawaii: Hawaii Agricultural Experiment Station, 1957. 20p. (Hawaii Agricultural Experiment Station Circular, No. 52).

This circular contains information about 140 foods, providing data on calories, carbohydrates, fat, protein, calcium, phosphorus, iron, vitamin A, thiamin, riboflavin, niacin, and ascorbic acid.

294.   Miller, Carey D., B. Branthoover, N. Seguchi, H. Denning, and A. Bauer. **Vitamin Values of Foods Used in Hawaii**. Honolulu, Hawaii: Hawaii Agricultural Experiment Station, 1956. 94p. (Hawaii Agricultural Experiment Station Technical Bulletin, No. 30).

Moisture, carotene, thiamin, riboflavin, niacin, and ascorbic acid in over 450 foods are included, with detailed information on handling of samples and analysis.

295.   Murai, Mary, Carey D. Miller, and Florence Pen. **Some Tropical South Pacific Island Foods: Description, History, Use, Composition, and Nutritive Value**. Honolulu, Hawaii: University of Hawaii Press, 1958. 159p. (Hawaii Agricultural Experiment Station Bulletin, No. 110).

Information on breadfruit, coconut, pandanus, starchy root vegetables, and foods made from these items is included, as well as a seafood supplement and detailed description of items analyzed, with analytical procedures.

296.   Norgan, N. G., J. V. G. A. Durnin, and A. Ferro Luzzi. "The Composition of Some New Guinea Foods." **Papua New Guinea Agricultural Journal** 30 (September 1979): 1-3.

Protein, water, fiber, ash, and energy values for 87 foods are given.

297. Peters, Frank E. **Chemical Composition of South Pacific Foods: An Annotated Bibliography**. Noumea, New Caledonia: South Pacific Commission, 1957. 106p. (South Pacific Commission. Technical Paper No. 100).

A French-language version has also been published (*La Composition Chimique des Aliments du Pacifique Sud*, Noumea, New Caledonia, January 1957). Some of this information appeared in the journal *Qualitas Plantarum* (5 [1959]: 313-43). This bibliography of 326 references is arranged by author with some tabular data excerpted from sources. There is an index of authors and plant names.

298. Peters, Frank E. **The Chemical Composition of South Pacific Foods**. Noumea, New Caledonia: South Pacific Commission, 1958. 56p. (South Pacific Commission. Technical Paper No. 115).

This paper provides data on proximate composition, amino acids, carotene, thiamin, niacin, and ascorbic acid of major plant foods and human milk. Detailed information on analytical procedures and samples is included.

299. Rody, Nancy, and Francis M. Pottenger. **Nutrition Island Style: The Nutrition Planning Book for Hawaii and the Pacific**. Honolulu, Hawaii: Curriculum Research and Development Group, University of Hawaii, 1983. 119p.

Intended as a workbook for analyzing diets, most of this volume consists of charts providing information in terms of percentage of the RDAs in foods. Nutrient standard forms in the book permit correlating and adding the percentage of RDAs for different foods consumed.

300. South Pacific Commission, Fiji National Food and Nutrition Committee and Fiji School of Medicine. **Food Composition Tables for Use in the South Pacific**. Noumea, New Caledonia: The Commission, 1983. 33p.

This is a revised edition of a work by the same title issued in the 1960s by the Nutrition Department of the South Pacific Health Service. It provides data on energy values, protein, fat, carbohydrates, calcium, iron, vitamin A, thiamin, riboflavin, niacin, and vitamin C in nearly 200 foods per 100 grams of edible portion. The table is arranged by broad food groups. Values were converted from imperial to metric measures and vitamin A is now expressed in micrograms, but there has been no major revision of the nutrient composition data. Additional material provided is a table indicating the weight of common measures or units of food, directions for use, sources of data, an abbreviated, simplified table, and recommended daily intakes of nutrients.

301. Standal, B. R., D. R. Bassett, P. B. Policar, and M. Thom. **Fatty Acids, Cholesterol, and Proximate Composition of Certain Prepared and Unprepared Foods in Hawaii**. Honolulu, Hawaii: Hawaii Agricultural Experiment Station, 1975. 69p. (Hawaii Agricultural Experiment Station. Research Bulletin No. 146).

Data on 17 fatty acids, food energy, water, protein, fat, carbohydrate, fiber, ash, and cholesterol in 220 foods eaten in Hawaii are provided, with a description of some of the foods. Data on many mixed dishes are included. The appendix includes conversion of household measurements to weight in grams.

302.   Wenkam, Nao S. **Foods of Hawaii and the Pacific Basin: Vegetables and Vegetable Products—Raw, Processed, and Prepared. Volume 1: Composition**. Honolulu, Hawaii: Hawaii Institute of Tropical Agriculture and Human Resources, College of Tropical Agriculture and Human Resources, University of Hawaii at Manoa, 1983. 172p. (Hawaii Institute of Tropical Agriculture and Human Resources. Research Extension Series, No. 38).

"This publication is the first of a series designed to revise and expand composition data on foods of consequence to Hawaii and the Pacific Basin. It makes available under one cover the nutrient profile of foods scattered in several sources.... Contains values for 183 foods in the raw, prepared and processed forms. The data in the tables are from laboratory analysis and do not contain estimated, derived, or imputed values from another form of the food or a similar food. Some data are taken from previous publications. Single values are provided for energy, proximate constituents (water, protein, total lipid, total carbohydrate, fiber, ash), minerals (calcium, iron, magnesium, phosphorus, potassium, sodium), and vitamins (ascorbic acid, thiamin, riboflavin, niacin, vitamin A)." Amounts are for a 100-gram edible portion, edible portion of common measure, and edible portion of one pound as purchased. Appendix A contains a detailed description of how the samples were treated and how the analyses were made.

303.   Wenkam, Nao S. **Foods of Hawaii and the Pacific Basin: Vegetables and Vegetable Products—Raw, Processed, and Prepared. Vol. 2: Percentage of U.S. Recommended Daily Allowances**. Honolulu, Hawaii: Hawaii Institute of Tropical Agriculture and Human Resources, College of Tropical Agriculture and Human Resources, University of Hawaii at Manoa, 1986. 28p. (Research Extension Series, No. 065).

This publication presents data on protein, vitamin A, vitamin C, thiamin, riboflavin, niacin, calcium, and iron for 183 vegetables and vegetable products contained in the first volume expressed as a percentage of the RDA supplied in specified amounts of food. Table 2 identifies those foods which are important sources of specific nutrients. Tables 3 and 4 are tables of the RDAs. An errata sheet showing a revised table 3 is inserted.

304.   Wenkam, Nao S., and Carey D. Miller. **Composition of Hawaii Fruits**. Honolulu, Hawaii: Hawaii Agricultural Experiment Station, 1965. 87p. (Hawaii Agricultural Experiment Station Bulletin, No. 135).

"From chemical analyses and vitamin assays originating in the Department of Foods and Nutrition, University of Hawaii."

Data are included on 64 fruits per 100 grams edible portion, in common household units, and in 100-calorie portions. Covered are moisture, food energy, protein, fat, carbohydrate, fiber, ash, calcium, phosphorus, iron, vitamin A, thiamin, riboflavin, niacin, and ascorbic acid. Some values are taken from Hawaii Agricultural Experiment Station Technical Bulletin, No. 30 (entry 294).

305.   Wenkam, Nao S., and Flora L. Thong. **Sodium and Potassium in Some Hawaii Foods**. Honolulu, Hawaii: Hawaii Agricultural Experiment Station, 1969. 4p. (Hawaii Agricultural Experiment Station. Technical Paper No. 987).

"Reprinted from the *Hawaii Medical Journal* 28 (Jan.-Feb. 1969): 209-212." Information on some 30 foods is provided.

306. Yang, Goang-Yean, and Bluebell R. Standal. **Sodium and Potassium in Ready-to-Eat Foods in Hawaii**. Honolulu, Hawaii: Hawaii Agricultural Experiment Station, 1973. 4p. (Agricultural Experiment Station. Journal Series, No. 1522).

This is reprinted from the *Hawaii Medical Journal* 32 (September/October 1973). It covers approximately 100 foods.

Latin America and the Caribbean

307. Caribbean Food and Nutrition Institute. **Food Composition Tables for Use in the English-Speaking Caribbean**. Kingston, Jamaica: The Caribbean Food and Nutrition Institute, 1974. 115p.

This publication contains data on over 1,200 foods, principally from published food composition tables. Included are data on water content, protein, fat, carbohydrate, energy value, fiber, calcium, iron, vitamin A, thiamin, riboflavin, niacin, and ascorbic acid. The arrangement is by food groups. Indexes to common and scientific names of plants and animals are provided.

308. Colbon de Reguero, Lillian, and Sylvia M. Rodriguez de Santiago. **Tabla de Composición de Alimentos de Uso Corriente en Puerto Rico**. Rio Piedras, Puerto Rico: Editorial Universitaria, 1975?. 31p.

In Spanish and in English, this table is arranged by broad food groups, and provides data on the following nutrients: water, caloric value, protein, fat, carbohydrates, fiber, calcium, iron, sodium, potassium, thiamin, vitamin A, riboflavin, niacin, and ascorbic acid. An appendix lists botanical, English, and Spanish names of foods. An alphabetical index lists foods in English and in Spanish.

309. Colombia. Instituto Colombiano de Bienestar Familiar. **Tabla de Composición de Alimentos Colombianos**. 4. ed. Bogotá, Colombia: Instituto Colombiano de Bienestar Familiar, 1978. 93p.

This table is in Spanish.

310. Fundaçaõ Instituto Brasileiro de Geografia e Estatística. Secretaria de Planejamento da Presidencia da Republica. **Tabelas de Composiçaõ dos Alimentos**. Rio de Janeiro: Fundaçaõ Instituto Brasileiro de Geografia e Estatístico, 1977. 201p.

This table is in Portuguese.

311. Hernandez, Mercedes, Adolfo Chavez, and Hector Bourges. **Valor Nutritivo de los Alimentos Mexicanos: Tablas de Uso Practico**. 7a. ed. Mexico City, Mexico: Instituto Nacional de la Nutrición, Division de Nutricion, 1977. 34 leaves. (Publicaciones de la Division de Nutrición v. L-12).

These tables are in Spanish.

312. Leung, Woot-tsuen Wu. **Food Composition Table for Use in Latin America**. Washington, D.C.: Government Printing Office, 1961. 145p.

Arranged by major food groups, this table provides nutrient values for over 700 foods. Covered are energy, moisture, protein, fat, carbohydrates, fiber, ash, calcium, phosphorus, iron, vitamin A, thiamin, riboflavin, niacin, and ascorbic acid. Foods are identified with both English and Spanish names. Included are a glossary of common names of edible plants, an index of scientific names for plants, and a bibliography of sources.

313.   McDowell, Lee R., et al. **Latin American Tables of Feed Composition: Nutritional Data for Argentina [and Other Nations]**. Gainesville, Fla.: University of Florida, 1974. 509p.

This table is a worthwhile source for unusual plant foods. It is organized by genus and species and contains data from most countries in Latin America. Foods are identified as to variety and part of plant or animal used. A chart converts common names to the appropriate scientific name. An abbreviated edition is available in Spanish (*Tablas de Composición de Alimentos de America Latina: Datos Nutricionales*, Gainesville, Fla., University of Florida, 1974).

314.   Venezuela. Instituto Nacional de Nutrición. **Tabla de Composición de Alimentos para Uso Practico**. rev. ed. Caracas, Venezuela: Instituto Nacional de Nutrición, 1964. 40p. (Publicación No. 23).

This table is in Spanish.

Middle East

315.   Food and Agriculture Organization of the United Nations. Food Policy and Nutrition Division. **Food Composition Tables for the Near East**. Rome: Food and Agriculture Organization, 1982. 265p. (FAO Food and Nutrition Paper, No. 26). ISBN 9251012776.

"This joint FAO/USDA publication provides basic information on the nutrient content of foods consumed in the following countries: Afghanistan, Bahrain, Cyprus, Egypt, Iran, Iraq, Jordan, Kuwait, Lebanon, Libya, Oman, Pakistan, Qatar, Saudi Arabia, Somalia, Sudan, Syria, and Yemen. It contains food composition tables covering proximate composition, mineral and vitamin content, amino acid content, and fatty acid content for 14 groups of foods. Appendixes include an index of common names of foods and an index of scientific names of plants and fish" (*Food Science and Technology Abstracts*, 1984, 2A120).

316.   Pellet, P. L., and Sossy Shadarevian. **Food Composition: Tables for Use in the Middle East**. 2nd ed. Beirut, Lebanon: American University of Beirut, 1970. 116p.

This publication contains much new information obtained by direct analysis with detailed description of analytical procedures. It is divided into four parts, each arranged by major food groups: major nutrients with entries accompanied by Arabic names and plant foods accompanied by genus and species; iodine, potassium, and sodium; amino acids, with 18 amino acids plus total sulphur-containing amino acids; composite dishes with recipes. Appendixes include an index of scientific names with Arabic and Turkish names, an index of composite dishes, and glossaries of common Arabic names for foods, etc.

NUTRIENT DATABASES
AND PROGRAMS

USDA

The Human Nutrition Service of the U.S. Department of Agriculture is charged with maintaining an up-to-date database of information on the nutrient composition of foods and with making this information available in both published and machine-readable form. It is estimated that there are now over 700,000 individual nutrient values stored in the National Nutrient Data Bank (NDB). One of the major purposes of this database is to produce and constantly revise the various sections of *Composition of Foods* (Agriculture Handbook No. 8). This same database is also used to produce *Nutritive Value of American Foods* (Home and Garden Bulletin, No. 72) and *Nutritive Value of American Foods in Common Units* (Agriculture Handbook No. 456).

A number of different subsets of this database can be purchased from the National Technical Information Service (5285 Port Royal Road, Springfield, VA 22161). The most extensive of these subsets is *USDA Nutrient Data Base for Standard Reference*. It corresponds to data published in Agriculture Handbook No. 8 plus imputed values where there are none available and where sections of the handbook have not been completed. This database is available on floppy diskettes for the IBM PC.

Other sets available correspond to Agriculture Handbook No. 456 (also available on floppy diskettes for the IBM PC), Home and Garden Bulletin, No. 72, special databases created for use in the USDA *Nationwide Food Consumption Survey, 1977-78*, and a number of additional special purpose sets.

Other Major Databases

Most other nutrient databases in the United States use data from the National Nutrient Data Bank and supplement these with information from other sources. An example of this is the University of Michigan data bank. It consists of data from the National Nutrient Data Bank supplemented by data from manufacturers.

An effort is now being made to set up an international organization to acquire and disseminate reliable, evaluated food composition data. International Network of Food Data Systems (INFOODS) resulted from a planning conference held in Rome in 1983 and is expected to incorporate a worldwide network of nutrient databases with accurate and compatible data. INFOODS has helped to sponsor regional conferences on nutrient database compatibility to help achieve these goals. So far ASIAFOODS, EUROFOODS, LATINFOODS, and NOAFOODS (North America) conferences have been held or are planned. Denmark, Sweden, Norway, Finland, and Iceland are establishing a common database called NORFOODS. LINDAS (Lebensmittel-Inhaltstoff-Daten-System) is the major database in the Federal Republic of Germany.

Nutrient Analysis Programs

Numerous nutrient analysis programs are now available to anyone with a personal computer. Many of these are geared to the nutrition professional, but a surprisingly large number are intended for the general public. Some are designed to be used as nutrition education tools. Many have data on no more than 700 to 800 foods, and are based on USDA Home and Garden Bulletin, No. 72. Considering the ethnic diversity of the U.S. population, this number seems hardly adequate to provide data on the number of foods most Americans encounter on a daily basis. In addition to the number and diversity of foods, other considerations in the purchase of such programs are number of nutrients, sources of the data, and the types of calculations that can be performed.

Information is available in the form of articles or reviews in magazines or professional journals. Advertisements in nutrition, health, and microcomputer periodicals are sometimes the only source of information on a new program. An entire journal, the *Journal of Dietetic Software*, focuses on this subject, though it is not limited to microcomputer software. Unfortunately, because most of this software is frequently revised, this information is out-of-date almost as soon as it is printed. Nonetheless, these sources provide access to software and describe basic features of programs, even if they do not have information on the latest revisions.

USDA's Food and Nutrition Information Center (FNIC) is collecting microcomputer software in food and nutrition for on-site preview. These packages deal with consumer education, nutrition information, and dietary analysis.

Sources of Information on
Nutrient Databases and Programs

317.   Byrd-Bredbenner, Carol, Suzanne Pelican, and P. J. Long. "Software Programs." **Journal of Nutrition Education** 16 (June 1984): 77-117.

The extensive article includes checklists for the evaluation of nutrition education and nutrient analysis software with extensive reviews or listings of programs. These are primarily for microcomputers, but some are for mainframes. Included are a list of distributors and an index by type of machine.

318.   Hoover, Loretta W., ed. **Nutrient Data Bank Directory**. 1st ed.- . Columbia, Mo.: Department of Human Nutrition, College of Home Economics, University of Missouri, 1981- . annual.

The most recent edition of this directory (1986) contains nonevaluative data on 99 nutrient databases and nutrient analysis programs. The first part of the directory has basic data on the systems, such as whether quantities are in household units or other units of measurement, number of foods, number of nutrients, the computers these systems are designed to run on, etc.

The second part has more detailed charts on database characteristics, including food constituents, missing value schemes, target audience, data sources, etc. It does not include information on the various USDA nutrient data sets available.

319.   **Softwhere, Health Care**. Minneapolis, Minn.: Moore Data Management Services, 1984- . semi-annual. ISSN 8756-1077. (available from Moore Data Management Services, 1660 S. Highway 100, Minneapolis, MN 55416).
Brief descriptions of over 1,000 programs in all areas of health care, including nearly 60 in diet and nutrition, are included in this software catalog. Some of the listings do not contain recent revisions of the programs, nor are prices current. There are alphabetical package and vendor indexes.

GENERAL SOURCES ON COMPUTER PROGRAMS

Occasionally, it is necessary to consult more general software directories. These fall into two categories: directories listing programs regardless of the type of machine, and those listing software for a specific machine (e.g., Apple, IBM, etc.). Directories for specific machines are unfortunately too numerous for listing in this guide.

320.   **Datapro Directory of Microcomputer Software**. Delran, N.J.: Datapro Research Corporation, 1983- . ISSN 0730-8795.
This looseleaf service provides brief descriptions of currently available programs. The arrangement is by broadly defined applications category. Each entry includes purchasing information, data on required memory and hardware, source language, as well as a brief description of the program ranging from a sentence or two to 20 lines or so. Available are applications, product name, vendor/product, and computer systems indexes.

321.   **Directory of Software**. Delran, N.J.: Datapro Research Corporation, 1975- . ISSN 0730-8779.
This looseleaf (for updating) directory is identical in format to the *Datapro Directory of Microcomputer Software*, but with programs for mainframes. Included are applications, product name, vendor/product, and hardware indexes.

322.   **The Software Encyclopedia**. New York: R. R. Bowker, 1985- . 2v. ISBN 0835221558.
This is an extensive listing of over 22,000 microcomputer programs currently available for purchase. Volume 1 has an alphabetical list of programs by title with information on version, compatible hardware, required memory, drives, and number of disks. A separate directory of 3,000 software publishers in the back of the volume provides address information. Volume 2, *The Expanded Applications Index*, lists programs by application (e.g., word processing, accounting, database management) along with a description of the programs and purchasing information.

SELECTED REFERENCES
ON FOOD COMPOSITION TABLES

Cooke, J. R. "Food Composition Tables—Analytical Problems in the Collection of Data." *Human Nutrition: Applied Nutrition* 37A (1983): 441-47.

"Food Composition Data: Problems and Plans." *Journal of the American Dietetic Association* 85 (September 1985): 1080-83.

Greenfield, H., and R. B. H. Wills, eds. "Tables of Food Composition: An Australian Perspective. Proceedings of a Workshop held at the University of New South Wales, 27 June 1980." *Food Technology in Australia* 33 (1981): 101-30.

Klein, Barbara P. "Nutrient Analysis Information for Decision Making." *Food Technology* 37 (December 1983): 37-39+.

Murphy, Elizabeth, Bernice K. Watt, and Robert L. Rizek. "Tables of Food Composition: Availability, Uses and Limitations." *Food Technology* 27 (January 1973): 40-51.

Perisse, J. "Heterogeneity in Food Composition Table Data." *Food and Nutrition* (FAO), 9 (1983): 14-17.

Polachi, Wanda. "Food Composition Tables: Recommended Method for Deriving Nutrient Values in Their Preparation." *Journal of the American Dietetic Association* 85 (1985): 1134-36.

· Southgate, D. A. T. "Availability of and Needs for Reliable Analytical Methods for the Assay of Foods." *Food and Nutrition Bulletin* 5 (July 1983): 30-39.

Southgate, D. A. T. *Guide Lines for the Preparation of Tables of Food Composition.* New York: B. S. Karger, 1974. 57p. ISBN 3805517807.

Stewart, K. K. "The State of Food Composition Data: An Overview with Some Suggestions." *Food and Nutrition Bulletin* 5 (July 1983): 55-68.

SELECTED REFERENCES
ON NUTRIENT DATABASES

Butrum, Ritva R., and Susan E. Gebhardt. "Nutrient Data Bank: Computer-Based Management of Nutrient Values in Foods." *Journal of the American Oil Chemists Society* 53 (December 1976): 727A-730A.

Cook, R. A., P. A. Quatromoni, and C. M. Cook. "Use of Two Short Data Bases Adapted to the Microcomputer." *Nutrition Reports International* 32 (December 1985): 1303-9.

Dwyer, Johanna, and Carol West Suitor. "Caveat Emptor: Assessing Needs, Evaluating Computer Options." *Journal of the American Dietetic Association* 84 (March 1984): 302-12.

Hepburn, Frank N. "The USDA National Nutrient Data Bank." *American Journal of Clinical Nutrition* 35 (May 1982): 1297-1301.

Hoover, Loretta W. "Computerized Nutrient Data Bases I: A Comparison of Nutrient Analysis Systems." *Journal of the American Dietetic Association* 82 (May 1983): 501-5.

Hoover, Loretta W., and Betty P. Perloff. "Computerized Nutrient Data Bases II: Development of a Model for Appraisal of Nutrient Data Base System Capabilities." *Journal of the American Dietetic Association* 82 (May 1983): 506-8.

Hoover, Loretta W., and Betty P. Perloff. *Model for Review of Nutrient Data Base Systems Capabilities.* Columbia, Mo.: Curators of the University of Missouri, 1981. 76p.

National Nutrient Data Bank Conference, 1st- . *Proceedings.* Alexandria, Va.: National Technical Information Service, 1976- . annual.
     1st, PB85-245207/XAB.
     3rd, PB85-245215/XAB.
     5th, PB85-245223/XAB.
     6th, PB85-245231/XAB.
     7th, PB85-245249/XAB.
     8th, PB84-159151.

Rand, William M., and Vernon R. Young. "International Network of Food Data Systems (INFOODS): Report of a Small International Planning Conference." *Food and Nutrition Bulletin* 5 (July 1983): 15-22.

Rand, William M., and Vernon R. Young. "Report of a Planning Conference Concerning an International Network of Food Data Systems (INFOODS)." *American Journal of Clinical Nutrition* 39 (1984): 144-51.

Rand, William M., et al., eds. *Proceedings of the First ASIAFOODS Conference.* Bangkok, Thailand: Prayurawong Co., 1985. 106p.

Rizek, Robert L., et al. "USDA's Nutrient Data Bases." In *Agricultural Outlook Conference, 60th, 1983, Washington, D.C. Proceedings: Outlook '84,* 292-98. Washington, D.C.: U.S. Department of Agriculture. 1984?. A1.2:Ag8/23/984. (Microfiche).

West, C. E., ed. "Eurofoods: Towards Compatibility of Nutrient Data Banks in Europe." *Annals of Nutrition and Metabolism* 29 (Supplement No. 1, 1985). 72p. ISBN 3805542097.

12
Nutrition and Food Consumption Surveys

This chapter is devoted to a discussion of nutrition and food consumption surveys that provide data representative of the populations of entire countries. Such surveys are generally conducted by government agencies both here and abroad. Less extensive diet surveys of particular groups (e.g., vegetarians or adolescents) are usually published in journals and are located by using an indexing/abstracting service such as *Nutrition Abstracts and Reviews*, *Index Medicus*, or *Food and Nutrition Quarterly Index*. Data from the national surveys may also be reported in the journal literature. Very often they undergo additional analysis.

The two major U.S. government surveys of food consumption and nutrition status are the Nationwide Food Consumption Survey (NFCS), conducted by the USDA, and the National Health and Nutrition Examination Survey (NHANES or HANES) conducted by the U.S. Department of Health and Human Services. Both are planned as periodic surveys and both use a statistically designed sample representative of the population as a whole. The surveys provide different, but complementary information. The results are made available to researchers in machine-readable form. Such surveys are important for a number of reasons: They are useful in planning food and health programs and nutrition education efforts, and they frequently help researchers formulate hypotheses for further research.

NATIONWIDE FOOD CONSUMPTION SURVEYS (NFCS) AND OTHER USDA SURVEYS

The USDA has conducted food consumption surveys at approximately 10-year intervals since 1935/36. Recent surveys have examined the foods eaten by families in different regions of the country over a one-week period. In the last two surveys data were also collected on food eaten by different household members. Many nutritionists now feel the 10-year interval is too long to measure food consumption in an environment where dietary patterns are changing very rapidly because of the introduction of new foods, new methods of processing, and other trends such as increased number of meals away from home. The long time lag between the collection and the publication of these data is also a problem. The information is virtually out-of-date by the time it is made available to researchers and professionals. For instance, some of the reports from the 1977/78 Nationwide Food Consumption Survey were still being published in 1985. Fortunately, the publication of preliminary reports from the 1977/78 food consumption survey has made some of these data available much earlier.

Publications reporting the results of the Nationwide Food Consumption Surveys since 1955 are listed below. For citations to the older surveys, consult the article by P. B. Swann cited at the end of this chapter.

Nationwide Food Consumption Surveys

1955

323. United States. Agricultural Research Service. **Household Food Consumption Survey, 1955. Report.** No. 1-17. Washington, D.C.: Government Printing Office, 1956-1963. A1.86.

1. *Food Consumption of Households in the United States.* 1956. 196p.

2. *Food Consumption of Households in the Northeast.* 1956. 195p.

3. *Food Consumption of Households in the North Central Region.* 1956. 196p.

4. *Food Consumption of Households in the South.* 1956. 196p.

5. *Food Consumption of Households in the West.* 1956. 194p.

6. *Dietary Levels of Households in the United States.* 1957. 68p.

7. *Dietary Levels of Households in the Northeast.* 1957. 68p.

8. *Dietary Levels of Households in the North Central Region.* 1957. 68p.

9. *Dietary Levels of Households in the South.* 1957. 68p.

10. *Dietary Levels of Households in the West.* 1957. 64p.

11. *Home Freezing and Canning by Households in the United States by Region.* 1957. 72p.

12. *Food Production for Home Use by Households in the United States by Region.* 1958. 88p.

13. *Home Baking by Households in the United States by Region.* 1958. 130p.

14. *Food Consumption and Dietary Levels of Households as Related to the Age of the Homemakers, United States by Region.* 1959. 134p.

15. *Food Consumption and Dietary Levels of Households as Related to Employment of Homemaker, United States by Region.* 1960. 130p.

16. *Dietary Evaluation of Food Used in Households in the United States.* 1961. 55p.

17. *Food Consumption and Dietary Levels of Households of Different Sizes, United States by Region.* 1963. 168p.

1965-66

324. United States. Agricultural Research Service. **Household Food Consumption Survey, 1965-66: Report.** No. 1-18. Washington, D.C.: Government Printing Office, 1968-1974. A1.86.

1. *Food Consumption of Households in the United States, Spring 1965.* 1968. 212p.

2. *Food Consumption of Households in the Northeast, Spring 1965.* 1968. 213p.

3. *Food Consumption of Households in the North Central Region, Spring 1965.* 1968. 213p.

4. *Food Consumption of Households in the South, Spring 1965.* 1968. 213p.

5. *Food Consumption of Households in the West, Spring 1965.* 1968. 213p.

6. *Dietary Levels of Households in the United States, Spring 1965.* 1970. 117p.

7. *Dietary Levels of Households in the Northeast, Spring 1965.* 1970. 117p.

8. *Dietary Levels of Households in the North Central Region, Spring 1965.* 1970. 117p.

9. *Dietary Levels of Households in the South, Spring 1965.* 1970. 117p.

10. *Dietary Levels of Households in the West, Spring 1965.* 1970. 117p.

11. *Food and Nutrient Intake of Individuals in the United States, Seasons and Year, 1965-66.* 1972. 291p.

12. *Food Consumption of Households in the United States, Seasons and Year, 1965-66.* 1972. 217p.

13. *Food Consumption of Households in the Northeast, Seasons and Year, 1965-66.* 1972. 215p.

14. *Food Consumption of Households in the North Central Region, Seasons and Year, 1965-66.* 1972. 215p.

15. *Food Consumption of Households in the South, Seasons and Year, 1965-66.* 1973. 215p.

16. *Food Consumption of Households in the West, Seasons and Year, 1965-66.* 1973. 215p.

17. *Food Consumption of Households by Money Value of Food and Quality of Diet, United States, North and South.* 1972. 217p.

18. *Dietary Levels of Households in the United States, Seasons and Year, 1965-66.* 1974. 191p.

PRELIMINARY REPORTS, 1977-78

325. United States. Department of Agriculture. Science and Education Administration. **Nationwide Food Consumption Survey, 1977-78. Preliminary Report.** No. 1- . Washington, D.C.: Government Printing Office, 1979- . A111.9/2.

1. *Money Value of Food Used by Households in the United States, Spring 1977.* 1979. 17p.

2. *Food and Nutrient Intakes of Individuals in 1 Day in the United States, Spring 1977.* 1980. 121p.

3. *Nutrient Levels in Food Used by Households in the United States, Spring 1977.* 1981. 16p.

4. *Food Consumption and Dietary Levels of Households in Hawaii, Winter, 1978.* 1981. 29p.

5. *Food and Nutrient Intakes of Individuals in 1 Day in Hawaii, Winter, 1978.* 1981. 66p.

6. *Food and Nutrient Intakes of Individuals in 1 Day in Alaska, Winter, 1978.* 1981.

7. *Food Consumption and Dietary Levels of Households in Alaska, Winter, 1978.* 1981. 25p.

8. *Food Consumption and Dietary Levels of Low-Income Households, November, 1977-March, 1978.* 1981. 33p.

9. *Food Consumption and Dietary Levels of Households in Puerto Rico, Summer and Fall, 1977.* 1982. 38p.

10. *Food Consumption and Dietary Levels of Low-Income Households, November 1979-March, 1980.* 1982. 48p.

11. *Food and Nutrient Intakes of Individuals in 1 Day, Low-Income Households, November, 1977-March, 1978.* 1982. 200p.

12. *Food and Nutrient Intakes of Individuals in 1 Day in Puerto Rico, Summer and Fall, 1977.* 1982. 94p.

13. *Food and Nutrient Intakes of Individuals in 1 Day, Low-Income Households, November, 1979-March, 1980.* 1982. 209p.

— *Eating Patterns and Food Frequencies of Children in the United States.* 1980. 18p. (unnumbered).

1977-78

326.   United States. Department of Agriculture. Human Nutrition Information Service. **Nationwide Food Consumption Survey, 1977-78.** Washington, D.C.: Government Printing Office, 1982- . A111.9: .

> No. H-1. *Food Consumption: Households in the United States, Spring 1977.* 1982. 297p.
>
> No. H-2. *Food Consumption: Households in the Northeast, Spring 1977.* 1982. 301p.
>
> No. H-3. *Food Consumption: Households in the North Central Region, Spring 1977.* 1982. 303p.
>
> No. H-4. *Food Consumption: Households in the South, Spring 1977.* 1982. 301p.
>
> No. H-5. *Food Consumption: Households in the West, Spring 1977.* 1982. 301p.
>
> No. H-6. *Food Consumption: Households in the United States, Seasons and Year 1977-78.* 1983. 309p.
>
> No. H-7. *Food Consumption: Households in the Northeast, Seasons and Year 1977-78.* 1983. 312p.
>
> No. H-8. *Food Consumption: Households in the North Central Region, Seasons and Year.* 1983. 311p.
>
> No. H-9. *Food Consumption: Households in the South, Seasons and Year 1977-78.* 1983. 311p.
>
> No. H-10. *Food Consumption: Households in the West, Seasons and Year 1977-78.* 1983. 312p.
>
> No. H-11. *Dietary Levels: Households in the United States, Spring 1977.* 1985. 190p.
>
> No. H-12. *Dietary Levels: Households in the Northeast, Spring 1977.* 1985. 190p.
>
> No. H-13. *Dietary Levels: Households in the North Central Region, Spring 1977.* 1985. 190p.
>
> No. H-14. *Dietary Levels: Households in the South, Spring 1977.* 1985. 190p.
>
> No. H-15. *Dietary Levels: Households in the West, Spring 1977.* 1985. 190p.
>
> No. I-1. *Food Intakes: Individuals in 48 States, Year 1977-78.* 1983. 617p.
>
> No. I-2. *Nutrient Intakes: Individuals in 48 States, Year 1977-78.* 1984. 437p.
>
> No. I-3. *Food and Nutrient Intakes: Individuals in Four Regions, 1977-78.* 1985. 544p.

Other USDA Surveys

327. Allen, Joyce E., and Kenneth E. Gadsdon. **Nutrient Consumption Patterns of Low-Income Households**. Washington, D.C.: Government Printing Office, 1983. 46p. (U.S. Department of Agriculture. Technical Report, No. 1685). A1.36:1685.

328. Manchester, Alden C., and Richard A. King. **U.S. Food Expenditures, 1954-78**. Washington, D.C.: Government Printing Office, 1979. 23p. (Agricultural Economics Report, No. 41). A1.107.

329. Pao, Eleanor M. **Foods Commonly Eaten by Individuals: Amount Per Day Per Eating Occasion**. Washington,·D.C.: Government Printing Office, 1982. 431p. (Agricultural Research Report, No. 44). A1.87:44.

This report is based on data from the 1977-1978 Nationwide Food Consumption Survey, but not officially published as a part of it. "Data on 3-day intakes of 200 commonly used foods and food groups by individuals."

330. Salathe, Larry E. **Household Expenditure Patterns in the United States**. Washington, D.C.: Government Printing Office, 1979. 23p. (U.S. Department of Agriculture. Technical Bulletin, No. 1603). A1.36:1603.

331. Salathe, Larry E., and Reuben C. Buse. **Household Food Consumption Patterns in the United States**. Washington, D.C.: Government Printing Office, 1979. 27p. (U.S. Department of Agriculture. Technical Bulletin, No. 1587). A1.36:1587.

332. United States. Department of Agriculture. Economic Research Service. **Food Consumption, Prices, and Expenditures**. (1960-1979-). Washington, D.C.: Government Printing Office, 1980- .

Through 1977, this appeared as Agricultural Economic Report, No. 138, with annual supplements. Subsequently it has been included in issues of the *Statistical Bulletin* as follows: No. 656, 1960-1979; No. 672, 1960-1980; No. 694, 1960-1981; No. 701, 1962-1982; No. 713, 1963-1983; No. 736, 1964-1984. It contains per capita consumption figures for various foods as well as supply and utilization figures and percentage of nutrients contributed by major food groups. Some of the data are from the early 1900s.

333. United States. Department of Agriculture. Food and Nutrition Service. **Food Consumption and Nutrition Evaluation, the National School Lunch Program**. Washington, D.C.: U.S. Department of Agriculture, 1979. 129p.

NHANES AND THE TEN-STATE SURVEY

The Department of Health and Human Services first conducted a National Health Survey in the 1950s. In 1968 this was expanded to include data on nutrition and was called the Ten-State Nutrition Survey. The first major survey of nutritional status in the country, it emphasized data on low-income groups likely to be at risk nutritionally.

The National Health and Nutrition Examination Survey (HANES I or NHANES I) was conducted between 1971 and 1974 by the National Center for Health Statistics and was designed to assess health status of individuals with emphasis on dental health, vision, and nutritional status. It collected data on food intake and from medical and dental exams. Included were anthropometric data and various biochemical measurements. The survey was intended to provide the means of assessing nutritional status and to evaluate diet in relation to nutritional status. It also included surveys of high risk groups. NHANES II was conducted between 1976 and 1980. Some of the data from NHANES I were still being published in 1983 and only a small amount of the data from NHANES II have been published thus far.

Data from the National Health Survey and the NHANES surveys are published in *Vital and Health Statistics: Series 11*. Computer tapes are also made available to researchers with the expertise to use the data in this form. In early 1984 over 230 separate publications had been issued in this series. As indicated by the titles listed below, the scope of these publications is incredibly broad. Basic data on intake of major nutrients for both NHANES I and II were issued in publications entitled *Dietary Intake Source Data*.

Publications from these surveys are accessible selectively through *Nutrition Abstracts and Reviews*. They are indexed more completely in the *Monthly Catalog of U.S. Government Publications* and the following publications.

334.   United States. Department of Health and Human Services. **Publications Catalog of the United States Department of Health and Human Services** (1979-). Washington, D.C.: Government Printing Office. 1980- . annual. ISSN 0278-0143. HE1.18/3: .

335.   United States. National Center for Health Statistics. **Catalog of Publications**. Hyattsville, Md.: National Center for Health Statistics, 1980- . irregular. HE20.6216. (*1977-1981* — 1977-1981; *1981* — 1976-1980; *1983* — 1978-1982).

Ten-State Nutrition Survey

336.   United States. Centers for Disease Control. **Ten-State Nutrition Survey, 1968-1970**. Atlanta, Ga.: U.S. Department of Health, Education and Welfare, 1972?. 6v. in 5. (United States. Department of Health, Education and Welfare. DHEW Publication, No. (HSN) 72-8130-72-8134). HE20.2302:N95/968-70.

"The first comprehensive attempt to assess the nutritional status of the American people.... The Survey was designed to examine the nutritional status and dietary practices of low-income groups. However, ... data on middle and upper income groups was also obtained." The ten states sampled were California, Kentucky, Louisiana, Massachusetts, Michigan, New York (including New York City), South Carolina, Texas, Washington, and West Virginia.

NHANES I: Selected Publications

337.   Abraham, Sidney, et al. **Dietary Intake Source Data, United States 1971-74**. Hyattsville, Md.: U.S. National Center for Health Statistics, 1979. 404p. (DHEW Publication, No. (PHS) 79-1221). HE20.6202:D56/971-74.

This was not issued as part of the series Vital and Health Statistics.

338. United States. Center for Health Statistics. **Vital and Health Statistics: Series 11**. Hyattsville, Md.: Center for Health Statistics, 1977- . HE20.6209:11/.

No. 202. *Dietary Intake Findings, United States 1971-74.* 1977. 74p.

No. 203. *Blood Pressure Levels of Persons 6-74 Years, United States, 1971-74.* 1977. 103p.

No. 205. *Total Serum Cholesterol Levels of Adults 18-74 Years, United States, 1971-74.* 1978. 31p.

No. 208. *Weight by Height and Age for Adults 18-74 Years, United States, 1971-74.* 1979. 56p.

No. 209. *Caloric and Selected Nutrient Values for Persons 1-74 Years, United States, 1971-74.* 1979. 88p.

No. 210. *Food Consumption Profiles for White and Black Persons 1-74 Years, United States, 1971-74.* 1979. 103p.

No. 211. *Weight and Height of Adults 18-74 Years, United States, 1971-74.* 1979. 49p.

No. 217. *Serum Cholesterol Levels of Persons 4-74 Years of Age by Socioeconomic Characteristics, United States, 1971-74.* 1980. 49p.

No. 220. *Total White Blood Cell Counts for Persons Ages 1-74 Years with Differential Leukocyte Counts for Adults Ages 25-74 Years, United States, 1971-1975.* 1982. 36p.

No. 221. *Hypertension in Adults 25-74 Years of Age, United States, 1971-1975.* 1981. 107p.

No. 223. *Decayed, Missing and Filled Teeth among Persons 1-74 Years, United States.* 1981. 55p.

No. 224. *Height and Weight of Adults Ages 18-74 Years, by Socio-economic and Geographic Variables, United States.* 1981. 62p.

No. 225. *Diet and Dental Health: A Study of Relationships, United States, 1971-74.* 1982. 85p.

No. 226-227. *Dietary Intake and Cardiovascular Risk Factors: United States, 1971-75.* 1983. 2v.

No. 229. *Diet and Iron Status, a Study of Relationships, United States, 1971-74.* 1983. 83p.

No. 230. *Obese and Overweight Adults in the United States.* 1983. 93p.

NHANES II: Selected Publications

339. United States. Center for Health Statistics. **Vital and Health Statistics: Series 11**. Hyattsville, Md.: Center for Health Statistics, 1983- . HE 20.6209:11/.

No. 231. *Dietary Intake Source Data: United States, 1976-80.* 1983. 483p.

No. 232. *Hematological and Nutritional Biochemistry Reference Data of Persons 6 Months-74 Years of Age: United States, 1976-80.* 1983. 173p.

No. 233. *Blood Lead Levels for Persons Ages 6 Months-74 Years, United States, 1976-80.* 1984. 61p.

No. 234. *Blood Pressure Levels in Persons 18-74 Years of Age in 1976-80 and Trends in Blood Pressure from 1960 to 1980 in the United States.* 1986. 68p.

No. 236. *Total Serum Cholesterol Levels of Adults 20-74 Years of Age, United States, 1976-1980.* 1986. 59p.

Other DHHS Surveys

340. United States. Centers for Disease Control. **Nutrition Surveillance**. Washington, D.C.: Department of Health and Human Services, 1978- . annual. ISSN 0193-1377. HE20.7011/24: .

"Summarizes information including selected indices of nutritional status, received from 22 states which comprise a group of contributors to a developing program of nutrition surveillance in the United States. Data are for children and adolescents less than 18 years of age. Includes hemoglobin and hematocrit, height and weight for age, and weight for height."

341. United States. Environmental Protection Agency. Office of Toxic Substances. **Dietary Consumption Distributions of Selected Food Groups for the U.S. Population**. Washington, D.C.: Environmental Protection Agency, 1980. 63p. EP5.2:D56.

Data on consumption of certain foods to determine possible exposure of the population to toxic substances are presented.

342. Heller, Christine A., and Edward M. Scott. **The Alaska Dietary Survey 1956-1961**. Washington, D.C.: Government Printing Office, 1967. 281p. (Public Health Service Publication, No. 999-AH-2; Environmental Health Series. [AH] Arctic Health No. 2).

FOREIGN AND INTERNATIONAL SURVEYS

Bibliographies and Guides

343. Food and Agriculture Organization of the United Nations. **Review of Food Consumption Surveys**. Rome: Food and Agriculture Organization of the United Nations, 1958- . irregular.

Individual reviews have appeared in 1958, 1962, 1970, 1977, 1981, and 1985. Since 1977 they have been issued as FAO Food and Nutrition Papers. The 1977 review was number 1 in this series; the 1981 review was number 27; and the 1985 review was number 35.

This publication "presents data from selected surveys, in which household food consumption is classified by income, total expenditure, or some other indicators of economic status." The 1981 survey (published in 1983) contains lists of surveys from previous publications. It lists and describes surveys by country and contains tabular data for individual countries.

344.　Food and Agriculture Organization of the United Nations. Statistics Division, Economic and Social Policy. **Bibliography of Food Consumption Surveys**. Rome: Food and Agriculture Organization of the United Nations, 1984. 46p. (FAO Food and Nutrition Paper, No. 18 Rev. 1). ISBN 9251014949.

"The purpose of this bibliography is ... to catalogue, as briefly as possible, some of the main features of the content and results of recent household budget and food consumption surveys conducted in different countries. The surveys covered are those conducted from 1972-1982.... The objective is to present in a single publication, the sources of this information.... Methodological and tabulated results of some of the surveys listed in this bibliography have already been presented in various issues of the *Review of Food Consumption Surveys*."

345.　Organization for Economic Co-operation and Development. **Food Consumption Statistics = Statistiques de la Consommation des Denrées Alimentaires**. 1st ed.- (1954-1966-). Paris: Organization for Economic Co-operation and Development, 1968- .

Included are production and per capita consumption statistics for agricultural commodities in Australia, Austria, Canada, Denmark, Finland, France, Germany, Ireland, Italy, Japan, the Netherlands, New Zealand, Norway, Portugal, Spain, Sweden, Switzerland, Turkey, the United Kingdom, the United States, and Yugoslavia.

Australia and New Zealand

346.　Australian Bureau of Statistics. **Apparent Consumption of Food Stuffs and Nutrients**. Canberra, Australia: Australian Bureau of Statistics, 1972/73- . ISSN 0312-6226.

347.　New Zealand. Department of Statistics. **New Zealand Household Expenditure and Income Survey**. Wellington, New Zealand: Department of Statistics, 1974- . annual. ISSN 0112-6601. (Previous titles: *Household Sample Survey*; *New Zealand Household Survey*).

Canada

GENERAL

348.　Canada. Bureau of Nutritional Sciences. Health Protection Branch. **Food Consumption Patterns Report: A Report from Nutrition Canada**. Ottawa, Ont.: Health and Welfare Canada, 1977. 247p.

Includes "part of the data from the Canadian National Survey of Nutritional Status in 1970-1972" (*Nutrition Abstracts and Reviews A*, 1978, #3675).

349. Canada. Bureau of Nutritional Sciences. **Anthropometry Report**. Prepared by A. Demirjian. Ottawa, Ont.: Information Canada, 1980. 133p.

350. Canada. Department of Consumer and Corporate Affairs. **Report on Food Consumption and Nutrition**. Ottawa, Ont.: Department of Consumer Affairs and Nutrition, 1978. 92p.

351. Canada. Statistics Canada. Family Expenditure Section. **Urban Family Food Expenditure. Dépenses Alimentaires des Familles Urbaines**. Ottawa, Ont.: Minister of Industry, Trade and Commerce, 1974?- .

352. Watts, T. A., et al. **Canadian Food Consumption Patterns and Nutritional Trends**. Ottawa, Ont.: Food Policy Group, Consumer and Corporate Affairs, Canada, 1977. 152p.

PROVINCES

353. Canada. Bureau of Nutritional Sciences. **The Alberta Survey Report: A Report from Nutrition Canada**. Ottawa, Ont.: Information Canada, 1974. 150, 125p.

354. Canada. Bureau of Nutritional Sciences. **The British Columbia Survey Report: A Report from Nutrition Canada**. Ottawa, Ont.: Information Canada, 1974. 152, 125p.

355. Canada. Bureau of Nutritional Sciences. **The Manitoba Survey Report: A Report from Nutrition Canada**. Ottawa, Ont.: Information Canada, 1974. 150, 125p.

356. Canada. Bureau of Nutritional Sciences. **The New Brunswick Survey Report: A Report from Nutrition Canada**. Ottawa, Ont.: Information Canada, 1974. 150, 93p.

357. Canada. Bureau of Nutritional Sciences. **The Newfoundland Survey Report: A Report from Nutrition Canada**. Ottawa, Ont.: Information Canada, 1974. 150, 125p.

358. Canada. Bureau of Nutritional Sciences. **The Nova Scotia Survey Report: A Report from Nutrition Canada**. Ottawa, Ont.: Information Canada, 1974. 150, 125p.

359. Canada. Bureau of Nutritional Sciences. **The Ontario Survey Report: A Report from Nutrition Canada**. Ottawa, Ont.: Information Canada, 1974. 152, 125p.

360. Canada. Bureau of Nutritional Sciences. **The Quebec Survey Report: A Report from Nutrition Canada**. Ottawa, Ont.: Information Canada, 1974. 152, 125p.

361.   Canada. Bureau of Nutritional Sciences. **The Saskatchewan Survey Report: A Report from Nutrition Canada**. Ottawa, Ont.: Information Canada, 1974. 150, 125p.

Europe

362. · Deutsche Gesellschaft für Ernährung. **Ernährungsbericht**. Frankfurt am Main, W. Germany: Deutsche Gesellschaft für Ernährung, 1964?- . quadrennial.
   This is a survey of foods and nutrients consumed. The third report was issued in 1976 and is 480 pages long.

363.   Great Britain. Ministry of Agriculture, Fisheries, and Food. National Food Survey Committee. **Household Food Consumption and Expenditures: Annual Report of the National Food Survey Committee**. 1st- . London: H.M.S.O., 1951?- . ISSN 0304-3273.
   Great Britain has conducted a national food consumption survey since 1940. In the beginning, it surveyed only the lower socio-economic groups, but was later expanded to groups more representative of the population as a whole. It is now primarily an economic survey. Its purpose is to monitor changes in food consumption, rather than survey nutritional status. However, it does reflect information of nutritional importance. Every fifth year since 1965 the report has been enlarged to show trends in food consumption and quality of diet.

HISTORICAL INFORMATION

   Most systematic nutrition or food consumption surveys by government bodies date from the 1930s and 1940s. Reliable data prior to that period are difficult to locate. Information for the United States is contained in the volumes of *The Changing American Diet* or *Food Consumption Prices Expenditures* listed below.

364.   Brewster, Letitia, and Michael F. Jacobson. **The Changing American Diet**. Washington, D.C.: Center for Science in the Public Interest, 1978. 80p. ISBN 0893290076.
   Based on USDA statistics, this compilation provides data on changes in the consumption of specific foods and nutrients. Some of the data go back to the early 1900s.

365.   Colburn, Mary, and Michael F. Jacobson. **The Changing American Diet: Update 1982**. Washington, D.C.: Center for Science in the Public Interest, 1982. 8p.
   This updates the CSPI's *Changing American Diet* for the period 1976-1981.

366.   United States. Department of Agriculture. Economic Research Service. **Food Consumption Prices Expenditures**. Washington, D.C.: Government Printing Office, 1968. 193p. (Agricultural Economic Report, No. 138). A1.107:138.
   This title contains per capita food consumption statistics back to 1909 and supply and utilization data for major agricultural commodities.

SELECTED REFERENCES

Brown, George E. "National Nutrition Monitoring System: A Congressional Perspective." *Journal of the American Dietetic Association* 84 (1984): 1185-88.

Clark, F. "Recent Food Consumption Surveys and Their Uses." *Federation Proceedings* 33 (1974): 2270-74.

Davis, Thomas R. A., Dean F. Gamble, and Stanley N. Gershoff. "Review of Studies of Vitamin and Mineral Nutrition in the United States (1950-1968)." *Journal of Nutrition Education* 1 (Supplement 1, 1969): 39-57.

Habicht, J-P., J. M. Lane, and A. J. McDowell. "National Nutrition Surveillance." *Federation Proceedings* 37 (1978): 1181-87.

Hegsted, David Mark. "The Classic Approach—The USDA Nationwide Food Consumption Survey." *American Journal of Clinical Nutrition* 35 (1985): 1302-5.

Hegsted, David Mark. "Nationwide Food Consumption Survey: Implications." In *1980 Agricultural Outlook: Papers Presented at the Agricultural Outlook Conference—Held in Washington, D.C., November 5-8, 1979,* 539-42. Washington, D.C.: Government Printing Office, 1979. Y4.Ag8/3Ou81980.

Lowenstein, F. W. "The Health and Nutrition Examination Survey in the USA." *Bibliotheca Nutritio et Dieta* 20 (1974): 62-68.

Murphy, R. S., and G. A. Michael. "Methodologic Consideration of the National Health and Nutrition Examination Survey." *American Journal of Clinical Nutrition* 35 (1982): 1255.

National Academy of Public Administration. *Improving the Health and Nutrition Examination Survey: An Evaluation by a Panel of the National Academy of Public Administration.* Washington, D.C.: National Academy of Public Administration, 1980. 120p.

"National Nutrition Monitoring System." *Journal of the American Dietetic Association* 84 (1984): 1171-80.

National Research Council. Food and Nutrition Board. *National Survey Data on Food Consumption: Uses and Recommendations.* Washington, D.C.: National Academy Press, 1984. 133p.

Ostenso, Grace L. "National Nutrition Monitoring System: A Historical Perspective." *Journal of the American Dietetic Association* 84 (1984): 1181-85.

Pao, Eleanor M., and S. J. Mickle. "Problem Nutrients in the United States." *Food Technology* 35 (September 1981): 58-69, 79.

Rizek, Robert L., and Elizabeth M. Jackson. *Current Food Consumption Practices and Nutrient Sources in the American Diet*. Hyattsville, Md.: U.S. Consumer Nutrition Center, 1980. 34p.

Schwerin, H. S., et al. "Food Coding Patterns and Health: A Reexamination of the Ten State and HANES Surveys." *American Journal of Clinical Nutrition* 34 (1981): 568-80.

Schwerin, H. S., et al. "How Have the Quantity and Quality of the American Diet Changed during the Past Decade?" *Food Technology* 35 (September 1981): 50-57.

Swann, P. B. "Food Consumption by Individuals in the United States: Two Major Surveys." *Annual Review of Nutrition* 3 (1983): 413-32.

United States. Congress. Senate. Committee on Agriculture, Nutrition and Forestry. *Trends in the American Diet*. Washington, D.C.: Government Printing Office, 1980. 66p. Y4.AG 8/3:D56/2.

United States. General Accounting Office. *Nationwide Food Consumption Survey: Need for Improvement and Expansion: Report to the Select Committee on Nutrition and Human Needs*. Washington, D.C.: Government Printing Office, 1977. 39p. GA1.13:CED-77-56.

Welsh, S. O., and R. M. Marston. "Review of Trends in Food Use in the United States, 1909 to 1980." *Journal of the American Dietetic Association* 81 (1982): 120-25.

13
Dietary Standards, Recommendations, and Guidelines

Dietary standards are official recommendations on dietary intakes. Most larger countries have such recommendations, which in the United States are called the *Recommended Dietary Allowances* and are revised every five to six years by the Food and Nutrition Board of the National Research Council.

Such standards are different from less official dietary goals, guidelines, or recommendations, which often serve as nutrition education tools to improve the diet of the population at large. They are also distinguished from the position papers of professional organizations defining their officially held views on nutrition matters.

Official recommendations such as the RDAs have many different functions. They can be used in diet surveys, to plan diets to include adequate amounts of essential nutrients, to plan for an adequate food supply, label food products, etc.

The listing of dietary standards included in this chapter is deliberately selective. To locate information on the dietary standards of other countries, use the bibliography in this chapter. For position papers of professional organizations, consult the appendix of *Manual of Nutrition and Diet Therapy*, edited by Norma Jean Grills and Marcia Vermaire Bosscher (Macmillan, 1981). The listing here of dietary guidelines and recommendations is extensive for the United States, but selective for other countries.

It should be noted that some of these recommendations are shrouded in controversy. In one instance two official American bodies published recommendations which contrasted markedly on a number of points, much to the confusion of the American public. The U.S. Department of Agriculture recommended reducing dietary cholesterol and fat in its *Dietary Guidelines for Americans* while the Food and Nutrition Board of the National Research Council ignored these concerns.

BIBLIOGRAPHIES AND GUIDES

367. International Union of Nutritional Sciences. Committee Y5. "Recommended Dietary Intakes around the World, 1982," Part I, **Nutrition Abstracts and Reviews A** 53 (1983): 939-1015; Part II, **Nutrition Abstracts and Reviews A** 53 (1983): 1076-1119.

This useful report provides actual reproductions of dietary standards from throughout the world with notes and citations to original publications. It includes comparative data on individual nutrients on a country-by-country basis.

FAO/WHO

368. Passmore, R., et al. **Handbook on Human Nutritional Requirements**. Food and Agriculture Organization of the United Nations and World Health Organization. Rome: Food and Agriculture Organization of the United Nations, 1974. 66, 4p. (FAO Nutritional Series, No. 28; WHO Monograph Series, No. 61).

Individual Countries

369. Australia. National Health and Medical Research Council. Nutrition Committee. **Dietary Allowances for Use in Australia**. Canberra, Australia: Australian Government Publishing Service, 1979. 25p. ISBN 0642041180.

370. Canada. Department of National Health and Welfare. Bureau of Nutritional Sciences. **Dietary Standard for Canada**. rev. ed. Ottawa, Ont.: Information Canada, 1975. 110p.

371. Caribbean Food and Nutrition Institute. **Recommended Dietary Allowances for the Caribbean**. Kingston, Jamaica: Caribbean Food and Nutrition Institute, 1979. 47p.

372. Centre National de Coordination des Études et Recherches sur l'Alimentation et de la Nutrition (CNERNA). Commission: Apports Nutritionels. **Apports Nutritionels Conseillés pour la Population Française**. 2e. tirage rev. [par] Henri Dupin et les Membres de la Commission. Lavoisier, France: Technique et Documentation, 1982. 101p. ISBN 0285206163.

373. Deutsche Gesellschaft für Ernährung. **Empfehlungen für die Nährstoffzufur**. 3. Aufl. Frankfurt am Main, W. Germany: Umschau Verlag, 1975. 64p.

Previous editions were published under the title: *Die Wünschenswerte Höhe der Nährungszufur*.

374. Gopalan, C., and B. S. Narasinga Rao. **Dietary Allowances for Indians**. Hyderabad, India: National Institute of Nutrition, Indian Council of Medical Research, 1980. 87p. (Special Report Series, No. 60).

375. Great Britain. Committee on Medical Aspects of Food Policy. **Recommended Daily Amounts of Food Energy and Nutrients for Groups of People in the United Kingdom**. London: H.M.S.O., 1979. 27p. ISBN 011520342X.

376. National Research Council. Committee on Dietary Allowances. **Recommended Dietary Allowances**. 9th rev. ed. Washington, D.C.: National Academy of Sciences, 1980. 185p. ISBN 0309024914.

  Since the tenth revised edition, scheduled to appear in 1985, has been postponed, this ninth edition may serve as the standard for several years to come.

377. New Zealand. Nutrition Advisory Committee. **Recommendations for Selected Nutrient Intakes of New Zealanders**. Wellington, New Zealand: The Committee, 1983. 26p.

DIETARY GUIDELINES AND RECOMMENDATIONS

Australia

378. Australia. Commonwealth Department of Health. **Dietary Guidelines for Australians**. Canberra, Australia: Australian Government Publishing Service, 1982. 20p. ISBN 0642065411.

Canada

379. Canada: Health and Welfare Canada. **Canada's Food Guide. Handbook**. Ottawa, Ont.: Health and Welfare Canada, 1983. 56p. ISBN 0662119479.

United States

380. American Dietetic Association. **Dietary Guidelines to Lower Cancer Risk**. Chicago: American Dietetic Association, 1984. 12p.

381. National Research Council. Committee on Diet, Nutrition, and Cancer. **Diet, Nutrition, and Cancer**. Washington, D.C.: National Academy Press, 1982. 1v. (various paging). ISBN 0309032806.

382. National Research Council. Food and Nutrition Board. **Toward Healthful Diets**. Washington, D.C.: National Academy Press, 1980. 24p. ISBN 0309030773.

383. United States. Congress. Senate. Select Committee on Nutrition and Human Needs. **Dietary Goals for the United States**. Washington, D.C.: Government Printing Office, February 1977. 79p. Y4.N95:D56.

384. United States. Congress. Senate. Select Committee on Nutrition and Human Needs. **Dietary Goals for the United States**. 2nd ed. Washington, D.C.: Government Printing Office, December 1977. 83p. Y4.N95:D56/977-2.

385.   United States. Department of Agriculture. **Nutrition and Your Health: Dietary Guidelines for Americans**. 2nd ed. Washington, D.C.: U.S. Department of Agriculture, 1985. 23p. (Home and Garden Bulletin, No. 232). A1.77:232/ 985.

386.   United States. Office of the Assistant Secretary of Health and Surgeon General. **Healthy People: The Surgeon General's Report on Health Promotion and Disease Prevention**. Washington, D.C.: United States Department of Health, Education and Welfare, 1979. 1v. (various paging). (DHEW Publication No. (PHS) 79-55071). HE20.2:H34/5.

SELECTED REFERENCES

Bush, M. B., and M. Ballantyne. "An Evaluation of Canada's Food Guide and Handbook." *Journal of the Canadian Dietetic Association* 40 (1979): 321.

Canada. Health and Welfare Canada. *A Look at the Dietary Standard for Canada*. Ottawa, Ont.: Health and Welfare Canada, 1977. 4p. (Dispatch No. 39).

Council for Agricultural Science and Technology. *Dietary Goals for the United States: A Commentary*. Ames, Iowa: Council for Agricultural Science and Technology, 1977. 18p. (Council for Agricultural Science and Technology. Report No. 77).

Harper, A. E. "Dietary Goals—A Skeptical View." *American Journal of Clinical Nutrition* 31 (1978): 310-21.

Harper, A. E. "Recommended Dietary Allowances—1980." *Nutrition Reviews* 38 (1980): 290-94.

Harper, A. E. "U.S. Dietary Goals: Against." *Journal of Nutrition Education* 9 (1977): 154-56.

Hegsted, D. M. "The Development of National Dietary Guidelines." *Proceedings of the Nutrition Society of Australia* 4 (1979): 96-106.

Hegsted, D. M. "Dietary Goals—A Progressive View." *American Journal of Clinical Nutrition* 31 (1978): 1504-9.

Hegsted, D. M. "Dietary Standards." *Journal of the American Dietetic Association* 66 (1975): 13-21.

Hollingsworth, D. F. "Dietary Standards." In *Nutrition Reviews' Present Knowledge in Nutrition*, 5th ed., Robert E. Olson, et al., eds., 711-23. New York: The Nutrition Foundation, 1984. ISBN 093536840X.

International Union of Nutritional Sciences. "Recommended Dietary Intakes and Allowances around the World." *Food and Nutrition Bulletin* 4 (1982): 34-45.

Irwin, M. Isabel, et al. *Nutritional Requirements of Man: A Conspectus of Research*. New York: The Nutrition Foundation, 1980. 592p. ISBN 093536823X.

Kris-Etherton, P. M., ed. *Proceedings of the Conference on the Implementation of the U.S. Dietary Goals and Guidelines, May 18-19, 1981*. University Park, Pa.: Pennsylvania State University, 1981?. 85p.

Latham, M. C., and L. S. Stephenson. "U.S. Dietary Goals: For." *Journal of Nutrition Education* 9 (1977): 152-54.

Leverton, R. M. "The RDA's Are Not for Amateurs." *Journal of the American Dietetic Association* 66 (1975): 9-11.

Masek, J. "Recommended Nutrient Allowances." *World Review of Nutrition and Dietetics* 25 (1976): 1-107.

McNutt, K. W. "An Analysis of Dietary Goals for the United States, Second Edition." *Journal of Nutrition Education* 10 (1978): 61-62.

Munro, H. N. "How Well Recommended Are the Recommended Dietary Allowances?" *Journal of the American Dietetic Association* 71 (1977): 490-94.

Murray, T. K., and J. Rae. "Nutrition Recommendations for Canadians." *Canadian Medical Association Journal* 120 (1979): 1241-42.

National Dairy Council. *Statement on Dietary Goals for the United States: Submitted to the Select Committee on Nutrition and Human Needs, United States Senate*. Rosemont, Ill.: National Dairy Council, 1977. 6p.

National Research Council. Food and Nutrition Board. *Research Needs for Establishing Dietary Guidelines for the U.S. Population*. Washington, D.C.: National Academy of Sciences, 1979. 41p.

"Round Table on Comparison of Dietary Recommendations in Different European Countries." *Nutrition and Metabolism* 21 (1977): 210-79.

Swenerton, H., and W. L. Dunkley. "Recent Activities of Public Agencies to Assure Healthful Diets for Americans." *Journal of Dairy Science* 65 (1982): 484-87.

Truswell, A. S. "Recommended Dietary Intakes—Difficulties and Trends." *Proceedings of the Nutrition Society of Australia* 6 (1981): 9-20.

Turner, Michael, and Juliet Gray, eds. *Implementation of Dietary Guidelines: Obstacles and Opportunities*. London: British Nutrition Foundation, 1982. 44p. (BNF Monograph Series). ISBN 0907667015.

United Fresh Fruit and Vegetable Association. *Dietary Goals for the United States*. Washington, D.C.: United Fresh Fruit and Vegetable Association, 1978. 10p.

United States. Congress. House. Committee on Science and Technology. Subcommittee on Domestic and International Scientific Planning, Analysis, and Cooperation. *The Scientific Adequacy and Usefulness of the Recommended Dietary Allowance (RDA) Standards: Hearings before the Subcommittee on Domestic and International Scientific Planning, Analysis and Cooperation.* Washington, D.C.: Government Printing Office, 1978. 595p. Y4.Sci2: 95/88.

United States. Congress. Senate. Committee on Appropriations. Subcommittee on Agriculture, Rural Development, and Related Agencies. *Dietary Guidelines for Americans: Hearing before a Subcommittee of the Committee on Appropriations.* Washington, D.C.: Government Printing Office, 1980. 306p. Y4.AP6/2:D56/981.

United States. Congress. Senate. Select Committee on Nutrition and Human Needs. *Dietary Goals for the United States: Supplemental Views.* Washington, D.C.: Government Printing Office, November 1977. 869p. Y4.N95: D56/Supp.

United States. General Accounting Office. *What Foods Should Americans Eat?: Better Information Needed on Nutritional Quality of Foods: Report to the Congress.* Washington, D.C.: General Accounting Office, 1980. 92p. GA1.13:CED-80-68.

United States. Office of the Assistant Secretary of Health and Surgeon General. *Healthy People: The Surgeon General's Report on Health Promotion and Disease Prevention: Background Papers: Report to the Surgeon General on Health Promotion and Disease Prevention.* Washington, D.C.: Government Printing Office, 1979. 484p. (DHEW Publication No. (PHS) 79-55071A). HE20.2:H34/5/papers.

Weil, W. B. "National Dietary Goals: Are They Justified at This Time?" *American Journal of Diseases of Children* 133 (1979): 368-70.

Whitehead, R. G. "Dietary Goals—Past and Present." *Royal Society of Health Journal* 101 (1981): 58-62.

Wolf, Isabel, and Betty B. Peterkin. "Dietary Guidelines: The USDA Perspective." *Food Technology* 38 (July 1984): 80-86.

Woodruff, C. W. "Dietary Goals for the United States." *American Journal of Diseases of Children* 133 (1979): 371-72.

14
Nutrition Assessment

The concept of nutrition assessment includes various methods of determining nutrition status of individuals and groups or populations. It encompasses diet or food consumption surveys, anthropometric measurements, biochemical tests, and clinical signs and symptoms of deficiency. This chapter is a highly selected list of materials relating to these subjects, as well as methods for conducting nutrition and food consumption surveys.

BIBLIOGRAPHIES AND GUIDES

387.   Krantzler, Nora J., et al. "Methods of Food Intake Assessment—An Annotated Bibliography." **Journal of Nutrition Education** 14 (1982): 108-19.
   Krantzler's bibliography contains 87 items with abstracts on food intake assessment.

DICTIONARIES

388.   Bennington, James, ed. **Saunders Dictionary & Encyclopedia of Laboratory Medicine and Technology**. Philadelphia, Pa.: W. B. Saunders, 1984. 1674p. ISBN 072161714X.
   This dictionary attempts to provide comprehensive coverage of terms related to currently used methods and techniques for laboratory analysis in the area of biochemistry, clinical chemistry, toxicology, hematology, mycology, electron microscopy, cytology, and other fields.

HANDBOOKS, MANUALS,
AND OTHER DATA COMPILATIONS

389.   American College of Obstetricians and Gynecology. **Assessment of Maternal Nutrition**. Chicago: American College of Obstetricians and Gynecologists, 1978. 25p.

390. Bayer, Leona M., and Nancy Bagley. **Growth Diagnosis: Selected Methods for Interpreting and Predicting Physical Development from One Year to Maturity**. 2nd ed. Chicago: University of Chicago Press, 1976. 240p. ISBN 0226039587.

"It is the intent of this book to convert selected segments of developmental data into simple techniques for appraising growth. The emphasis is on practical application not on describing the research behind it."

391. Buckler, J. M. H. **A Reference Manual of Growth and Development**. Oxford: Blackwell Scientific, 1979. 104p. ISBN 0632001852.

Normal values are given for height, weight, stages of puberty, skeletal maturity, head circumference, dental development, etc., for children and adolescents of various ages.

392. Burk, Marguerite C. **Analysis of Food Consumption Survey Data for Developing Countries**. Rome: Food and Agriculture Organization of the United Nations, 1980. 139p. (Food and Nutrition Paper, No. 16). ISBN 9251009686.

"This manual on analysis of food consumption surveys complements other FAO manuals on the planning and conducting of such surveys."

393. Burk, Marguerite C., and Eleanor M. Pao. **Methodology for Large-Scale Surveys of Household and Individual Diets**. Washington, D.C.: Government Printing Office, 1976. 88p. (Home Economics Research Report, No. 40). A1.87:40.

"Summarizes technical information relevant to planning large-scale surveys of food consumption of households and food intakes of individuals from which data on nutrient content can be calculated."

394. Graitcer, Philip L. **A Manual for the Basic Assessment of Nutrition Status in Potential Crisis Situations**. Atlanta, Ga.: Nutrition Division, Bureau of Smallpox Eradication, Centers for Disease Control, U.S. Public Health Service, 1980. 22, 10 leaves. HE20.7008:N95. Microfiche.

This is a brief manual on the assessment of nutrition in crisis situations, such as famine or war. The emphasis is on protein-calorie malnutrition.

395. Hartog, Adel P. den, and Wija A. van Staveren. **Manual for Social Surveys on Food Habits and Consumption in Developing Countries**. Wageningen, Netherlands: PUDOC, 1983. 114p. ISBN 902200838X.

"This guide provides advice and background information on collecting data on food habits and food consumption for small scale surveys."

396. Henry, John Bernard. **Clinical Diagnosis and Management**. 17th ed. Philadelphia, Pa.: W. B. Saunders, 1984. 1502p. ISBN 0721646573.

This revised edition contains 57 individually authored chapters in the following sections: "The Clinical Laboratory," "Clinical Chemistry," "Medical Microscopy," "Hematology and Coagulation," "Immunology and Immunopathology," "Medical Microbiology," and "Administration of the Clinical Laboratory." There are appendixes and a subject index.

397. Jacobs, David, et al. **Laboratory Test Handbook with DRG Index**. St. Louis, Mo.: Mosby/Lex-Comp, 1984. 848p. ISBN 0801629969.

"The authors have attempted to present each of the common and many of the less common laboratory tests. Points of information pertinent to the major aspects of the tests [include] test name and synonyms, patient care, specimen interpretation and references." Includes tests used for the laboratory assessment of nutritional status.

398.   Jelliffe, Derrick Brian. **The Assessment of Nutritional Status of the Community**. Geneva: World Health Organization, 1966. 271p. (World Health Organization. Monograph Series, No. 53).
"With special reference to field surveys in developing regions of the world."

399.   Jensen, Terri G., DeAnn Englert, and Stanley J. Dudrick. **Nutritional Assessment: A Manual for Practitioners**. Norwalk, Conn.: Appleton-Century-Crofts, 1983. 210p. ISBN 083857078X.
This manual provides the procedures and forms developed at Hermann Hospital, University of Texas Medical School, to identify patients with clinical and subclinical malnutrition and to provide guidelines for dietary care. It includes guidelines for interpreting nutritional assessment data.

400.   McLaren, Donald S. **Color Atlas of Nutritional Disorders**. Chicago: Year Book Medical Publishers, 1981. 109p. ISBN 0815158335.
The *Color Atlas* contains color and black-and-white photographs with brief commentary illustrating deficiency diseases, food toxin disorders such as ergotism and fetal alcohol syndrome, and disorders of uncertain etiology, such as osteoporosis and diverticular disease. An index is included.

401.   Pao, Eleanor M., and Marguerite C. Burk. **Portion Sizes and Day's Intakes of Selected Foods**. Washington, D.C.: U.S. Department of Agriculture, Agricultural Research Service, Northeastern Region, 1975. 70p. (ARS-NE No. 67). A77:NE-67.
Prepared for the nutrition labeling program at the FDA, this publication contains information on portion sizes of various foods consumed. It is useful for diet studies because it contains the weights of various household measures of foods.

402.   Reh, Emma. **Manual on Household Food Consumption Surveys**. Rome: Food and Agriculture Organization of the United Nations, 1962. 103p. (FAO Nutritional Studies, No. 18).
This manual deals with all aspects of conducting national and local surveys on household food consumption in developing countries.

403.   Roche, Alex F., and Robert M. Malina. **Manual of Physical Status and Performance in Childhood**. New York: Plenum, 1983. 2v. in 3. ISBN 0306411369 (vol. 1); 0306411377 (vol. 2).
Volumes 1A and 1B are extensive compilations of anthropometric and growth data for children from different geographic areas in the United States. Also included are data from Canada, the United Kingdom, and Australia. Many of the tables from the United States have data on black children and a few have data on other races.

404. Simko, Margaret D., Catherine Cowell, and Judith A. Gilbride, eds. **Nutrition Assessment: A Comprehensive Guide for Planning Intervention**. Rockville, Md.: Aspen, 1984. 396p. ISBN 0894438514.

This practical guide to assessing individual and group nutrition needs includes information on the nutrition profile; anthropometric techniques; physical examination; methods of collecting dietary data; laboratory assessment of nutritional status; and planning, implementation, evaluation, and monitoring of nutrition intervention. The appendix includes an extensive bibliography, height and weight tables, growth charts, and various anthropometric measurements. There is an index.

405. Sonnenwirth, Alex C., and Leonard Jarett, eds. **Gradwohl's Clinical Laboratory Methods and Diagnosis**. 8th ed. St. Louis, Mo.: C. V. Mosby Co., 1980. 2339, 201p. (in 2v.). ISBN 080164741X.

This voluminous standard work has been extensively revised to include newer laboratory methods. It is intended to serve as a work of reference, a text, and a laboratory manual. It covers the full range of chemical, hematological, immunological, bacteriological, virological, mycological, parasitological, and serological tests. An outstanding feature of this book is the extremely detailed index of 201 pages; another is its discussion of underlying physiological mechanisms. There are 748 illustrations, with 50 in color. Included are tests used for the laboratory assessment of nutritional status.

406. United States. Centers for Disease Control. **Weighing and Measuring Children: A Training Manual for Supervisory Personnel**. Atlanta, Ga.: Department of Health and Human Services, Public Health Service, Centers for Disease Control, 1980. 1v. (various paging). HE20.7008:W42.

407. United States. Interdepartmental Committee on Nutrition for the National Defense. **Manual for Nutrition Surveys**. 2nd ed. Washington, D.C.: Government Printing Office, 1964. 327p. Y3In8/13:6-2:Su7.

Now somewhat dated, this manual was developed to standardize methods and techniques for surveys in developing countries using survey teams. An index is included.

408. Webb Associates. Anthropology Research Project. **Anthropometric Source Book**. Washington, D.C.: National Aeronautics and Space Administration, Scientific and Technical Information Office, 1978. 3v. (NASA Reference Publication, No. 1024). NAS1.61:1224/v.1-3.

Some of the anthropometric data presented in these volumes are for the weightless state. These volumes include difficult to locate material for adult males and females of various nationalities. For instance, there are data on muscle strength, height, weight, hip breadth, chest breadth, waist circumference, etc.

409. Wright, Richard A., Steven Heymsfield, and Clifford B. McManus. **Nutritional Assessment**. Boston: Blackwell Scientific Publications, 1984. 290p. ISBN 0865420165.

This volume discusses nutrition assessment of the hospitalized patient. The appendix includes reference values based on mortality statistics and population surveys as well as anthropometric measurements. There is an index.

SELECTED REFERENCES

Beal, Virginia A., and Mary Jane Laus, eds. *Proceedings of the Symposium on Dietary Data Collection, Analysis, and Significance*. Amherst, Mass.: Massachusetts Agricultural Experiment Station, College of Food and Natural Resources, University of Massachusetts at Amherst, 1982. 164p. (Massachusetts Agricultural Experiment Station. Bulletin No. 675).

Bigwood, Edouard Jean. *Guiding Principles for Studies on the Nutrition of Populations*. Geneva: Health Organization, League of Nations, Technical Commission on Nutrition, 1939. 281p. (Series of League of Nations Publications, III. Health. 1939. III.).

Chumlea, W. C., A. F. Roche, and D. Mukherjee. *Nutritional Assessment of the Elderly through Anthropometry*. Columbus, Ohio: Ross Laboratories, 1984. 44p.

Food and Agriculture Organization of the United Nations. *Methodology of Nutritional Surveillance: Report of a Joint FAO/UNICEF/WHO Expert Committee*. Geneva: World Health Organization, 1976. 66p. (WHO Tech. Report Series, No. 593). ISBN 9241205938.

Mason, John B., et al. *Nutritional Surveillance*. Geneva: World Health Organization, 1984. 194p. ISBN 9241560789.

National Research Council. Committee on Food Consumption Patterns. *Assessing Changing Food Consumption Patterns*. Washington, D.C.: National Academy Press, 1981. 284p. ISBN 0309031354.

Sauberlich, H. E., J. H. Skala, and R. P. Dowdy. *Laboratory Tests for the Assessment of Nutritional Status*. Cleveland, Ohio: CRC Press, Inc., 1974. 136p. ISBN 0849301211.
This publication originally appeared in *CRC Critical Reviews in Clinical Laboratory Sciences*, volume 4, number 3.

Simopoulos, Artemis P., ed. "Conference on the Assessment of Nutritional Status, Bethesda, Maryland, September 16-18, 1981: Selected Papers." *American Journal of Clinical Nutrition (Supplement)* 35 (May 1982): 1089-1325.

Somogyi, J. C., and A. Szczyiel, eds. *Assessment of Nutritional Status and Food Consumption Surveys: Proceedings of the Eleventh Symposium of the Group of European Nutritionists, Warsaw, April 9-13*. Basel, Switzerland: S. Karger, 1974. 197p. (Bibliotheca "Nutritio et Dieta," No. 20). ISBN 3805516851.

Underwood, Barbara, ed. *Methodologies for Human Population Studies in Nutrition Related to Health; Proceedings of the U.S. Japan Malnutrition Panels, Bethesda, Maryland, July 24-25, 1979*. Bethesda, Md.: National Institutes of Health, 1982. 195p. (NIH Publication, No. 82-2462). HE20. 3002:M56. Microfiche.

15
Nutrition Education
and Community Nutrition

INDEXING/ABSTRACTING SERVICES

For material on nutrition education, it is sometimes necessary to consult the major indexing/abstracting services in the field of education. Sources such as *Index Medicus* or *Nutrition Abstracts and Reviews* frequently do not yield satisfactory results, because they focus on nutrition science literature. *Index Medicus*, for instance, does not index the *Journal of Nutrition Education*.

The *Food and Nutrition Quarterly Index* and its predecessor, *Food and Nutrition Bibliography*, provide extensive coverage of nutrition education materials, including audiovisual materials, for the years they are available. However, they have had a history of gaps and delayed publication.

New information in the field of education is collected, abstracted, and indexed by the Educational Resources Information Center (ERIC) in the U.S. Department of Education. This is a nationwide network of 16 clearinghouses, each of which has responsibility for a specific subject area (e.g., elementary and early childhood education). Much of the information collected and indexed is also disseminated to libraries on microfiche. Many libraries receive ERIC documents on microfiche. Copies may be ordered in microfiche or paper format from the ERIC Document Reproduction Service (EDRS) (3900 Wheeler Avenue, Alexandria, VA 22304).

The two major indexing and abstracting services produced from indexing done by the Educational Resources Information Center are listed below.

410. **Current Index to Journals in Education**. Vol. 1- . Phoenix, Ariz.: Oryx Press, 1969- . monthly. ISSN 0011-3565.

"*Current Index to Journals in Education* (*CIJE*) is a monthly guide to current periodical literature in education, covering articles in approximately 750 major education and education related journals." Included in this number is the

Journal of Nutrition Education. Together with *Resources in Education* (*RIE*), *CIJE* provides coverage of the whole range of education-related literature. It is an excellent source for material on food and nutrition education. As with *RIE*, subject terms are selected from the *Thesaurus of ERIC Descriptors* (also published by Oryx Press).

Online Equivalent: ERIC.

Arrangement: The main entry section lists articles with abstracts by item number. The index section lists articles by subject and also by author. Both sections are cumulated on a semi-annual basis.

411.   **Resources in Education**. Vol. 10- . Washington, D.C.: U.S. Department of Education, 1975- . monthly. ISSN 0098-0897. (Volumes 1-9 were issued as *Research in Education*).

Resources in Education (*RIE*) is the major abstracting service for nonjournal literature in the field of education. When used in conjunction with *Current Index to Journals in Education*, it covers the whole spectrum of education literature. A variety of nutrition and food education materials is abstracted, including curriculum materials, reports of research, and bibliographies. Index terms are selected from the *Thesaurus of ERIC Descriptors*. Topics included are nutrition, nutrition education research, nutrition instruction, food, food production, food service, and foods instruction.

Online Equivalent: ERIC.

Indexes: Subject, author, institution, publication type, clearinghouse number/ED number cross-reference. Cumulative indexes are issued semi-annually.

Oryx Press publishes an easy-to-use annual cumulation of both the abstracts section and the indexes, entitled *Resources in Education* (*RIE*) *Annual Cumulation* (ISSN 0197-9973).

ONLINE DATABASES

412.   **AGRICOLA**

A detailed description of this database appears in chapter 5. It covers nutrition education materials extensively, by virtue of the fact that materials from *FNIC* are included with abstracts.

413.   **ERIC**

The most extensive database in education, ERIC originates from the National Institute of Education and consists chiefly of the journal articles in over 700 education-related periodicals indexed in *Current Index to Journals in Education* (*CIJE*) and reports, curriculum materials, books and other types of non-journal publications found in *Resources in Education* (*RIE*). The database goes back to 1966 and now contains over 550,000 records. It is updated on a monthly basis.

BIBLIOGRAPHIES AND GUIDES

414.   Buckle, Roxanne, Rosemary Berardi, and Donna MacDonald. **Food and Nutrition Posters: A Guide to Sources**. Toronto: Nutrition Information Service, Ryerson Polytechnical Institute Library, 1983. 47p. ISBN 0919351093.

Intended for nutritionists, dietitians, and educators, this guide provides information on where to obtain 243 free or inexpensive food, nutrition, and health posters. Information for ordering is included.

415. California. State Department of Education. Nutrition Education and Training Program (NET). **Nutrition Education Materials Developed by NET Programs**. Sacramento, Calif.: California State Department of Education, 1985. 144p. (Available from Coordinator, Nutrition Education and Training Program, Office of Child Nutrition Services, California State Department of Education, 721 Capitol Mall, Sacramento, CA 95814-4785).

This annotated bibliography describes nutrition education materials by state nutrition education and training programs throughout the country. It includes print and nonprint materials. Entries provide information on availability and cost.

416. Chicago Nutrition Association. **Nutrition References and Book Reviews**. 5th ed. Chicago: Chicago Nutrition Association, 1981. 76p. (8158 S. Kedzie Avenue, Chicago, IL 60652).

Books described in this annotated bibliography are divided into five categories: recommended, recommended for special purposes, recommended for advanced reading, recommended only with reservations, and not recommended. Also listed are books included in previous editions and organizations and govern ment agencies which distribute nutrition materials. Included are citations to book reviews and guidelines for evaluating materials. Names and addresses of publishers are appended. This book is suitable for the general public and professionals in other fields.

417. Gordon, Kathleen, Marilyn Chedu, and Donna MacDonald. **Index of Free and Inexpensive Nutrition Information Materials**. Toronto: Nutrition Information Service, Ryerson Polytechnical Institute Library, 1981. 269p. ISBN 0919351018.

Organized by subject, this directory lists about 2,000 pamphlets or brochures available free of charge or costing $3.00 or less. Although materials from the United States are included, the emphasis is on Canadian materials. Entries include title, publisher, date, pagination, cost, and intended level of material. Indexes included are subject, title, and source (with addresses).

418. Israel, Ronald C., and Peter Lamptey, eds. **Nutrition Training Manual Catalogue for Health Professionals, Trainers and Field Workers in Developing Countries**. Newton, Mass.: International Nutrition Communication Service, 1982?. 102p. ($6.00, Education Development Center, 55 Chapel Street, Newton, MA 02160).

Prepared under a grant from the Agency for International Development, this catalog of "training manuals" reviews 116 health and nutrition "manuals" for use by health professionals in developing countries. The term "manual" includes textbooks, curriculum guides, course outlines, and other materials. In addition to bibliographic information and critical annotations, each entry includes information on language, location, target group, type of emphasis, and sponsor. Appendixes provide definitions of subject categories and addresses where materials may be obtained. Included are title, author, and area indexes.

419. Israel, Ronald C., and Joanne P. Nestor Tighe. **Nutrition Education: State of the Art: Review and Analysis of the Literature**. Paris: Division of Science, Technical, and Vocational Education, United Nations Educational, Scientific, and Cultural Organization, 1984. 115p. (Nutrition Education Series, No. 7).

This publication was also issued as *Nutrition Education* (Paris: United Nations Educational, Scientific, and Cultural Organization, 1984, 96p. [Educational Documentation and Information; Bulletin of the International Bureau of Education, No. 232]).

This annotated bibliography of nearly 400 items contains an "Introduction to the Literature of the Last Five Years" and covers material on policy issues, conceptual approaches, food habits, case studies relating to different geographic regions, and evaluation. Nutrition education materials from nutrition education campaigns in a number of countries and an author and editor index are also included. The authors are associated with the Education Development Center in Newton, Massachusetts. "It is not a state-of-the-art review as claimed in the title.... Indexed by country and topic, it provides Unesco readership with a wealth of useful information that does not appear in established journals" (*Food and Nutrition Bulletin* 7 [June 1985]: 74-75).

420. McLaughlin, Elaine Casserly, et al. **Nutrition Education Resource Guide: An Annotated Bibliography of Educational Materials for the WIC and CSF Programs**. Washington, D.C.: Government Printing Office, October 1982. 146p. (Bibliographies and Literature Guides of Agriculture, No. 24). A1.60/3.

"This resource guide to evaluated print and audiovisual nutrition education materials has been developed to assist state and local staff of the Special Supplemental Food Program for Women, Infants and Children (WIC) and the Commodity Supplemental Foods Program (CSFP) in selecting, acquiring and developing accurate and appropriate material for nutrition education of WIC/CSFP participants."

The 340 items listed in this bibliography deal with pregnancy, breastfeeding, infant feeding, preschool children, general nutrition, specific nutrients, dental care, meal planning, and food buying. Information on availability, cost, reading level, and language is included.

421. National Nutrition Education Clearing House. **Audiovisuals for Nutrition Education**. rev. ed. Berkeley, Calif.: National Nutrition Education Clearing House, Society for Nutrition Education, 1979. 37p. (Nutrition Education Resource Series, No. 9).

This is an annotated bibliography of more than 250 audiovisual materials issued from 1974 to 1978 and reviewed in the *Journal of Nutrition Education*. A title index and an index to foreign-language materials are included. Each item is identified as to the educational level of the intended audience. Within subject areas, items are arranged by grade level.

422. Nutrition Foundation, New York. Office of Education and Public Affairs. **Index of Nutrition Education Materials**. rev. ed. Washington, D.C.: Office of Education and Public Affairs, The Nutrition Foundation, 1977. 237p.

"This updated and expanded index lists material under both subject matter headings and sources. More than two thousand booklets, pamphlets and audiovisual aids are included. Each listing includes audience level, information on how to order and single-copy price.... Foreign language and braille materials are listed according to subject in a special section.... A valuable source of information" (*Journal of the American Dietetic Association* 72 [1978]: 459).

423. Owen, Anita Yanochik. **Community Nutrition in Preventive Health Care Services: A Critical Review of the Literature**. Washington, D.C.: Government Printing Office, 1978. 320p. (Department of Health, Education and Welfare, Health Planning Bibliography Series, No. 7; DHEW Publication, No. (HRA) 78-14017). HE20.6112/2:7.

Included are reviews about 230 articles on nutrition and its role in preventive health care services from 1970-1977.

424. Pelican, Suzanne, and Marian I. Hammond. **Reviewed Clinical Nutrition Sources: Diabetes Education**. University Park, Pa.: Nutrition Information and Resource Center, Pennsylvania State University, 1983. 32p.

The books, teaching materials, and audiovisual resources in this bibliography have been evaluated according to the following criteria: accuracy, freedom from bias, technical quality, and appropriateness for target audience. It is especially useful for its materials on alternative eating styles and "cultural cuisines."

425. Rhea, Harold C. **Nutrition Education: Selected Resources. Bibliographies**. Washington, D.C.: ERIC Clearinghouse on Teacher Education, 1981. 56p. (microfiche). (Available from EDRS as ED 200 521).

Intended chiefly for instructors of nutrition at the elementary, secondary, and college level, this bibliography has separate sections devoted to books, documents, and journal articles selected from the ERIC database. Films, multimedia programs, organizations, and miscellaneous sources are included. Topics covered are general nutrition, food preparation, nutrition for athletes, weight control, etc. Much of the material was published within five to six years prior to inclusion. Emphasis is on nutrition education programs that deal with physical development.

426. Rubey, Jane A., comp. **Nutrition for Everybody: An Annotated List of Resources**. Berkeley, Calif.: Society for Nutrition Education, 1981. 24p. (Nutrition Information Resource Series).

This excellent annotated list of nutrition reference sources for the lay public covers general nutrition materials, guidelines for eating, food composition tables, nutrition throughout the life cycle, consumer health and education, special diets, weight control, etc.

427. Schurch, Beat, and Luce Wilquin. **Nutrition Education in Communities of the Third World**. Lausanne, Switzerland: Nestle Foundation for the Study of Nutrition Problems in the World, 1982. 208p.

Prepared for health professionals and nutritionists working in developing countries, this bibliography contains some 180 references with abstracts in English and French. A prefatory table lists the references, with an elaborate system of codes describing content.

428. Society for Nutrition Education. **Nutrition Information for the Whole Family**. rev. ed. Berkeley, Calif.: Society for Nutrition Education, 1979. 11p.

Provided here are annotated lists of recommended books, pamphlets, and periodicals with purchasing information and guidelines for evaluating materials.

429.   Society for Nutrition Education. SNE Resource Center. **Aging and Nutrition**. rev. ed. Berkeley, Calif.: SNE Resource Center, 1980. 16p. (Nutrition Education Resource Series, No. 5).

430.   Society for Nutrition Education. SNE Resource Center. **Elementary Teaching Materials**. rev. ed. Berkeley, Calif.: Society for Nutrition Education, 1979. 36p. (Nutrition Education Resource Series, No. 1).
    This annotated bibliography of selected printed and audiovisual materials for elementary teaching includes materials used as actual teaching tools as well as teacher reference materials. A title index and a Spanish-language materials index are included.

431.   Society for Nutrition Education. SNE Resource Center. **Infant Nutrition and Feeding**. rev. ed. Berkeley, Calif.: SNE Resource Center, 1980. 24p. (Nutrition Education Resource Series, No. 11).
    "A compilation of selected printed and audiovisual education materials useful to people concerned with the nutritional care of infants. Each item has been evaluated by a qualified nutritionist.... Information [is] provided on source, cost, and availability of materials."

432.   Society for Nutrition Education. SNE Resource Center. **Pregnancy and Nutrition**. rev. ed. Oakland, Calif.: SNE Resource Center, 1982. 20p. (Nutrition Education Resource Series, No. 2).
    This revised and expanded edition of the 1978 bibliography contains selected print and audiovisual materials for professionals and the lay public. It includes a list of Spanish-language materials and a title index.

433.   Society for Nutrition Education. SNE Resource Center. **Secondary Nutrition Education Materials and References**. rev. ed. Berkeley, Calif.: Society for Nutrition Education, 1981. 33p. (Nutrition Education Resource Series, No. 4).
    This annotated bibliography describes selected print, audiovisual, and teacher reference materials for secondary schools. A title and a Spanish-language materials index are included.

434.   Sprug, Joseph W. **Index to Nutrition and Health: A Selected Bibliography of 239 Titles with a Cumulative Index**. Westwood, Mass.: Faxon, 1981. 170p. (Useful Reference Series, No. 119). ISBN 0873051254.
    "This subject index to 239 books in the field of health is well organized and easy to use.... The majority of titles included received at least one favorable review.... Sprug, however, cautions that 'inclusion does not constitute a recommendation of a particular work.' This is not an index to the technical literature of biochemistry and nutrition sciences; rather it is an index to books from popular presses, a few university presses, and U.S. government reports and commissions" (*Choice* 19 [December 1981]: 492).

435.   United Nations Educational, Scientific, and Cultural Organization. **Show and Tell; Disciplines d'Éveil; Mostrar y Contar; A Worldwide Directory of Nutrition Teaching-Learning Resources.** Paris: Division of Science, Technical and Environmental Education, United Nations Educational, Scientific, and Cultural Organization, 1985. 269p. (Nutrition Education Series).

"Part of the UNESCO Resource Pack for Nutrition Teaching-Learning." The result of a worldwide search for nutrition education materials, this directory describes nearly 800 items and is divided into four sections: "In-School," "Out-of-School," "Nutrition — Other Topics and Information," and "Additional Resources." Material is arranged by language and by educational level where appropriate. "Nutrition — Other Topics and Information" includes references to selected food composition tables. The last section includes bibliographies, newsletters, periodicals, and organizations. Indcxcs arc by rcgion, country, and title.

436.   United States. Food and Drug Administration. **FDA Consumer Information. A Catalog of Food and Drug Administration Publications, Slide Shows, and Films.** Rockville, Md.: Department of Health and Human Services, Public Health Service, Food and Drug Administration, 1985. 21p. (HSS Publication No. (FDA) 85-1108). HE20.4016:C76.

Published annually, this brief catalog lists general materials and materials on food, nutrition, drugs, medical devices, and radiation.

437.   United States. National Agricultural Library. Food and Nutrition Information and Education Resources Center. **Audiovisual Resources in Food and Nutrition.** Phoenix, Ariz.: Oryx Press, 1979- . ISSN 0743-9318.

Volume 1, 1979 (not numbered), covers the years 1973-1978. Volume 2, 1984, covers the years 1979-1982. This is an annotated bibliography of audiovisual materials held by FNIC and available on loan. Covered are materials on food, human nutrition, and food service in all types of audiovisual formats including kits, games, cassette tapes, dioramas, filmstrips, models, flash cards, videorecordings, motion pictures, film loops, charts, and transparencies. Volume 1 includes personal and corporate author indexes, a title index, a media index, and a detailed subject index. Volume 2 contains an intellectual level index in addition to the other indexes.

438.   United States. National Agricultural Library. Food and Nutrition Information Center. **Promoting Nutrition through Education: A Resource Guide to the Nutrition Education and Training Program (NET).** Washington, D.C.: Food and Nutrition Information Center, National Agricultural Library, 1985. 269p. (Bibliographies and Literature of Agriculture, No. 31). A1.60/3:31. (Microfiche available from EDRS, ED 256 741).

Compiled by the Food and Nutrition Information Center as a resource guide for the Nutrition Education and Training Program (NET), part 1 of this annotated bibliography of print and audiovisual materials contains a description of 400 items developed with NET funds, arranged by level of audience. FNIC numbers, description of format and language, and purchasing information are included. Part 2 consists of citations from the literature relating to NET programs. The appendix contains names and addresses of regional and state NET coordinators. Title, state, and language indexes are included.

439.   United States. Public Health Service. Centers for Disease Control. **Source Book for Health Education Materials and Community Resources**. Atlanta, Ga.: Department of Health and Human Services, Public Health Service, Centers for Disease Control, Center for Health Promotion and Education, 1982. 92p. HE20.700:H34/7.

"A guide and resource directory to health education materials in 10 nationally recognized health risk areas. The guide is intended to help people who deliver health education/risk reduction services and who want to find books, filmstrips, brochures, and other materials that might help their clients." Topics covered are stopping smoking, improving nutrition, controlling high blood pressure, modifying alcohol intake or drinking habits, increasing physical activity, reducing stress, detecting cancer early, controlling diabetes mellitus, improving or maintaining wellness, and preventing traffic accidents.

440.   University of Michigan Medical School. Michigan Diabetes Research and Training Center. **Audiovisual Resources for Diabetes Education**. 5th ed. Ann Arbor, Mich.: Learning Resource Center, Office of Educational Resources and Research and Michigan Diabetes Research and Training Center, University of Michigan Medical Center, 1984. 328p. ($25.00 prepaid, Learning Resource Center, University of Michigan Medical School, 1135 E. Catherine, Box 38, Ann Arbor, MI 48109-0010).

This is a guide to information on over 400 videorecordings, films, slides, and filmstrips issued from 1974 on intended for professionals, patients, and general audiences. Audiocassettes are also included, but these are limited to items appropriate for patients. Individual sections are: "Subject Index," "Title or Main Section" and "Audience Index." The appendix lists American Diabetes Association local affiliates.

441.   Vandenberg, Lela, and Crissy Kateregga. **Nutrition and Food—Education, Policy and Practice: A Selected Annotated Bibliography**. East Lansing, Mich.: Non-Formal Education Information Center, College of Education, Michigan State University, 1982. 76p. (Annotated Bibliography. Non-Formal Education Information Center, No. 9).

"This bibliography—the ninth in a series for those who are working in or who are beneficiaries of nonformal education—consists of the Non-Formal Education Center's literature on nutrition and development. The 293 materials have been gathered from worldwide sources and include full information on where to obtain documents" (*Nutrition Planning* 6 [1983/84]: 23). Included are sections on nutrition education and training, food and nutrition policy and programs, food production, consumption and preparation, newsletters and periodicals, and organizations working to solve food and hunger problems.

HANDBOOKS, MANUALS, AND OTHER DATA COMPILATIONS

442.   American Association of Diabetes Educators. **Reference Manual for Evaluation of Diabetes Education Programs**. Pitman, N.J.: American Association of Diabetes Educators, 1982. 26p. ($4.00, American Association of Diabetes Educators, N. Woodbury Road, Box 56, Pitman, NJ 08070).

This is a brief manual "to clarify and condense existing evaluation theories and methods, to provide new educators with a chronological process for conducting patient and program evaluation." References and bibliography are included.

443. Barclay, Ellen J., and Susan Van der Vynckt. **Easy-to-Make Teaching Aids**. Paris: Division of Science, Technical and Vocational Education, United Nations Educational, Scientific and Cultural Organization, 1984. 138p. (Nutrition Education Series, No. 10).
Instructions and suggestions for creating simple, inexpensive teaching aids such as flannel boards with flannelgraphs, flip charts, games, puzzles, posters, skits, and plays are provided. A bibliography of materials used is included.

444. Caldwell, Lynn. **Nutrition Education for the Patient: A Handout Manual**. Philadelphia, Pa.: George F. Stickley Co., 1984. 135p. ISBN 0893130435.
This was designed as a series of fact sheets for patient handouts covering basic nutrition principles, diabetes, therapeutic diet instruction aids, weight control and calories, exercise and nutrition, as well as popular nutrition topics such as food additives, cholesterol, caffeine, fiber, alcohol, natural or organic foods, vitamins, etc. Some of the information is presented in tabular form. A bibliography and an index are included.

445. Holmes, Alan C. **Visual Aids in Nutrition Education: A Guide to Their Preparation and Use**. Rome: Food and Agriculture Organization of the United Nations, 1969. 145p.
"This manual is a practical guide to the selection and preparation of audio-visual aids for use in nutrition education programs. The media materials are concerned with food and nutrition problems in developing countries" (*FNIC Catalog 1973*, 1095-73).

446. IOX Assessment Associates. **A Program Evaluation Handbook for Health Education Programs in Diabetes: (Preliminary Version)**. Atlanta, Ga.: Department of Health and Human Services, Public Health Service, Centers for Disease Control, 1982. 403p. HE20.7008:H34/diabetes.
This handbook presents measurement tools for the evaluation of diabetes education programs and is intended as a possible resource for health educators. It discusses evaluation generally, presents information on various measures and on how to use them, and includes measures developed specifically for this purpose, but which have not been empirically verified. One of a series of seven handbooks prepared for the Centers for Disease Control, Center for Health Promotion and Education, it includes bibliographies.

447. IOX Assessment Associates. **A Program Evaluation Handbook for Health Education Programs in Nutrition: (Preliminary Version)**. Atlanta, Ga.: Department of Health and Human Services, Public Health Service, Centers for Disease Control, 1982. 339p. HE20.7008:H34/nutrition.
The purpose of this handbook is to present a range of measurement tools intended to serve as a resource in evaluating nutrition education programs. It includes general information on evaluation, a description of various kinds of measures, directions for using the handbook, and specific measures developed

for the book which were not empirically verified. It is one of a series of seven handbooks developed by the CDC.

448.   National Association of College and University Food Services. **Nutrition Education Sourcebook**. n.p.: National Association of College and University Food Services, 1980. 3v.

"Guidelines and ideas to incorporate nutrition education into college and university food services are presented. Nutrition education programs developed by various colleges and universities are described. A bibliography of books, leaflets, and pamphlets concerning dietary patterns, basic nutrition, special nutrients, diet and calories, vegetarianism, food composition, and other topics is provided. Key companies and organizations providing printed nutrition information are listed."

449.   New Jersey. State Department of Health. Nutrition Consultation Services. **New Jersey Guide for Developing Nutrition Services in the Community**. Trenton, N.J.: New Jersey State Department of Health, Office of Local Health and Regional Operations, Nutrition Consultation Services, 1982. 99p.

With cuts in federally funded programs, more local agencies will provide nutrition programs to fill the gap. This guidebook is designed to assist local health agencies and organizations in implementing nutrition programs, with the view of coordinating and integrating services. Topics addressed are nutrition assessment of individuals and the community; counseling techniques; diets; cultural, religious, and ethnic influences; food budgeting; drug and food interactions; vitamin supplements; and methods of teaching nutrition. A section entitled "Nutritional Resources and Services" lists organizations which can provide further information, audiovisual aids, and a brief list of professional books.

450.   Oliver, Shirley Doten, and Katherine Ogilvie Musgrave. **Nutrition: A Teacher Sourcebook of Integrated Activities**. Boston: Allyn and Bacon, 1984. ISBN 0205080308.

This is a teacher's guide to integrating basic nutrition information into the curriculum. Part 1 of this book, "The Nutrition Curriculum," contains an introductory chapter on curriculum design and twelve chapters on major content areas (e.g., classifying food into groups, associating health and food intake, teaching nutrients). Each has teacher goals, student objectives, related key concepts and teaching strategies (including learning activities), lists of materials, and information on evaluation and testing. When activities include food preparation, recipes are included. Activities and teaching methods are coded for appropriate grade levels, (kindergarten and grades 1-8). Part 2, "Extending and Enriching Nutrition Education," contains four chapters dealing with teacher planning and organization to ensure successful food experiences, extending nutrition beyond the classroom, meeting the needs of special students, and school meals. Appendixes include the RDAs, growth charts, and a glossary of terms. A bibliography and an index are appended.

451.   United States. Food and Nutrition Service. Nutrition and Technical Services Division. **The Idea Book: Sharing Nutrition Education Experiences**. Washington, D.C.: Nutrition Information Service, 1981. 90p. (FNS 234). A98.9:234.

Developed for nutritionists in the Special Supplemental Food Program for Women, Infants and Children, this book is not intended as a manual on how to plan, deliver, and evaluate nutrition education programs, but as a way of sharing ideas. The chapter headings are in question form, for example, "What Should I Consider When Planning a Nutrition Program?" A final chapter provides sources of nutrition information materials.

452. United States. Health Services Administration. Bureau of Community Health Services. **Guide for Developing Nutrition Services in Community Health Programs**. Rockville, Md.: U.S. Department of Health, Education and Welfare, Public Health Service, Health Services Administration, Bureau of Community Health Services, 1978. 43, [45]p. (DHEW Publication, No. (HSA) 78-5103). HE20.5108:N95.

"A guide to assist health planners, program administrators, health care providers including nutrition personnel, develop and implement nutrition services.... The guide is intended as an authoritative resource.... It is not intended as a detailed methodology."

453. United States. National Institutes of Health. **Foods for Health: Report of the Pilot Program**. Bethesda, Md.: Department of Health and Human Services, Public Health Service, National Institutes of Health, 1983. 219p. (NIH Publication No. 83-2036). HE20.3202:F73.

" 'Foods for Health,' a nutrition education research project, was designed to increase consumer awareness and knowledge about nutrition as it relates to cardiovascular risk factors." It was a pilot program conducted by Giant Foods in cooperation with the National Heart, Lung, and Blood Institute and is included here because it has an extensive appendix of promotional nutrition education materials which can be copied freely. Negatives and paper positives are available for printing or photocopying at no extra cost. It also contains radio spot announcements and newspaper ads.

454. Van der Vynckt, Susan, and Ellen Barclay. **The UNESCO Resource Pack for Nutrition Teaching-Learning: An Introduction to Volume 1**. Paris: United Nations Educational, Scientific, and Cultural Organization, Division of Science, Technical and Vocational Education, 1984. 74p. (Nutrition Education Series, No. 8).

"The purpose of this volume is to introduce the new *Unesco Resource Pack for Nutrition Teaching-Learning*." Some of the projected volumes have already appeared, but under somewhat different titles in the Nutrition Education Series. Individual items may not be labeled as belonging to the *UNESCO Resource Pack for Nutrition Teaching-Learning*.

455. Virginia Polytechnic Institute and State University. Cooperative Extension Service. **Nutrition Education Manual: Designed for Use by Principals, Teachers, and School Food Service Managers**. Blacksburg, Va.: Cooperative Extension Service, Department of Human Nutrition and Foods, Virginia Polytechnic Institute and State University, 1979?. 336p.

456. Weiss, Ellen, et al. **Community Food Education Handbook**. Nashville, Tenn.: Agricultural Marketing Project; distr., Nashville, Tenn.: Cooperative

Food Education Program, 1980. 65p. ($5.55, Cooperative Food Education Program, 2606 Westwood Drive, Nashville, TN 37204).

This handbook for those involved in community nutrition programs describes some food education programs in existence, target groups, agencies which provide assistance in running programs, materials, funding, evaluation, working in the schools, teacher training, and parent involvement.

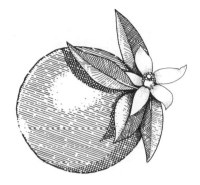

Part IV

DIETETICS

16
General Reference Sources and Diet Manuals

INDEXING/ABSTRACTING SERVICES

As a health professional providing nutrition care, the dietitian needs access to both the nutrition literature and the medical literature. This means becoming familiar with major indexing/abstracting services in both of these fields: *Index Medicus* for the health sciences literature and *Nutrition Abstracts and Reviews* for the nutrition science literature, both discussed in previous chapters. There are also other specialized materials sources which occasionally may prove useful, such as the *Bibliography of Hotel and Restaurant Administration*, which includes coverage of food service materials; and *Hospital Literature Index*, which indexes a wide range of materials on hospital food and dietetic services. Individual non-periodic bibliographies on specialized topics are additional resources.

457. **Hospital Literature Index**. Vol. 1- . Chicago: American Hospital Association, 1957- . quarterly. ISSN 0018-5736.

"The primary guide to literature on hospital and health care facility administration, including multi-institutional systems, health planning, and administrative aspects of health care delivery." This index is essentially a subject and author index to English-language articles on hospitals and other health care facilities. Useful for dietitians working in health care institutions, it indexes material on dietetic services, parenteral feeding, hospital food service, diet therapy, etc. It covers journals in all fields of health care administration indexed by the American Hospital Association as well as citations from the MEDLARS database.

Online Equivalent: HEALTH PLANNING & ADMIN.

Indexing Vocabulary: From 1978 on, subject headings are selected from *MeSH*. Prior to that time, the AHA published its own *Hospital Literature Subject Headings*.

List of Periodicals Indexed: A key to journal abbreviations and list of periodicals appear in each issue.

BIBLIOGRAPHIES AND GUIDES

458.   De Cristofaro, Joanne, et al. **A Selected Bibliography in Nutrition Support: Nutrition Assessment, Enteral and Parenteral Nutrition, and Other Related Topics**. Chicago: Dietitians in Critical Care, American Dietetic Association, 1983. 59p.

Covers books and articles on clinical nutrition support, nutrition assessment of adults and children, anthropometric and biochemical measurements, as well as nutrition support for special conditions and enteral and parenteral nutrition.

459.   Hoover, Loretta W. **Computers in Nutrition, Dietetics and Foodservice Management: A Bibliography**. 2nd ed. Columbia, Mo.: Curators of the University of Missouri, 1983. 47p.

Organized chronologically, this bibliography covers primarily journal articles and conference literature from 1958 to 1983. It has content codes describing subjects of articles (e.g., *DS* stands for "diet surveys" and *PC* stands for "patient care"). No index is provided.

DIRECTORIES

460.   American Dietetic Association. **Directory of Dietetic Programs: Accredited and Approved: Directory of Accredited and Approved Dietetic Programs**. Chicago: American Dietetic Association, 198?- . annual.

"Provides individuals seeking membership in the American Dietetic Association or registration by the Commission on Dietetic Registration of the American Dietetic Association with information about dietetic education programs accredited and approved by the American Dietetic Association, as well as advanced degree programs in nutrition and related areas."

DIET MANUALS

Diet manuals are important sources of reference for health care professionals responsible for the nutrition care of patients. They are vital not only to physicians prescribing specific diets and to dietetic staffs carrying out these instructions, but also to nurses, food service personnel, pharmacists, and others who may in some measure be responsible for helping to implement them.

Diet manuals introduce standardization into a process that might otherwise be open to subjective interpretation. All personnel involved must be absolutely clear what is meant by a specific type of diet, and diet manuals provide a needed frame of reference. Diet manuals are also frequently used as teaching tools for hospital dietitians and food service staffs.

Throughout the country individual health care institutions or state and local dietetic associations have produced manuals standardizing local dietetic practice while preserving local and regional diet patterns important for patient adherence to prescribed diets. A number of specialized manuals have been produced to fill specific needs (e.g., the nutritional care of vegetarians, renal patients, etc.).

The *Handbook of Clinical Dietetics* was produced by the American Dietetic Association to inject a degree of national standardization into this local and regional diversity. This handbook defines terminology and diet contents and is intended to serve as a model for the preparation of diet manuals.

The section below provides a selected list of diet manuals. Many local or state manuals are not represented in this section because information about their availability was not widely disseminated. Some manuals are listed without annotations because examination copies were not available.

General

461. American Dietetic Association. **Handbook of Clinical Dietetics**. New Haven, Conn.: Yale University Press, 1981. 517p. ISBN 0300022565.

This diet manual was developed by the American Dietetic Association to standardize diet contents and terminology, which have been subject to a great deal of regional variation. "This handbook, with its many references, should serve as a guide for the current practice of diet therapy and as a basis for the preparation of diet manuals.... One of the unique aspects of the handbook is that it delineates what not to do as well as what to do and lists those practices in diet therapy which are obsolete and should be discarded." It is well documented with references to the literature. An extensive appendix includes RDAs, normal laboratory values of clinical importance, height-weight tables, growth charts, osmolality of common foods, caffeine content of foods, cholesterol and fatty acid composition of foods, folacin content of foods, and composition of nutritional supplements. An index is appended.

462. Alpers, David H., Ray E. Clouse, and William F. Stenson. **Manual of Nutritional Therapeutics**. Boston: Little, Brown, 1983. 457p. ISBN 0316085092.

"Designed to conveniently provide current information in the diagnosis and treatment of nutritional problems.... The book is not intended to be a textbook of nutrition." Major sections are: "Assessment and Oral Management of Micronutrient Deficiency," "Assessment and Management of Macronutrient Deficiency," "Management by Use of Diets," and "Special Needs During Growth." The appendix includes nutritional analysis of fast foods and a disease specific reference index. A general index is also included.

463. Bernard, Marie A., Danny O. Jacobs, and John L. Rombeau. **Nutritional and Metabolic Support of Hospitalized Patients**. Philadelphia, Pa.: W. B. Saunders, 1986. 324p. ISBN 0721612040.

A reference book in which "members of the nutritional support team can find out the facts they need to know to make responsible decisions for their patients," this work contains general information on nutritional requirements; material on nutrition assessment; information on metabolic response to starvation, stress, or injury; indications for nutrition support, enteral, parenteral and central venous feeding, and nutrition support in specific diseases. There is an index.

464. Kelts, Drew G., and Elizabeth Jones, eds. **Manual of Pediatric Nutrition**. Boston: Little, Brown, 1984. 292p. ISBN 0316486353.

"A source of basic and practical information on current pediatric nutritional practices." Contains information on normal infant feeding, milks and formulas, general nutrition in childhood and adolescence, dental nutrition, nutrition assessment, supplements, enteral and parenteral nutrition, diet in various digestive and gastrointestinal problems, nutrition for specific disorders, and vegetarian diets. The appendix contains growth charts. There are numerous tables and bibliographies throughout, as well as an index.

465. Morrissey, Barbara G. **Quick Reference to Therapeutic Nutrition**. Philadelphia, Pa.: Lippincott, 1984. 608p. ISBN 0397544162.

Aimed at nurses, this is an extensive compilation of information relevant to nutrition therapy. It covers such topics as assessment of nutritional status, nutrition care plans, cardiovascular system, cancer, diabetes, obesity, gastrointestinal tract, gastrointestinal accessory organs and kidneys, and special disorders such as epilepsy. Appendixes include height and weight tables, nutrient composition of selected enteral formulas and parenteral solutions, RDAs, exchange lists, and ideal urinary creatinine levels for adults. An index is included.

466. Schatz, Pauline. **Manual in Clinical Dietetics**. 3rd ed. Redondo Beach, Calif.: Plycon Press, 1983. 190p. ISBN 068647144X.

This manual was written for students of dietetics who are about to enter internships. It is designed to introduce basic information on clinical conditions requiring diet modifications. There are case studies with questions and exercises. Appendixes include medical abbreviations, glossary, laboratory values, RDAs, food composition table, height-weight table, food exchanges, cholesterol values of selected foods, purine content of foods, food equivalents for low phenylalanine diets, etc.

467. Walker, W. Allen, and Kristy M. Hendricks. **Manual of Pediatric Nutrition**. Philadelphia, Pa.: W. B. Saunders, 1985. 160p. ISBN 0721691013.

Intended as a guide for dietitians, pediatricians, and others in managing the nutritional problems of pediatric patients, this manual covers nutrition assessment, estimation of energy needs, enteral and parenteral nutrition, nutrition support for patients with altered gastrointestinal function, and care of patients with normal gastrointestinal function but abnormal requirements. It contains extensive tables and charts: growth charts, height-weight tables, and other anthropometric data, data on formulated foods, common carbohydrates in foods, etc. There is an index.

State, Local, and Regional

ALABAMA

468. Campbell, Sheila M., ed. **Practical Guide to Nutritional Care for Dietitians and Other Health Care Professionals**. Birmingham, Ala.: Department of Dietetics, University of Alabama Hospitals, 1984. 57p. ($13.95, Marketing Department, University of Alabama Hospitals, 619 S. 19th Street, Birmingham, AL 35282-9885).

This volume highlights such topics as "nutrient content of selected products, medical record review and documentation, nutrition assessment, parenteral nutrition support, basic guidelines and standard patterns for modified diets, tube feedings and supplements, and metabolic effects of selected drugs.... Designed to serve as a quick reference book for dietitians, physicians, nurses, pharmacists, and other members of the nutrition support team" (*Journal of the American Dietetic Association* 85 [June 1985]: 270).

469. Mellen, Carol, and Rosario Garza. **The Children's Hospital of Alabama Diet Manual.** Birmingham, Ala.: Dietetics Department, The Children's Hospital, 1984. 200p. ($25.00, The Children's Hospital of Alabama, 1700 7th Avenue, South, Birmingham, AL 35233).

"A diet manual for use by nutritionists, physicians, and nurses who care for pediatric patients." It includes information on "diet therapies for numerous diseases in pediatric practice and patient information in an easy to copy form for distribution to patients."

470. University of Alabama Hospitals. Department of Dietetics. **Manual for Nutritional Management.** Birmingham, Ala.: The University, 1981. 346p. ($21.00, Department of Dietetics, University Hospitals/VAR, 619 S. 19th Street, Birmingham, AL 35233).

This diet manual for use by all health professionals and students contains sections on diet ordering, criteria for nutrition support, and an extensive 61-page section of appendixes.

ARKANSAS

471. Arkansas Dietetic Association. **Arkansas Diet Manual.** 5th ed. Little Rock, Ark.: Arkansas Dietetic Association, 1981. 1v. (looseleaf).

DISTRICT OF COLUMBIA

472. Roth, Johanna H., and Dorothea L. Slater, eds. **Diet Handbook.** Washington, D.C.: District of Columbia Dietetic Association, 1977. 452p.

FLORIDA

473. Florida Dietetic Association. **Diet Manual: Manual of Clinical Dietetics.** rev. ed. n.p.: Florida Dietetic Association, 1983. 1v. (looseleaf).

474. University of Florida. Shands Hospital. Department of Food and Nutrition Services. **Guide to Normal Nutrition and Diet Modification.** 3rd ed. Gainesville, Fla.: Tri-graphics Inc., 1983. 398p. ($18.50, University of Florida, Shands Hospital, Food and Nutrition Services, Box J-325, Gainesville, FL 32610).

This useful and extensive guide covers normal diets, special modification of consistency, diet therapy in various diseases, parenteral and enteral nutrition, nutrition assessment, drug-nutrient interactions, various test diets, allergy diets, diets for hereditary metabolic disorders, and special diets in pediatric disease. An extensive appendix contains height and weight tables, growth charts, nutrient composition of supplemental commercial products and infant formulas, dietary fiber content of foods, and caffeine content of selected beverages and drugs. A bibliography and a subject index are included.

GEORGIA

475.   Georgia Dietetic Association. Clinical Dietetics and Research Section. **Diet Manual of the Georgia Dietetic Association**. 2nd ed. Stone Mountain, Ga.: Georgia Dietetic Association, 1982. 1v. (looseleaf). ($20.00, Georgia Dietetic Association, 3833 Whitney Place, Duluth, GA 30136).

This extensive manual covering normal and therapeutic nutrition contains a section on enteral and parenteral nutrition with data on formulas and another section dealing with renal and hepatic nutrition. An index is included and appendixes include growth charts for infants and children; a table of sodium, potassium, and magnesium values; and information on foods containing caffeine.

HAWAII

476.   Hawaii Dietetic Association. **Hawaii Diet Manual**. 5th ed. Honolulu, Hawaii: Hawaii Dietetic Association, 1979. 1v. (looseleaf).

"The diets are planned around a normal meal pattern which takes into account the patient's food habits and needs. As a result of Hawaii's geographic location and multi-cultural composition, a unique cross-cultural eating pattern evolved and it is especially important for dietitians to have knowledge of the many ethnic foods." Unique features are suggestions for integrating cultural mixed dishes into the hospital diet; a glossary of local food terms; and lists of foods that are important sources of protein, calcium, phosphorus, iron, potassium, magnesium, vitamin A, thiamin, riboflavin, niacin, and ascorbic acid. Also included are a table of cholesterol values, height-weight tables, and an index.

ILLINOIS

477.   Chicago Dietetic Association and South Suburban Dietetic Association of Cook and Will Counties. **Manual of Clinical Dietetics**. 2nd ed. Philadelphia, Pa.: W. B. Saunders, 1981. 292p. ISBN 0721625371.

This manual contains sections dealing with general diets, pediatric nutrition, modified consistency diets, gastrointestinal diets, nutrition support during illness with an extensive table of approximate analysis of commercial tube feedings and nutritional supplements, calorie-controlled diets for diabetes, glycosuria, and hyperglycemia with basic exchange lists, protein-controlled diets, fat modified diets, cholesterol values, sodium-controlled diets, and miscellaneous test diets.

An extensive appendix includes growth charts, desirable weights, a food-drug interaction chart, a food composition table, caffeine content of selected beverages, and composition of vegetable protein foods. A detailed index is provided. Included as a separate pamphlet is a "Physicians Guide for Ordering Diets."

478.   Veterans Administration West Side Medical Center, Chicago, Illinois. **Diet Manual**. 2nd ed. Chicago: Veterans Administration, 1982. 114p. VA1.10: D56/982.

"Prepared for the Veterans Administration West Side Center, Chicago, Illinois by the Dietetic Service, with the approval of the Nutrition Committee and the medical staff." Very brief descriptions with sample menus of nearly 40 diets. Exchange lists are included.

479.   Veterans Administration Hospital, Hines, Illinois, and Foster G. McGaw Hospital. **Diet Manual**. 2nd ed. Washington, D.C.: Government Printing Office, 1981. 178p. VA1.10:D56/981.

This is the result of a collaborative effort between Hines Veterans Administration Hospital and Foster G. McGaw Hospital, Loyola University. It contains information on a large number of hospital diets, with rationale for use, proximate composition, and critical nutrients.

INDIANA

480.   Saint Elizabeth Hospital Medical Center. Dietetics Committee. **Manual of Applied Nutrition**. Lafayette, Ind.: Saint Elizabeth Hospital Medical Center, 1978- . 1v. (looseleaf).

IOWA

481.   Iowa Dietetic Association. **Simplified Diet Manual with Meal Patterns**. 5th ed. Ames, Iowa: Iowa State University Press, 1984. ISBN 0813814308.

"The fifth edition of the *Simplified Diet Manual* retains the basic purpose of earlier editions. In a simplified manner it provides a guide for the prescription and interpretation of diets and nutrition plans." Included are material on the *Daily Food Guide* and the *Dietary Guidelines*; general diets; soft diets; liquid diets; diabetic and calorie-controlled diets; fat and sodium-restricted diets; and protein- and purine-restricted diets. An appendix includes desirable weights and potassium content of food. There is an index.

KANSAS

482.   Stein, Patricia Gardner, and Norma Jean Winn Neufield, eds. **Kansas Diet Manual**. Topeka, Kans.: Kansas Dietetic Association, 1981. 298p.

This manual was prepared in cooperation with the Department of Dietetics and Nutrition, University of Kansas Medical Center, College of Health Sciences and Hospital.

KENTUCKY

483. Kentucky Dietetic Association. Louisville District. Diet Therapy Committee. **Diet Manual**. 3rd ed. Louisville, Ky.: Kentucky Dietetic Association, 1979- . 1v. (looseleaf).

LOUISIANA

484. Louisiana Dietetic Association. **Diet Manual: A Guide for Small Hospitals, Nursing Homes, and Other Health Care Facilities in Louisiana**. Baton Rouge, La.: Louisiana Dietetic Association, 1984. 200p. (Louisiana Dietetic Association, 7395 Exchange Place, Baton Rouge, LA 70806).

"This manual has been written primarily for use in small hospitals, nursing homes, and health care facilities staffed by consultant dietitians in Louisiana.... Designed to be used as a reference and for additional instruction for food service supervisors and clients." Written in a readable format, with pen and ink graphics, this volume includes current information regarding fiber in the diet, use of the prudent diet, nutrition assessment forms, and a large section on weight control management principles and techniques.

MARYLAND

485. Walser, MacKenzie, et al. **Nutritional Assessment: The Johns Hopkins Handbook**. Philadelphia, Pa.: W. B. Saunders, 1984. 403p. ISBN 0721613195.

The authors' aim was to produce a book containing information about specific diets as well as a discussion of major dietary principles, the goals and rationale for specific diets, and criteria for their selection. The book covers both normal and therapeutic nutrition, with chapters and subsections on specific disorders and their dietary management. Each section has a bibliography for further reading. Appendixes include mean heights and weights and energy intakes, amino acid requirements, essential vitamins and minerals and their function, exchange lists, etc. Also included are data useful for specific diets (e.g., tables of sodium values with material on sodium restricted diets). There is an index.

MASSACHUSETTS

486. Beth Israel Hospital. Nutrition Services Department. **Beth Israel Hospital Diet Manual**. Lexington, Mass.: Collamore Press, 1982. 192p. ISBN 0669055239.

487. Massachusetts Dietetic Association. **Diet Manual for Long Term Care Facilities**. rev. ed. Boston: Massachusetts Dietetic Association, 1983. 49 leaves. ($10.50, Massachusetts Dietetic Association, 140 Richdale Road, Needham, MA 02149).

The purpose of this manual is to provide general information and guidelines related to diet modifications which are frequently prescribed for the geriatric resident in long-term care facilities. It contains information on sodium and potassium content of foods and a low tyramine diet.

488. Massachusetts General Hospital. Dietary Department. **Diet Reference Manual**. 2nd ed. Boston: Little, Brown, 1984. 217p. ISBN 0316549479.

The first edition of this book was published under the title *Diet Manual* in 1976. This revised edition is based on the *Handbook of Clinical Nutrition* and is the collaborative work of clinical dietitians and medical staff of the Massachusetts General Hospital. Topics or types of diets covered are normal diets; transitional diets (e.g., clear liquid diets, soft diets, etc.); enteral and parenteral nutrition; modifications for energy, fiber, fat, protein, food sensitivities, and minerals; and special diets for pregnancy, lactation, and children. Extensive appendixes contain food composition information, including a special table on alcoholic beverages, caffeine and purine content of foods, data on infant formulas, and test diets.

MICHIGAN

489. Grills, Norma Jean, and Marcia Vermaire Bosscher, eds. **Manual of Nutrition and Diet Therapy**. 10th ed. New York: Macmillan, 1981. 483p. ISBN 0023472804.

This is the diet manual of the University of Michigan Hospital. The tenth edition of this extensive manual has been produced to meet the expanded role of the dietitian in modern health care. Its purposes are to present standards based on expanding knowledge of the field and advances in technology, to provide for nutrition care of patients, and to serve as a text for dietitians. References to the literature appear at the end of each section. Also included are brief lists of books suitable for the lay public. The appendix includes food composition tables, various nutrient intake recommendations, and a list of position papers on nutrition issues from health and nutrition organizations. There is an index.

MINNESOTA

490. Mayo Clinic, Rochester Methodist Hospital, and St. Mary's Hospital. **Mayo Clinic Diet Manual: A Handbook of Dietary Practices**. 5th ed. Philadelphia, Pa.: W. B. Saunders, 1981. 320p. ISBN 0721662129.

Provided is information on normal nutrition and a large number of therapeutic diet modifications, diet during pregnancy and lactation, normal and therapeutic pediatric diets, formulas, food supplements, total parenteral nutrition, and special test diets. An extensive appendix includes mean heights and weights, growth charts, fatty acid and cholesterol content of food, sodium and potassium, calcium and phosphorus content of food, nutritive value of desserts, snack foods and alcoholic beverages, caffeine content of selected beverages, Dietary Guidelines for Americans, Dietary Goals, etc. There are numerous tables, bibliographies, and an index.

491. Twin Cities District Dietetic Association. **Manual of Clinical Nutrition**. 3rd ed. Minneapolis, Minn.: Twin Cities Dietetic Association, 1981. 1v. (looseleaf). ($16.00, Twin Cities District Dietetic Association, 2221 University Avenue, SE, Suite 300A, Minneapolis, MN 55414).

492. Twin Cities District Dietetic Association. **Manual of Pediatric Nutrition**. Minneapolis, Minn.: Twin Cities Dietetic Association, 1983. 343p. ($25.00, Twin Cities District Dietetic Association, 2221 University Avenue, SE, Suite 300A, Minneapolis, MN 55414).

In addition to diets which specify modifications in consistency and texture, control of calories, carbohydrates, fats, proteins and minerals, this manual is a useful source for therapeutic diets used in the treatment of numerous diseases and disorders of children. It includes a salicylate-free diet; lists of foods which contain and do not contain FD&C No. 5; and information on feeding children with cleft lip and palate, Prader-Willi Syndrome, etc. There is an entire section devoted to infant formulas and enteral and parenteral nutritional support, plus an appendix with numerous test diets, laboratory value deviation in disease, etc.

MISSISSIPPI

493. Mississippi Dietetic Association. Diet Therapy Section. **Diet Manual of the Mississippi Dietetic Association**. 7th ed. n.p.: Mississippi Dietetic Association, 1980. 1v. (looseleaf). (Cover title: *Mississippi Diet Manual*).

MISSOURI

494. Missouri. Division of Health. **Missouri Diet Manual**. 5th ed. St. Louis, Mo.: Missouri Division of Health, 1981. 154p.
    Previous editions were prepared by the Missouri Dietetic Association.

NEBRASKA

495. Nebraska Dietetic Association. **Nebraska Handbook of Diets: Normal and Therapeutic**. 3rd ed. Lincoln, Nebr.: Nebraska Dietetic Association, 1982- . 203p. (looseleaf). ($12.80, Nebraska Hospital Association, 1335 "L" Street, Box 94833, Lincoln, NE 68509).
    Prepared by the Nebraska Dietetic Association in cooperation with the Nebraska Hospital Association, this handbook is primarily intended for use by dietitians and food service supervisors in health care facilities. It includes menu patterns and special diets.

NEW JERSEY

496. New Jersey. State Department of Health. **New Jersey Diet Manual**. rev. ed. Trenton, N.J.: Department of Health, 1983. 135p. ($5.00, New Jersey State Dept. of Health CN364, Trenton, NJ 08625).
    This manual was compiled for use by physicians, dietitians, nurses, and food service supervisors in hospitals, nursing homes, extended care facilities and other institutions. "The intent ... is to provide basic information for the current practice of diet therapy."

NEW YORK

497. Central New York Dietetic Association. **Reference Diet Manual**. Syracuse, N.Y.: Central New York Dietetic Association, 1984. 184p. ($18.00, CNYDA Diet Manual, 11½ Onondaga Street, Skaneateles, NY 13152).
    "A reference for normal and clinical nutrition for dietitians, students and health-related professionals. [Includes a] guide for physicians in prescribing modified diets, extensive sections on long term care, renal disease nutrition, diet and heart disease, nutrition in pregnancy and lactation and pediatrics. [Includes many] tables."

498.   Genesee Dietetic Association. Long Term Care Dietitians Group. **Geriatric Diet Manual**. Rochester, N.Y.: Genesee Dietetic Association, 1984. 135p. ($18.00, Genesee Dietetic Association, 15 Shadow Dawn Court, Rochester, NY 14617).

"This manual ... is intended for use in long term care facilities.... The information provided in covering most therapeutic diets includes: purpose, goals, characteristics, adequacy, a listing of foods allowed and avoided or daily food plan, and a sample day's menu. However, for several frequently used diets such as bland, low protein, high protein, and sodium restricted, there are no dietary guidelines and/or sample day's menu" (*Journal of Nutrition for the Elderly* 4 [Winter 1984]: 92-93).

499.   Hudson Valley Dietetic Association. **Diet Manual**. rev. ed. Albany, N.Y.: Hudson Valley Dietetic Association, 1980. 1v. (looseleaf). ($15.00, Harmon Associates, 34 Elsmere Avenue, Delmar, NY 12054).

This guide provides relevant nutrition information for normal and therapeutic needs and is an easy-to-use reference for health care facilities, government agencies, educators, health care providers, nutritionists, and students. It covers modifications of normal diet (e.g., kosher diets, vegetarian diets), data on infant formulas, diet in pregnancy and lactation and therapeutic diets (e.g., modifications in consistency, in calories, carbohydrates, fat and protein), plus miscellaneous restricted diets, various low sodium diets, gluten-free diets, egg-free diets, and mineral contents of foods. The appendix contains information on intravenous solutions, height and weight tables, etc. A supplement to this manual appeared in 1982.

500.   Long Island Dietetic Association. **Long Island Diet Manual**. 4th rev. ed. Syosset, N.Y.: Long Island Dietetic Association, 1983. 199p. ($10.00 prepaid, P.O. Box 27, Syosset, NY 11791).

"Meant to be used in hospitals and to serve as a guide to other health care facilities." In addition to the standard dietary modification, this manual contains information on postoperative gastric diets, ulcer diets, high and low fiber diets, fluid diabetic diet, high fiber diabetic diet, medium chain trigylceride diet, diets for Type I-V hyperlipoproteinemia, and Type IV hyperlipidemia, as well as tube feeding, etc. The appendix includes food sources of minerals and vitamins, kosher dietary laws, and foods high in oxalate.

501.   Montefiore Medical Center. **Diet Manual, Nutrition Department**. rev. ed. Bronx, N.Y.: Montefiore Medical Center, 1985. 142p. (Montefiore Hospital and Medical Center, 111 E. 210th Street, Bronx, NY 10467).

NORTH CAROLINA

502.   North Carolina Dietetic Association. **Diet Manual**. 3rd ed. Charlotte, N.C.: North Carolina Dietetic Association, 1984. 300p. (looseleaf). ($26.00, NCDA, Inc., 5836 Gate Post Road, Charlotte, NC 28211).

This manual for small hospitals and nursing homes is appropriate for use by food service supervisors as well as dietitians, nurses, and physicians. In addition to the standard types of information on diet modifications and special diets, this manual covers food patterns and food items that are unique to North Carolina.

Such items as collards, corn bread, fat back, and opossum are foods included in some lists. Appendixes include information on sodium and potassium content of foods, nutritional analysis of fast foods, Dietary Guidelines, American Heart Association recommendations, height and weight tables, and guidelines for recording nutritional information in medical records.

OHIO

503.   Children's Hospital Medical Center. Dietary Department. **Diet Manual**. rev. 1983 ed. Cincinnati, Ohio: Children's Hospital Medical Center, 1983. 1v.

This is meant to be used as a supplement to the *Cincinnati Diet Manual*, third edition (1983).

504.   Children's Medical Center. **Children's Medical Center Handbook of Nutrition**. Dayton, Ohio: Children's Medical Center, 1980. 114p. ($10.00, Dietetic Services Department, Children's Medical Center, One Children's Plaza, Dayton, OH 45404).

"A reference for physicians, dietitians and allied health professionals in meeting the nutrition needs of the individual patient. Includes information on physical growth."

505.   Greater Cincinnati Dietetic Association. **Cincinnati Diet Manual**. 3rd ed. Cincinnati, Ohio: Greater Cincinnati Dietetic Association, 1983. 252p.

506.   Stark County Dietetic Association. **Stark County Dietetic Association Diet Manual**. 4th ed. Canton, Ohio: Daring Press, 1983. 350p. ($17.00 plus postage, Daring Press, 1308 Harrison Avenue, SW, Canton, OH 44706).

507.   Toledo Dietetic Association. Diet Therapy Section. **Diet Manual**. 5th ed. Toledo, Ohio: Toledo Dietetic Association, 1982. 110p. (looseleaf). ($15.00, The Graphics Group, Inc., 380 S. Erie Street, Toledo, OH 43602).

This guide for health care professionals in selecting appropriate diets for growth, health, maintenance, and therapeutic applications is also a reference source for nutrition assessment and nutritional management of disease. The appendix includes caffeine content of selected items and blood chemistry findings in health and disease.

OKLAHOMA

508.   Oklahoma Dietetic Association. **Oklahoma Diet Manual**. 7th ed. Norman, Okla.: Oklahoma Dietetic Association, 1982. 1v. (various paging).

PENNSYLVANIA

509.   University of Pennsylvania. Hospital. **Manual of Nutritional Care**. 4th ed. Philadelphia, Pa.: University of Pennsylvania Hospital, 1980. 196p.

This manual contains material on consistency modifications, diets for the management of cardiovascular disease, endocrine disorders, gastrointestinal disorders, liver disease, renal disease, nutrition during pregnancy and lactation, the prevention and treatment of malnutrition (including enteral nutrition), and miscellaneous test diets. The appendix includes foods high in specific vitamins and minerals; ideal weights; anthropometric data; laboratory criteria for nutritional assessment; normal serum lipid values; fat, sodium, potassium, calcium, and phosphorus values for selected foods; and total and supplemental feedings.

510.   University of Pennsylvania. Hospital. **1985 Supplement to the Manual of Nutritional Care**. Philadelphia, Pa.: Hospital of the University of Pennsylvania, 1985. 87p. ($16.00, Hospital of the University of Pennsylvania, Dept. of Food and Nutrition Services, 3400 Spruce Street, Philadelphia, PA 19104).

This supplement contains revisions of selected sections of the *Manual of Nutritional Care* as well as new sections dealing with acute renal failure, food sensitivity, diet for short bowel syndrome, ostomy diets, low tyramine diet, postoperative soft diet, etc. The appendix contains tables with nutrient composition of formulated foods.

TEXAS

511.   Lorenzen, Evelyn J., ed. **Dietary Guidelines**. Houston, Tex.: Gulf Publishing Co., Book Division, 1978. 182p. ISBN 0872011763.

Written by the Dietary Committee, Texas Children's Hospital, this volume includes bibliographical references and an index.

512.   Texas Dietetic Association. **A Diet Manual for Hospitals and Nursing Homes**. 4th ed. Austin, Tex.: Texas Dietetic Association, 1984. 1v. (various paging). ($25.00, Texas Dietetic Association, P.O. Box 15661, Austin, TX 78761).

"This diet manual ... has been planned for use primarily in small hospitals and nursing homes which frequently do not have their own manual.... Written to assist medical staff, dietitians, and food service supervisors." Appendixes include information on selected food sources of vitamins and minerals, caffeine content of selected beverages, oxalate and dietary fiber content of selected foods, and growth charts. An index is included.

WISCONSIN

513.   Wisconsin. Division of Health. Bureau of Community Health and Prevention. **Nutrition for Health Promotion and Prevention: Manual for Health Care Providers**. rev. ed. Madison, Wis.: Bureau of Community Health and Prevention, Division of Health, Wisconsin Department of Health and Social Services, 1984. 279p. ($6.00, Printing and Mailing Services Section, Document Sales and Distribution Unit, 202 S. Thornton Avenue, Madison, WI 53702).

"This manual for health care providers has been restructured to address a more comprehensive scope of nutrition and the delivery of nutrition services." It is divided into two sections. Part I discusses normal nutrition throughout the life cycle and emphasizes disease prevention and maintenance of good health. Part II includes the type of information usually presented in diet manuals dealing with modifications in texture, caloric content, fat, sodium content, etc. Also included are tables for magnesium, potassium, zinc, vitamin A, vitamin C, folacin, and vitamin B-6 in selected foods. There is an appendix.

Specialized Diet Manuals

514.   Council on Renal Nutrition of New England. **Renal Nutrition Handbook for Patients**. rev. ed. Brookline, Mass.: National Kidney Foundation of Massachusetts, 1983. 103p. ($12.00/set, $4.75/*Handbook for Patients* plus $1.50 postage, CRNNE, c/o National Kidney Foundation of Massachusetts, 344 Harvard Street, Brookline, MA 02146).

"Contains over 100 pages of in-depth information about protein, potassium, phosphorus, sodium, and fluid controlled diets. Includes rationale for diet modifications in renal failure; food lists; low sodium seasoning guides; and information on food labeling, dining out and menu planning."

515.   Council on Renal Nutrition of New England. **Renal Nutrition Handbook for Renal Dietitians**. rev. ed. Brookline, Mass.: National Kidney Foundation of Massachusetts, 1983. 111p. ($12.00/set, $8.50/*Handbook for Renal Dietitians* plus $1.50 postage, CRNNE Diet Handbook, c/o National Kidney Foundation of Massachusetts, 344 Harvard Street, Brookline, MA 02146).

"This handbook is a comprehensive supplement to *Renal Nutrition Handbook for Patients*, and has been devised as a resource ... for individual patient teaching. Sections may be copied and added to the patient's handbook as needed."

516.   De St. Jeor, Sachiko T., et al. **Low Protein Diets for the Treatment of Renal Failure**. Salt Lake City, Utah: University of Utah Press, 1970. 71p.

Diets containing the "minimum safe" quantities of essential amino acids for uremic patients are presented. Included is background information for the dietitian, physician, and patient. There are instructions for the patient which provide protein equivalencies of foods, menus, and recipes.

517.   Dreifke, Colleen, et al., eds. **Infant Formulas and Selected Nutritional Supplements**. Columbus, Ohio: Children's Hospital, Department of Dietetics, 1984. 26p.

"Designed to provide basic nutritional product information for physicians, dietitians, nurses and students.... Products included are infant formulas, electrolyte solutions, modular components and enteral supplements." Infant formula tables provide information on carbohydrate, protein, fat, sodium, potassium, iron, and osmolality. An index is included.

518.   Jones, Walretta O., comp. **Diet Guide for Patients with Chronic Dialysis**. Bethesda, Md.: National Institutes of Health, National Institute of Arthritis, Metabolism and Digestive Diseases, Artificial-Chronic Uremia Program, 1976. 24p. (DHEW Publication, No. (NIH) 76-685).

519.   Memorial Sloan-Kettering Cancer Center. Food Services Department. **Diet Manual for Memorial Sloan-Kettering Cancer Center and the Hospital for Special Surgery**. 2nd ed. New York: Memorial Sloan-Kettering Cancer Center, 1978. 146p. (looseleaf). ($12.00, Food Services Department, Memorial Hospital, c/o M. Fairchild, 1275 York Avenue, Box 12, New York, NY 10021).

520. Michigan Dietetic Association. **Dietary Formulas and Nutritional Supplements for Infants**. [Battle Creek, Mich.]: The Association, n.d. ($1.00, Evelyn Cole and Associates, 217 Oriole, Battle Creek, MI 49017).

"A 26-page booklet compiled to assist in translating diet prescriptions into appropriate kinds and quantities of nourishments."

521. Seventh-day Adventist Dietetic Association. **Diet Manual, including Vegetarian Meal Plan**. 6th ed. Margaret Kemmerer Heath, ed. Loma Linda, Calif.: Seventh-day Adventist Dietetic Association, 1982. 537p.

The Seventh-day Adventist Dietetic Association has developed this *Diet Manual* for use in its hospitals and health facilities where vegetarian diets are promoted for health purposes. "The primary purpose of this *Diet Manual* is to provide nutritionally adequate vegetarian meal patterns for normal and therapeutic dietary regimes." Especially useful are the sections on adapting vegetarian diets for pregnancy and lactation and for pediatric and geriatric age groups. Most sections include a brief discussion of related physiology to clarify the rationale for diet therapy, and references are included to provide substantiation and sources of additional information. There is an index.

522. United States. National Heart, Lung, and Blood Institute. **The Dietary Management of Hyperlipoproteinemia: A Handbook for Physicians and Dietitians**. Bethesda, Md.: National Institutes of Health, 1978. 95p. (DHEW Publication, No. (NIH) 78-110). HE20.2802:H99/973.

This volume comes with five types of diets, each issued in pamphlet form for patient use: Type I, Type IIa and b, Type III, Type IV, and Type V hyperlipoproteinemia.

STANDARDS

523. American Dietetic Association. Dietitians in Critical Care Practice Group. Quality Assurance Committee. **Suggested Guidelines for Nutrition Management of the Critically Ill Patient**. Chicago: American Dietetic Association, 1984. 99p. ISBN 0809100119.

Process related guidelines for quality assurance of nutrition care of the critically ill are given.

524. Colorado Dietetic Association and Denver Dietetic Association. **Standards of Practice: Nutritional Quality Assurance in Acute Care Hospitals**. Denver, Colo.: Colorado Dietetic Association, 1980. 20p.

525. Fischer, Kay Huskins, and Malcolm Olmsted. **Standards of Dietetic Care: A Foundation for Quality Assurance**. Loma Linda, Calif.: Seventh-day Adventist Dietetic Association, 1981. 115p.

"The standards in this manual are a basis for a quality assurance program. They are to be used as models for writing ... standards, not for information on clinical practice. They were written for the needs of Florida Hospital."

526. Rose, James C. **Policies and Procedures for Hospital Dietetic Services**. Rockville, Md.: Aspen Systems Corp., 1983. 497p. ISBN 0894438824.

This volume contains over 4,000 detailed procedures and policies relating to hospital dietetic services, including numerous forms. There are two major sections. The pages with blue tabs are the policy manual and the pages with red tabs are the procedures manual. In each, policies and procedures are grouped by broad areas. Policies include such things as the chain of command, records retention, telephone policy, interdepartmental and external communication, signs, visitors, etc. Procedures include activities such as ordering equipment and supplies and termination of employees. There is no index, but both sections have a detailed table of contents.

527. Walters, Farah M., and Sally J. Crumley. **Patient Care Audit: A Quality Assurance Procedure Manual for Dietitians**. Chicago: American Dietetic Association, 1978. 105p.

"Patient care audit is a process for retrospectively monitoring and improving the performance of the health care team." Included are sets of criteria of optimum nutritional care. The appendix includes patient care audit forms.

DRUG-NUTRIENT INTERACTIONS

528. Morgan, Brian L. G. **The Food and Drug Interaction Guide**. New York: Simon and Schuster, 1986. 335p. ISBN 0671524305.

Intended for the general public, this book is an alphabetically arranged compendium of information on over 300 generic drugs. It discusses action, side effects, foods to avoid, possible nutritional interactions, prevention and treatment, and identifies high risk groups where relevant. The appendix lists acidic and alkaline foods, goitrogenic foods, foods high in cholesterol, calcium, dietary fiber, fats, folacin, iron, magnesium, oxalate, phosphorus, potassium, purines, protein, sodium, complex carbohydrates, tyramine, vitamin A, thiamin, riboflavin, niacin, vitamin B-6, vitamin B-12, vitamin C, vitamin D, vitamin E, vitamin K, and zinc.

529. Powers, Dorothy E., and Ann O. Moore. **Food Medication Interactions**. 4th ed. Tempe, Ariz.: F-M I Publishing, 1983. 172p. ISBN 0960616403. ($7.95, Food-Medication Interactions, P.O. Box 44033, Phoenix, AZ 85064).

This extensive listing of medications with classification and nutritional significance also contains information on abnormal laboratory test values which may be of nutritional significance, effects of herbal teas, food and beverage sources of oxalates, tyramine, dopamine, phenylethylamine in foods and beverages, pH and acid content of various beverages, foods potentially causing changes in urinary pH, medications containing phosphates, and medications containing potassium. There is a bibliography but no index.

530. Roe, Daphne A. **Handbook, Interactions of Selected Drugs and Nutrients in Patients**. 3rd ed. Chicago: Publications Department, American Dietetic Association, 1982. 142p. ISBN 0880910046.

"This compilation is intended as a guide to potential drug-nutrient interactions, which may in susceptible patients, lead to varying degrees of nutritional depletion. It includes indications of prevalence; drug dosage-time relationships; associated predisposing factors; possible mechanisms of interaction; and when possible, recommendations for prevention and treatment. It is designed to serve as an up to date reference for drug-nutrient interactions reported in the scientific literature on human subjects. Results from animal experiments are included in several cases."

Arrangement is by type of drug according to the American Hospital Formulary Service (AHFS) classification. There are lists of nutrients showing known nutrient-drug interactions, dietary substances affecting nutrient and drug absorption, and prohibited foods and beverages by drug group and specifications. A list of cited literature is appended. An index is included.

PARENTERAL AND ENTERAL NUTRITION

Bibliographies and Guides

531.   Worthen, Dennis B., and Joan R. Lorimer. **Enteral Hyperalimentation with Chemically Defined Diets: A Source Book**. 2nd ed. Norwich, N.Y.: Information Services, Research Department, Scientific Affairs, Norwich-Eaton Pharmaceuticals, 1979. 276p.

"The new edition contains some 550 bibliographic citations of published articles on the subject of hyperalimentation — 200 more entries than the first edition" (*Journal of the American Dietetic Association* 75 [December 1979]: 725).

Directories

532.   Chernoff, Ronni, ed. **Directory of PEN Products and Services**. Silver Spring, Md.: American Society for Parenteral and Enteral Nutrition, 1985?. 188p. (ASPEN, 8605 Cameron Street, Suite 500, Silver Spring, MD 20910).

"This greatly expanded directory includes information from 118 companies providing products and/or services used in the practice of parenteral and enteral nutrition. Description of equipment, solutions, formulas, supplies, and additives, with new sections on computer software and home nutrition support services, along with names, addresses, and telephone numbers of suppliers are provided" (*American Dietetic Journal* 85 [June 1985]: 770).

Handbooks, Manuals, and Other Data Compilations

533.   DelRio, Deeann, Karen Williams, and Becky Miller Esvelt. **Handbook of Enteral Nutrition: A Practical Guide to Tube Feeding**. El Segundo, Calif.: Medical Specifics Publishing, 1982. 155p. (MSP Quick Reference Series).

This handbook includes individually authored sections on indications of tube feeding, malnutrition in hospitalized patients, nutrition assessment, formula selection, delivery systems, feeding techniques, complications of tube feeding, surgically placed feeding tubes, and nutrition support of the critically ill. There are references, but no index.

534. Fort Worth Dietetic Association. **Enteral Nutrition Formula Handbook**. Fort Worth, Tex.: Fort Worth Dietetic Association, 1986. 28p. ($2.50, Fort Worth Dietetic Association, P.O. Box 1748, Fort Worth, TX 76101).

Designed to assist health professionals providing nutritional care, this booklet contains an extensive table presenting nutritional analysis data for enteral formulas. Values are given per liter. Also included are information on equipment and supplies, a table showing the management of complications, a monitoring schedule, an enteral support decision tree, names and addresses of pharmaceutical companies, and selected references.

535. Grant, Andrew, and Elizabeth Todd, eds. **Enteral and Parenteral Nutrition: A Clinical Handbook**. Oxford: Blackwell Scientific Publications, 1982. 175p. ISBN 063200732X.

Basic background information, techniques for administering parenteral and enteral nutrition, nursing care of enteral patient, patient monitoring, metabolic complications, immunological effects of malnutrition, nutrition in malignancy, renal failure, liver disease, and for patients with burns is provided. Appendixes contain data on nutrient analysis of commercial solutions, formulas, and dietary supplements as well as manufacturers' addresses. There is an index.

536. Grant, John P. **Handbook of Total Parenteral Nutrition**. Philadelphia, Pa.: W. B. Saunders, 1980. 197p. ISBN 0721642101.

"Covers the salient features of parenteral nutrition beginning with an historical perspective and ending with discussions of the vitamin and trace elements and deficiencies related to total parenteral nutrition. Principles of patient selection, catheter insertion and longtime maintenance, preparation and administration of solutions, and recognition and management of all potential complications are presented.... The text is complemented by 24 tables, 83 figures and almost 1,000 references."

537. Kaminski, Mitchell V., ed. **Hyperalimentation: A Guide for Clinicians**. New York: Marcel Dekker, 1985. 719p. ISBN 0824773756.

Intended as a reference text for surgeons, gastroenterologists, nutritionists and pharmacists, this book consists of 26 chapters by individual contributors covering all facets of total nutritional support. It includes general material as well as information on nutritional support for specific diseases such as cardiac disease, cancer, respiratory failure, renal failure, burns, as well as chapters on ambulatory home support and new devices and techniques. There is a subject index.

538. Kerner, John A. **Manual of Pediatric Parenteral Nutrition**. New York: Wiley, 1983. 365p. ISBN 0471092916.

A practical guide to the use of parenteral feeding in infants and children, this book presents material on the indications for parenteral nutrition, techniques for nutrition assessment, nutrient requirements, etc. It contains numerous tables, not only on infant formulas and defined diets, but also on electrolyte and mineral abnormalities, amino acid profiles of solutions, and complications resulting from parenteral feeding. Extensive bibliographies appear at the ends of chapters. Appendixes include terminology, information on parenteral nutrition and drug compatibility, and home parenteral nutrition. There is an index.

539. Naguy, Judith, Carol Nartker, and Julia Koogler. **Enteral Nutrition; A Handbook for Health Care Practitioners**. Dayton, Ohio: Good Samaritan Hospital and Health Center, Clinical Dietetic Services, 1983. 40p. ($3.50, Dietary Department, Good Samaritan Hospital and Health Center, 2222 Philadelphia Drive, Dayton, OH 45406).

This booklet is designed as a reference on all aspects of enteral nutrition for health care practitioners. It includes information on indications for administration of tube feedings, recommended initial dilution for enteral feedings, complications of tube feedings, and nutritional analysis of available enteral products.

540. Rombeau, John L., and Michael D. Caldwell, eds. **Enteral and Tube Feeding**. Philadelphia, Pa.: W. B. Saunders, 1984. 610p. (Clinical Nutrition, Vol. 1). ISBN 0721676448.

This extensive reference text contains 30 individually authored chapters dealing with such topics as digestive physiology, human nutritional requirements, nutrition assessment, use of computers in nutrition support, formulated foods, enteral delivery systems, modular feeding, use of enteral nutrition for cancer, renal and liver patients, pediatric enteral nutrition, enteral nutrition for the aged, and pharmacologic aspects of enteral nutrition. Bibliographies are included throughout. There is an index.

541. Rombeau, John L., and Michael D. Caldwell, eds. **Parenteral Nutrition**. Philadelphia, Pa.: W. B. Saunders, 1986. 752p. (Clinical Nutrition, Vol. 2). ISBN 0721676456.

A companion volume to the authors' *Enteral and Tube Feeding*, this extensive collection of 43 individually authored chapters is useful both as a text and as a reference book. It covers a wide range of topics including metabolic aspects of parenteral feeding, equipment, parenteral nutrition for specific diseases and age groups, trace elements, and home parenteral nutrition. There is an index.

17
Books on Special Diets and Exchange Lists

GENERAL

542.   American Dietetic Association. **Resource Kit for Modified Diets: Nutrition Education Materials**. [Chicago]: American Dietetic Association, n.d. 125 leaves.

Prepared to assist the dietitian "in providing patients on modified diets with the tools to bridge the gap between their old and new ways of eating once they leave the hospital setting," this kit provides tips on graphics for patient education materials and comes with a booklet of illustrations that can be freely copied. It includes rationales for special diets; tables showing food-drug interactions; tips on meal planning; lists of foods high in sodium and potassium; charts on seasoning with herbs, spices and wine; a guide to foods high in fiber; and a bibliography of cookbooks for diabetic, low sodium, modified fat, weight loss, and high fiber diets. The blue pages are aimed at the dietitian and the white pages are for the patient. Also included are sources of additional information. There is no index.

543.   Casale, Joan T. **The Diet Food Finder**. New York: R. R. Bowker, 1975. 304p. ISBN 0835207838.

This is a bibliography of books on special diets plus recipe indexes. Appendixes include: "Directory of Publishers," "Retail Mail Order Suppliers for Special Dietary Foods," and "Brand Name Availability List." Author, title, and subject indexes are included.

544.   Goodman, Harriet Wilinsky, and Barbara Morse. **Just What the Doctor Ordered: Gourmet Recipes Developed with Boston's Beth Israel Hospital for Low-Calorie, Diabetic, Low Fat, Low-Cholesterol, Low-Sodium, Bland, High-Fiber, and Renal Diets**. New York: Holt, Rinehart and Winston, 1982. 697p.

This extensive cookbook contains an impressive selection of recipes and information on protein, fat, carbohydrate, sodium, potassium, cholesterol, and exchange values for each recipe. Also included are general information on nutrition, exchange lists, a seasonings chart showing which diets permit a specific seasoning, equivalents and substitutions, a glossary of nutrition, conversion factors, and an index.

545. Jacobson, Helen Saltz. **The Special Diet Foreign Phrase Book: Your Passport to Dining in Mexico, Spain, Germany, France, and Italy.** Emmaus, Pa.: Rodale Press, 1982. 293p. ISBN 0878574042.

This volume contains travel tips, useful names and addresses, telephone numbers, and other handy information in addition to the individual sections devoted to special diet terminology in Spanish, German, French, and Italian.

ALLERGIES

546. American Dietetic Association. **Food Sensitivity: A Resource Including Recipes.** Chicago: American Dietetic Association, 1985. 127p. (Food Sensitivity Series). ISBN 0880910127.

This work is designed to help dietitians and other health professionals counseling people with food sensitivities and allergies. Part 1 is a brief introduction to food sensitivities to eggs, wheat, milk, soy, etc. Part 2 includes recipes grouped by major categories ranging from appetizers to desserts. Recipes are clearly labeled as not containing milk, wheat, or eggs. Part 3 consists of useful tables of milk substitutes, families of food plants, classes of food animals, flour substitutes, foods containing soy, food sources of tartrazine and salicylates, and foods containing eggs. Part 4 contains the appendixes and includes additional sources of information, distributors of gluten-free products, packaged and prepared foods allowed on a modified gluten diet, a list of food companies providing product information with addresses, and lists of foods containing FD&C Yellow No. 5 (tartrazine) and sulfiting agents.

547. Rudoff, Carol. **The Allergy Gourmet.** Menlo Park, Calif.: Prologue Publications, 1983. 201p. ISBN 0930048113.

Milk-free, wheat-free, corn-free, egg-free, and soy-free recipes are included here, with an index. Some of the baked goods use barley flour and are therefore problematic for people on gluten-free diets.

CANCER

548. Birge, K. **Nutrition for Cancer Patients Undergoing Radiation and Chemotherapy.** Stanford, Calif.: Department of Dietetics, Stanford University Hospital, 1981. 24p. ($4.10, Department of Dietetics, Room C108, Stanford University Hospital, 300 Pasteur Drive, Stanford, CA 94305).

"Written for the cancer patient, this booklet covers basic nutrition facts and methods of increasing protein and energy intakes. The author suggests ways of coping with nausea, vomiting, mouth and throat problems, constipation, diarrhea, and loss of appetite" (*Journal of Nutrition Education* 14 [1982]: 161).

549.   Bukoff, Marilyn, et al. **Nutrition: Guidance for the Cancer Patient.** Iowa City, Iowa: University of Iowa, 1981. 37p. ($3.00, Campus Stores, Iowa Memorial Union, University of Iowa, Iowa City, IA 52242).

"Designed to assist patients and their families in maintaining an adequate diet." Includes information on ways of meeting nutrient needs and special problems that may affect the eating behavior of the cancer patient.

550.   Fishman, Joan, and Barbara Anrod. **Something's Got to Taste Good: The Cancer Patient's Cookbook.** Kansas City, Kans: Andrews and McMeel, 1981. 222p. ISBN 0836221036.

This cookbook was developed by a dietitian, a patient, and a writer as a result of a questionnaire eliciting information from patients. It provides recipes for appetizing, easy-to-prepare, easy-to-eat foods, and has basic information on nutrition as well as advice on taste blindness and other problems. An index is included.

551.   Margie, Joyce Daly, and Abby S. Bloch. **Nutrition and the Cancer Patient.** Radnor, Pa.: Chilton Book Co., 1983. 269p. ISBN 0801971209.

"Provides resources, references, and recipes for coping with cancer. For patients and health professionals." It includes over 300 recipes.

552.   Persigehl, C., Richard Ripple, and Connie Hill. **Nutritional Guide for Upper and Lower Abdominal Radiation Therapy.** Boise, Idaho: Mountain States Tumor Institute, 1982. 83p. ($2.00, Mountain States Tumor Institute, Department of Patient and Family Support, 151 E. Bannock, Boise, ID 83702).

This guide is designed to assist the patient in maintaining an adequate diet during radiation therapy.

553.   United States. National Cancer Institute. **Diet and Nutrition: A Resource for Parents of Children with Cancer.** Bethesda, Md.: U.S. Department of Health, Education and Welfare, Public Health Service, National Institutes of Health, 1979. 57p. HE20.3152:D56/3.

This booklet contains general advice and information on special diets which may be required.

554.   United States. National Institutes of Health. **Eating Hints: Recipes and Tips for Better Nutrition during Cancer Treatment.** Bethesda, Md.: U.S. Department of Health, Education and Welfare, Public Health Service, National Institutes of Health, 1980. 86p. (NIH) Publication, No. 80-2079). HE20.3152:Ea8.

This is a reprinting of a book originally written by members of the Yale-New Haven Medical Center (Marion E. Morra, Nancy Suski, and Bonny C. Johnson). It contains general advice plus recipes.

DIABETES

Bibliographies and Guides

555.   American Dietetic Association. Diabetes Care and Education Practice Group. **Diabetes Mellitus and Glycemic Response to Different Foods.** Chicago: American Dietetic Association, 1983. 17p.

This bibliography of 51 journal articles contains detailed abstracts based on MEDLINE, BIOSIS, and AGRICOLA searches. There is an author index.

556. United States. National Diabetes Information Clearinghouse. **Cookbooks for People with Diabetes, Selected Annotations**. Bethesda, Md.: Department of Health and Human Services, Public Health Service, National Diabetes Information Clearinghouse, 1981. 19p. (NIH Publication, No. 81-2177). HE20.3316C77 1981.

Described are 44 cookbooks for the diabetic. The text may be freely copied. Title and author indexes are included.

557. Wheeler, Madelyn L., et al. **Fiber and the Patient with Diabetes Mellitus: A Summary and Annotated Bibliography**. 2nd ed. Chicago: Diabetes Care and Education Practice Group, American Dietetic Association, 1983. 25p.

A revised and expanded edition of a bibliography first issued in 1980, this work contains over 100 references with abstracts as well as a summary of findings and an author index.

Handbooks, Manuals, and Other Data Compilations

558. Krall, Leo P., ed. **Joslin Diabetes Manual**. 11th ed. Philadelphia, Pa.: Lea & Febiger, 1978. 324p. ISBN 0812106075.

This manual is addressed specifically to the layperson and contains all of the information a diabetic needs for self-care—physiology, diet, treatment, testing, insulin, and hypoglycaemic agents, complications, etc.

Dietary Advice and Cookbooks

559. American Diabetes Association. **The American Diabetes Association, the American Dietetic Association Family Cookbook**. Englewood Cliffs, N.J.: Prentice-Hall, 1980-1984. 2v. ISBN 0130249017 (vol. 1).

Included is basic information on nutrition, meal planning and exchanges, obesity and diabetes, dining out, calculating exchanges from food labels and recipes, and meal plans for sick days with a full range of recipes accompanied by exchange values, carbohydrate content, calories, protein, fat, sodium, and potassium. Index.

560. Barbour, Pamela Gillispie, and Norma Green Spivey. **The Exchange Cookbook: Featuring Dessert & Casserole Recipes for Diabetic & Weight Control Programs**. Atlanta, Ga.: G&G Publishing Co., 1982. 179p. ISBN 0961002808.

Written by a dietitian and a home economist, this cookbook is based on the ADA exchange system. The emphasis is on mixed dishes and desserts, although a wide range of other recipes is included. It includes exchange lists, exchanges allowed in meal patterns with or without milk ranging from 1,000-3,000 calories, sample menus, storage times for a variety of frozen goods, a list of food additives, and an index by food groups.

561.   Cavaiani, Mabel. **The New Diabetic Cookbook**. Chicago: Contemporary Books, 1984. 303p. ISBN 0809255243.

The major portion of this book is devoted to over 200 recipes from soup to dessert, accompanied by the following information: calories, food exchanges, protein, fat, and sodium. It also contains information on food exchanges and on how to calculate them, menus for special occasions, suggestions for lowering cholesterol intake, cooking equipment and ingredients, and hints on canning and freezing. There is an index.

562.   Ķaplan, Dorothy J. **The Comprehensive Diabetic Cookbook**. completely rev. and updated ed. New York: F. Fell Publishers, 1981. 254p. ISBN 081190427X.

In addition to over 200 recipes listing exchange values per serving, this book has exchange lists and a brand-name list of prepared foods with exchanges. An index is appended.

563.   Little, Billie. **Recipes for Diabetics**. rev. and updated ed. New York: Grosset & Dunlap, 1981. 288p. ISBN 0448146207.

Approximately 200 recipes with exchange values from appetizers to chutney are provided. Also included are exchange lists, daily menu guides for various caloric intakes from 1,000 to 2,500, and an extensive brand-name product list with exchange values. There is an index.

564.   Middleton, Katharine, and Mary Abbott Hess. **The Art of Cooking for the Diabetic**. New York: New American Library, 1978. 386p. ISBN 0809282704.

General information is given about diabetes, exchange lists and tips on shopping, eating while traveling, sugar substitutes, as well as a full range of recipes including desserts with exchange values for carbohydrate, protein, fat, caloric, and sodium content. There is an index.

565.   Revell, Dorothy Tompkins. **Oriental Cooking for the Diabetic**. Tokyo: Japan Publications; distr., New York: Kodansha International through Harper & Row, 1981. 160p. ISBN 087040492X.

Written by a professional dietitian, this book contains about 175 recipes for all types of dishes from appetizers to desserts, with exchange values. It includes exchange lists and menu plans for 1,200-, 1,500-, and 1,800-calorie diets. A bibliography and an index are included.

566.   Smith, Elizabeth. **Dr. Elizabeth Smith's New World of Eating: Vegetarian Meal-Planning for Diabetic Persons: A Lacto-Ovo-Vegetarian Diet**. Winnipeg, Man.: Hyperion Press, 1979. 36p. ISBN 0920534058.

"Accompanied with sample menus, this easy-to-follow guide offers explicit nutrient information for the vegetarian with diabetes. However, the material may be too complicated and technical for many homemakers" (*Journal of the American Dietetic Association* 75 [1979]: 509).

567.   So, Betty. **Diabetes and Chinese Food**. [Toronto]: Canadian Diabetic Association, 1978. 33p.

"Written in English and Chinese, this manual will be welcomed by Chinese diabetics as well as dietitians working with them. Particularly useful is the inclusion of many traditional Chinese foods. The exchange lists roughly parallel the 1976 ADA version with some differences in vegetable classification and no breakdown within lists as to fat content" (*Journal of Nutrition Education* 11 [January/March 1979]: 52).

568. West, Betty M. **Diabetic Menus, Meals, and Recipes**. rev. ed. Garden City, N.Y.: Doubleday, 1978. 194p. ISBN 0385046510.

This revised edition of a book which has been in use for over 30 years has been greatly expanded by a registered dietitian. It contains general information about diabetes and some 120 recipes with data on carbohydrates, protein, fat, and calories. Also included are sample menus for a 1,500-calorie diet, exchange lists, and information on canning fresh fruits and vegetables. There is an index.

Exchange Lists

569. American Diabetes Association. **Exchange Lists for Meal Planning**. New York: American Diabetes Association; distr., Chicago: American Dietetic Association, 1976. 24p.

Common foods on six major exchange lists are included: milk, vegetables, fruits, bread, meat, and fat.

570. Arbogast, Karen Kramer. **Exchange Lists and Diet Patterns**. New York: Van Nostrand Reinhold, 1980. 340p. ISBN 0442256558.

This is an invaluable compendium of exchange lists, with meal patterns for low-potassium, high potassium, low-sodium, and adequate iron diets.

571. Barrett, Andrea. **The Diabetic's Brand-Name Food Exchange Handbook**. Philadelphia, Pa.: Running Press, 1984. 171p. ISBN 0894712373.

"Food exchanges for over 3,000 supermarket, grocery store and fast food products."

This is an invaluable reference source not only because of its completeness, but also for the added information preceding each group of foods (e.g., "sweets without sucrose" with its helpful preface and table of information on commonly used sweeteners). There is an index.

572. Birmingham District Dietetic Association. **A Guide to Meal Planning**. Birmingham, Ala.: Birmingham District Dietetic Association, 1981. 17p. ($0.55, Birmingham District Dietetic Association, P.O. Box 330, University Station, University of Alabama at Birmingham, Birmingham, AL 35294).

This guide uses the American Diabetes Association Exchange Lists for Meal Planning for diabetic or weight reduction diets. It also has brief exchange lists for kosher foods, Southern foods, and oriental foods.

573. Cinnamon, Pamela A., and Marilyn A. Swanson. **Everything about Exchange Values for Foods: How to Add – Mixed Dishes, Prepared Products, More Variety – To Your Diabetic Meal Plan**. Moscow, Idaho: University Press of Idaho, 1981. 60p. ISBN 0893010839.

"A supplement to the standard *Exchange Lists for Meal Planning*, 1976. Designed primarily for people with diabetes who want to incorporate mixed dishes into their diets."

574.   Franz, Marion J. **Exchanges for All Occasions: Meeting the Challenge of Diabetes**. Minneapolis, Minn.: International Diabetes Center, 1983. 210p.

This book is a treasure-trove of information for the diabetic. It includes the basic exchange lists; additional lists for specialized foods used in Chinese, Mexican, Italian, and Jewish cookery; lists suitable for camping trips; and a fast food list. Also included are hints about dining out, essential vocabulary while traveling abroad, holiday menus, food adjustments for exercise, information about alcoholic beverages, and hints for food preparation and recipe adjustments. Excellent!

575.   Franz, Marion J. **Fast Food Facts: Nutritive and Exchange Values for Fast-Food Restaurants**. Minneapolis, Minn.: International Diabetes Center, 1984. 31p.

Exchanges, caloric values, carbohydrate, protein, fat, and sodium in foods served at major fast food chains are given.

576.   Salmon, Margaret B. **Diabetic Diet Exchange Lists**. Demarest, N.J.: Techkits, Inc., 1984. 20p. ($1.50, Techkits, Inc., P.O. Box 105, Demarest, NJ 07627).

This booklet has been prepared "to assist professionals in the health field and diabetics to make appropriate selections of nutritious foods permitted on diabetic diets. Its emphasis is on portion size of foods permitted ... contains approximately 70 illustrations of the precise portion sizes of foods permitted on a diabetic diet." This booklet is also available in a Spanish-language edition.

577.   Salmon, Margaret B. **Diabetic Exchange Lists for Low Sodium Diets**. Demarest, N.J.: Techkits, Inc., 1980. 20p. ($1.50, Techkits, Inc., P.O. Box 105, Demarest, NJ 07627).

This booklet was prepared "to assist diabetic patients and health professionals in the selection of nutritious foods on low-sodium diets.... Information which is not contained in similar publications is the extensive use of illustrations of appropriate portion sizes."

578.   Swanson Center for Nutrition, Inc. **Diet Handbook**. Washington, D.C.: U.S. Department of Health, Education and Welfare, 1980. 23p. HE20.3308: D56/2.

Basic exchange lists with color photographs and quantities used are provided. The emphasis is on foods consumed by native peoples in the Southwest.

GLUTEN-FREE DIETS

579.   American Dietetic Association. **Gluten Intolerance: A Resource Including Recipes**. Chicago: American Dietetic Association, 1985. 99p. (Food Sensitivity Series). ISBN 0880910135.

This is intended as an aid for dietitians, health professionals, and people with gluten intolerance. Part 1 provides background information, including hints on baking with gluten-free flours and substitutes for wheat flour. Part 2 contains the recipes, which range from appetizers to desserts. Part 3 consists of appendixes and includes an extensive list of packaged and prepared food allowed on a modified gluten diet, food companies which serve as sources of product information, organizations which serve as a resource for people with celiac disease, and distributors for gluten-free products. All recipes included are wheat-free, but not all are completely gluten-free. Some recipes contain oats, rye, or barley and can be made gluten-free by substituting ingredients. Some of the recipes are milk and egg-free as well, and are also included in the other two titles in the Food Sensitivity Series.

580. Dunkley, Colleen R. **A Matter of Gluten: A Food Guide for Coeliacs**. Port Credit, Mississauga, Ont.: Nutrition Link, 1978. 31p. (Nutrition Link, P.O. Box 504, Port Credit, Mississauga, Ont. L5G 4M2).

This provides helpful information and advice for the celiac, including basic facts about the disease and lists of gluten-free and gluten-containing foods. Substitutes for wheat flour and thickeners, baking hints, and sources of information on gluten-free recipes and product lists are also provided.

581. Garst, Pat Murphy. **Celiac-Sprue and the Gluten Free Diet**. updated ed. Des Moines, Iowa: M. Stevens Agency, 1981. 147p. ($7.95, M. Stevens Agency, P.O. Box 3004, Frankfort, KY 40603).

Written for the patient, this book describes the disease and a gluten-free diet. It discusses foods to avoid and approved foods, hints for shopping, cooking and baking, and product sources but includes *no* recipes. There are a bibliography and an index.

582. Garst, Pat Murphy. **Gluten Free Cooking for Celiac Disease, Sprue and Gluten-Sensitive Enteropathy Diets**. Des Moines, Iowa: M. Stevens Agency, 1980. 169p. ($7.95, M. Stevens Agency, P.O. Box 3004, Frankfort, KY 40603).

Included is general information on a gluten-free diet and over 200 recipes ranging from soups to baked goods. Recipes use potato starch, wheat starch, rice flour, and cornmeal. It includes addresses for product sources and an index.

583. Hills, Hilda Cherry. **Good Food, Gluten Free**. New Canaan, Conn.: Keats Publishing, 1976. 239p. ISBN 0879831383.

"Over 300 recipes for gluten-free main dishes, breads, and biscuits, treats, desserts, and salads." Substituted for wheat flour are rice flour, cornmeal, soy flour, millet flour, and potato flour. Additional material provided is a brief history of celiac disease, information on feeding infants and young children, and miscellaneous suggestions for dining out, parties, and other eating occasions. There is an index.

584. Wood, Marion N. **Coping with the Gluten-Free Diet**. Springfield, Ill.: Charles C. Thomas, 1982. 150p. ISBN 0398047189.

Recipes in this book substitute rice flour as a thickener and in baking. An index is included.

HIGH FIBER DIETS

585.   Salmon, Margaret Belais. **A Professional Dietitian's Natural Fiber Diet Book**. West Nyack, N.Y.: Parker Publishing Co., 1979. 252p. ISBN 0137253338.

"The purpose of this book is to assist dieters who are overweight and need to lose weight safely and permanently, using the most acceptable guidelines for diet, exercise, and behavioral modification. This book contains the scientific explanation of several types of weight reduction diets, with emphasis on the use of foods containing fiber."

KOSHER DIETS

586.   Greenberg, Ruth R. **Handbook on Kosher Food: Information for Inservice Training**. New York: R. R. Greenberg, 1982. 57p. ($6.00, Ruth Greenberg, 4451 Tibbet Avenue, Riverdale, NY 10471).

"Designed as a tool for food service managers and supervisors, food and nutrition students and institutional inservice trainees.... Gives background information on ... the dietary laws or rules pertaining to Kosher food preparation."

LACTOSE INTOLERANCE

587.   American Dietetic Association. **Lactose Intolerance: A Resource Including Recipes**. Chicago: American Dietetic Association, 1985. 1v. (Food Sensitivity Series). ISBN 0880910143.

Designed as a resource for dietitians, health professionals, and individuals with lactose intolerance, this book is divided into three parts. Part 1 provides brief background information on lactose intolerance. Part 2 contains recipes from appetizers to desserts. Part 3 contains appendixes with information on the lactose content of milk products, sources of additional information including cookbooks, and sources of product information. It includes some of the same recipes as *Food Sensitivity: A Resource Including Recipes*. Some of the recipes are egg- and wheat-free as well. There is no index.

588.   Hamrick, Becky, and S. L. Wiesenfeld. **The Egg-Free, Milk-Free, Wheat-Free Cookbook**. New York: Harper & Row, 1982. 274p. ISBN 0060149787.

Coded recipes, lists of replacement ingredients for wheat flour and milk, instructions for reading labels, etc., are provided. To a large extent wheat flour is replaced by potato flour, corn flour, arrowroot, cornstarch, and rice flour. Nondairy creamer is used as a substitute for milk and nondairy whipped topping replaces cream. An index is appended.

589.   Hostage, Jacqueline E. **Living—Without Milk: A Cookbook and Nutritional Guide for Those Who Should Avoid Dairy Products**. 3rd ed. White Hall, Va.: Betterway Publications, 1981. 139p. ISBN 093262006X.

Provided are information on milk and butter substitutes and a full range of recipes, some of which use tofu as a cheese substitute, nondairy whipped topping for whipped cream, and nondairy creamer for milk. The volume includes a product information directory and other sources of information. An index is included.

590. Sainsbury, Isobel S. **The Milk-Free, Egg-Free Cookbook; How to Prepare Easy, Delicious Foods for People on Special Diets and Their Families**. Springfield, Ill.: Charles C. Thomas, 1974. 148p. ISBN 0398031088.

Milk-free and milk- and egg-free recipes using largely commercial milk substitutes such as soy milks are provided, as well as information on milk-free commercial products. There is an index.

591. Zukin, Jane. **Milk-Free Diet Cookbook: Cooking for the Lactose Intolerant**. New York: Sterling Publishing Co., 1982. 155p. ISBN 080695566X.

This book provides hints and recipes for lactose-free eating. Although recipes are free of dairy products, they do not stress alternative sources of calcium and many are recipes not ordinarily using milk products. A food composition table (USDA Home and Garden Bulletin, No. 72), is appended. There is an index.

LOW-OXALATE DIETS

592. Ney, Denise, et al., **The Low Oxalate Diet Book for the Prevention of Kidney Stones**. San Diego, Calif.: General Clinical Research Center of the University of California at San Diego, Medical Center, 1981. 30p. ($2.00, GCRC [H-203], University Hospital, 225 Dickinson Street, San Diego, CA 92101).

This volume contains general information about oxalate metabolism, patient guidelines, low-oxalate meal plan, low-oxalate and high-oxalate food lists, oxalate content of foods per 100 grams, oxalate in foods by food groups and by range of oxalate content. There is a bibliography.

LOW-SODIUM, LOW-CHOLESTEROL, LOW-FAT DIETS

593. American Heart Association. Northeast Ohio Affiliate. **Cooking without Your Salt Shaker**. Dallas, Tex.: American Heart Association, Northeast Ohio Affiliate, Inc., 1978. 145p.

594. Bagg, Elma W. **Cooking without a Grain of Salt**. Garden City, N.Y.: Doubleday, 1964. 224p.

Hints are given here for low-sodium eating, including alternative seasonings, suggestions for dining out, traveling, and sodium in selected municipal water supplies. Recipes include sodium and caloric values.

595. Baltzell, Kharin Bundesen, and Terry Martin Parsley. **Living without Salt**. Elgin, Ill.: Brethren Press, 1982. 240p. ISBN 0871785390.

This book contains about 300 recipes for all types of foods from appetizers to desserts and pickles. A chapter entitled "Salt Is Not the Only Seasoning" lists alternative seasonings and describes how to use them. It also discusses substitutes for baking powder and other high-sodium ingredients. There is an index.

596. Baskin, Rosemary M. **The Low-Sodium, Sugar, Fat Cookbook**. Oneonta, N.Y.: R. M. Baskin, 1984. 222p. ($11.95, P.O. Box 717, Oneonta, NY 13820).

Written by a registered dietitian, this cookbook contains a full range of recipes from appetizers to desserts. Each recipe has information on calories, carbohydrate, protein, fat, cholesterol, sodium, and exchanges. A variety of seasonings is used, but there is an emphasis on herbs and spices. Fructose and aspartame are used as sweeteners. Also included are a table of sodium values for selected foods; suggestions for adapting recipes; and information on herbs, spices, and seasonings. There is no index.

597. Birmingham District Dietetic Association. **A Guide to Low Sodium Meal Planning**. Birmingham, Ala.: Birmingham Dietetic Association, 1981. 17p. ($0.55, Birmingham Dietetic Association, P.O. Box 330, University Station, University of Alabama, Birmingham, AL 35294).

This pamphlet uses the American Diabetes Association's diabetic exchange lists incorporating low-sodium diet principles. It contains a spice chart showing how to season foods without salt and discusses label reading, salt substitutes, and food preparation techniques appropriate for weight control, diabetes, and sodium control.

598. Brenner, Eleanor P. **Gourmet Cooking without Salt**. Garden City, N.Y.: Doubleday, 1981. 432p. ISBN 0385148216.

A whole range of recipes from hors d'oeuvres and soups to desserts is included here. Many use a seasoned salt substitute of potassium chloride as a seasoning. There is an index.

599. Claiborne, Craig. **Craig Claiborne's Gourmet Diet**. New York: Times Books, 1980. 258p. ISBN 0812909143.

Gourmet-style, low-sodium, low-cholesterol recipes by the *New York Times* food editor are included here. A full range of recipes with information on calories, sodium, fat, and cholesterol per serving are offered. Wine is a commonly used seasoning. A brief food table listing calories, sodium, fat, and cholesterol of common foods is appended. An index is appended.

600. Eshleman, Ruthe, and Mary Winston. **The American Heart Association Cookbook**. 3rd ed. New York: David McKay Co., 1979. 519p. ISBN 067950902X.

A varied collection of recipes for low-fat, low-salt, and low-cholesterol dishes, ranging from appetizers to desserts, is included here. However, only caloric values are provided for each recipe. Also included is basic information on preferred cooking methods, herbs and spices, menus, eating out, and box lunches, as well as tables showing total fat, polyunsaturated fat, saturated fat, cholesterol, and calories for common foods. There is no index.

601. Hawaii Heart Association. **Salt — Who Needs It?** Honolulu, Hawaii: Hawaii Heart Association and Hawaii Dietetic Association, 1982. 63p.

Provided are low-sodium recipes for items ordinarily high in salt or sodium. Emphasis is on Hawaiian and Asian foods.

602. Margie, Joyce Daly, and James C. Hunt. **Living with High Blood Pressure: The Hypertension Cookbook**. Bloomfield, N.J.: HLS Press, 1978. 309p.

This *Hypertension Cookbook* provides information about high blood pressure, nutrition and drug therapy, menus for different levels of sodium intake, food groups arranged by sodium levels, plus a full range of low-sodium recipes with exchanges and caloric values. Extensive tables in the back provide sodium, potassium, cholesterol, total fat, and exchanges for the recipes. There is an index.

603.   Rodale Press. **No Salt Needed**. Emmaus, Pa.: Rodale Press, 1982. 96p. (Rodale's High Health Cookbook Series). ISBN 0878573933.
In addition to the 65 recipes, which range from soups to breads and desserts, this book provides hints on how to season foods, how to make low-sodium baking powder, and information on the sodium content of common foods. An index is appended.

604.   Schell, Merle. **The Chinese Salt-Free Diet Cookbook**. New York: New American Library, 1985. 348p. ISBN 0453004911.
Featured is a wide range of recipes made with a homemade soy sauce substitute, and substitutes for other popular sauces used in Chinese cooking. Each recipe has information on calories, sodium, carbohydrate, and fat.

605.   Wilson, Roger H. L., and Nancy Wilson. **Please Pass the Salt: A Manual for Low-Salt Eaters**. Philadelphia, Pa.: George F. Stickley, 1983. 182p. ISBN 0893130273.
This is an excellent book with recipes that include sodium, potassium, protein, and energy values for those on low-sodium diets.

SMOOTH DIETS

606.   Rosenthal, Gail. **Smoooth [sic] Food: For All with Dental Problems ... and Everyone Else**. Needham, Mass.: Galens, 1985?. 123p. ($7.95, Galens, 35 South Street, Needham, MA 02192).
These recipes for patients unable to chew include beverages, sauces, appetizers, salads and relishes, vegetables, main courses, and desserts. There is an index.

607.   Wilson, J. Randy. **Non-Chew Cookbook**. Glenwood Springs, Colo.: Wilson Publishing, Inc., 1985?. 200p. ($16.50, Wilson Publishing, Inc., P.O. Box 2190, Glenwood Springs, CO 81602-2190).
"The cookbook contains recipes for soups, beverages, main dishes, vegetables, and desserts. A nutrition computer analysis performed at Colorado State University, Fort Collins, provides nutrition information for each recipe. There is also a chapter of tips on how to adapt favorite recipes, how to eat a restaurant meal, and how to satisfy cravings. An index is also provided" (*Journal of the American Dietetic Association* 86 [1986]: 292).

VEGETARIAN DIETS

Bibliographies and Guides

608.   Dyer, Judith C. **Vegetarianism: An Annotated Bibliography**. Metuchen, N.J.: Scarecrow Press, 1982. 280p. ISBN 081081532X.

Dyer's book is the most extensive bibliography available on the subject of vegetarianism. It has a section on early works organized by time periods, and one on recent works, organized by subjects: general interest materials; history of vegetarianism; athletics; diet planning (even for pets); institutional food service; food technology; children's materials; reference sources; position papers; philosophical, ethical, and religious aspects; and medical aspects. An appendix lists vegetarian cookbooks. There are subject and author indexes.

609. Rose, Joel. **The Vegetarian Connection**. New York: Facts on File, 1985. 182p. ISBN 081601003X.

Judging from the title, this directory and guide should contain extensive information sources on vegetarian diets. However, many of the sections are filled with irrelevant material, some of it medically or scientifically questionable, much of it peripheral. For instance, a listing of newspapers and magazines omits *Vegetarian Times*, but includes *Nutrition Today*, a periodical which has on occasion been perceived as hostile to vegetarianism. "Filled with omissions, poor choices, and hopelessly out-of-date materials" (*Vegetarian Times* 98 [October 1985]: 56).

610. Schwartz, Diane. **Vegetable Cookery: A Selected Bibliography**. Bronx, N.Y.: Council on Botanical and Horticultural Libraries, 1978. 24p. (Plant Bibliography, No. 2).

This lists approximately 125 vegetarian and vegetable cookbooks selected because "they offer tasty, appealing and nutritious alternatives to the customary animal protein diet."

611. Society for Nutrition Education. Resource Center. **Vegetarians and Vegetarian Diets**. rev. ed. Oakland, Calif.: Society for Nutrition Education, 1982. 10p. (Nutrition Education Resource Series, No. 8).

Selected books, pamphlets, audiovisual aids, and periodical articles on vegetarian diets are listed in this pamphlet.

Handbooks, Manuals, and Other Data Compilations

612. Doyle, Rodger. **The Vegetarian Handbook: A Guide to Vegetarian Nutrition and Foods**. New York: Crown Publishers, 1979. 182p. ISBN 0517534703.

This basic book on vegetarian nutrition emphasizes good eating throughout the life cycle. It contains a few basic recipes for entrées, information on common food myths, a nutrient analysis of typical vegetarian menus, and tables with principal sources of calcium, iron, B-12, and sodium. There are notes and an index. "This well-researched and comprehensive guide to vegetarian living is a practical reference for anyone who is a vegetarian or contemplating this way of life" (*Life and Health* 95 [April 1980]: 27).

613. Nutrition Company. **Diet Planning for the Vegetarian**. Tallahassee, Fla.: Nutrition Company, 1984. 33p. ($4.50, Nutrition Company, P.O. Box 11102, Tallahassee, FL 32302).

This is a useful booklet for counseling patients on a vegetarian diet. It has exchange lists and sample menus for vegan and lacto-ovo-vegetarian diets as well as food composition information for foods frequently used by vegetarians.

614.   Robertson, Laurel, Carol Flinders, and Brian Ruppenthal. **The New Laurel's Kitchen: A Handbook for Vegetarian Cookery and Nutrition**. Berkeley, Calif.: Ten Speed Press, 1986. 511p. ISBN 0898151678; 089815166X (pbk).

A complete vegetarian cookbook and a handbook of nutrition, the tenth anniversary edition of this well-known volume has gone through substantial revision with a greater emphasis on health promotion through diet. One of the few cookbooks that actually complies with the dietary recommendations of the American Heart Association, the American Cancer Society, and the U.S. Dietary Goals, this edition contains many new recipes which are lower in fat with a greater percentage of calories from complex carbohydrates. The new "Food Guide" is primarily grain and vegetable based, with less emphasis on dairy products and legumes, which may make it difficult for certain groups of vegetarians, such as children and pregnant women, to receive an adequate amount of all the essential nutrients. This excellent resource includes numerous references to recent nutrition studies and an extensive food composition table which includes foods common to vegetarian and health enthusiasts' diets often difficult to locate elsewhere. An index is included.

615.   Smith, Elizabeth B. **Vegetarian Meal-Planning Guide: A Lacto-Ovo-Vegetarian Diet**. Winnipeg, Man.: Hyperion Press, 1979. 104p. ISBN 092053404X.

"Extensive information about the advantages of a vegetarian diet, explicit menu planning instructions, shopping tips, and thorough cooking techniques.... Basic nutrition, protein quality and protein composition in foods, and protein supplementation.... Includes many international, vegetable-protein-centered recipes. An appendix, a list of recommended books, and an index complete the book" (*Journal of the American Dietetic Association* 75 [1979]: 509).

Dietary Advice and Cookbooks

616.   Cottrell, Edyth Young. **The Oats, Peas, Beans & Barley Cookbook**. 2nd ed. Santa Barbara, Calif.: Woodbridge Press, 1980. 267p. ISBN 0912800852.

This is a totally from scratch, whole foods approach to vegetarian cooking, with nutrition as a major component. It includes recipes of all types for family-style meals ranging from breakfast foods and soyfoods to desserts, information on meal planning, and a nutrient analysis of recipes. Recipes tend to be labor intensive and may not be suited to those who demand convenience and speed. The author was a research nutritionist at Loma Linda University. The index is by categories of foods only.

617.   Lappé, Frances Moore. **Diet for a Small Planet**. 10th anniversary ed. New York: Ballantine Books, 1982. 496p. ISBN 0345306910.

Sometimes referred to as the book that started the "nutrition revolution," this is indeed a history making book. Lappé popularized the idea of complementing vegetable proteins to create a plant protein mix equivalent to the quality of animal protein. The book helped to shape the food attitudes of a whole generation, providing the philosophical and scientific framework for eating low on the food chain by stressing the wastefulness of meat production and by "proving" that it was possible to derive adequate nourishment from the plant kingdom. In this expanded tenth anniversary edition, Lappé has modified some of her views on complementing, stating that it is no longer necessary to complement proteins at each meal. As before, the book has numerous recipes, charts, and tables for combining complementary vegetable proteins. A bibliography and an index are included.

618.   Moore, Shirley R., and Mary P. Byers. **A Vegetarian Diet: What It Is: How to Make It Healthful and Enjoyable**. Santa Barbara, Calif.: Woodbridge Press, 1978. 120p. ISBN 0912800488.

"This book explains what a vegetarian diet is and how to make it healthful and enjoyable. Included are sample menus and some recipes" (*Your Life and Health* 96 [November 1981]: 30).

619.   Szilard, Paula, and Juliana J. Woo. **The Electric Vegetarian: Natural Cooking the Food Processor Way**. Boulder, Colo.: Johnson Publishing Co.; distr., Berkeley, Calif.: Ten Speed Press, 1980. 214p. ISBN 0933472501.

This nutrition-oriented vegetarian cookbook greatly simplifies from scratch, whole foods cooking by using the food processor (although many of the recipes can be prepared manually). A large number of the recipes are for the lacto-ovo vegetarian, but there are a substantial number suitable for the vegan. There is an emphasis on nutritious foods which taste good. A system of symbol codes greatly simplifies complementing proteins and a nutrition chapter discusses important nutrients likely to be deficient in a vegetarian diet. Recipes containing major protein foods include information on the number of grams of protein per serving. There are two indexes, one for subjects and recipe titles and one for major ingredients.

WEIGHT LOSS DIETS

Because of the large number of weight loss diet books on the market, and because so many are full of gimmickry, hyperbole, and unreliable information, this section lists only items that critically evaluate diets.

620.   Berland, Theodore. **Rating the Diets**. New York: Crown Publishers, 1983. 250p. ISBN 0517408392.

This is one of a series of periodic reviews of the latest weight loss diets. It includes criticisms of many currently used fad diets, with rebuttals by their proponents.

621.   Dazzi, Andrea, and Johanna Dwyer. "Nutritional Analysis of Popular Weight-Reduction Diets in Books and Magazines." **International Journal of Eating Disorders** 3 (Winter 1984): 61-79.

Critical evaluations of 12 current weight loss diets are provided.

622.   Fisher, Michelle C., and Paul A. Lachance. "Nutrition Evaluation of Published Weight-Reduction Diets." **Journal of the American Dietetic Association** 85 (1985): 450-54.

This is an evaluation of the nutritional adequacy of 14 popular diets.

623.   Storey, Rita, et al. **Popular Diets: How They Rate**. Santa Monica, Calif.: Los Angeles District, California Dietetic Association, 1982. 56p. ISBN 0943458005.
    Evaluations of 14 weight loss diets by professional dietitians are given here.

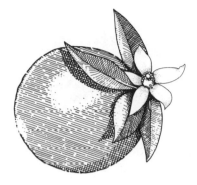

Part V

FOOD SCIENCE
AND
TECHNOLOGY

18
General Reference Sources

LOCATING RESEARCH —
INDEXING/ABSTRACTING SERVICES

The International Food Information Service (IFIS) is the major organization providing information services to food scientists and technologists on a worldwide basis. It was founded in 1968 in response to an acute need for an indexing/abstracting service specifically aimed at the food science and technology community. Currently there are four major partner organizations which share the role of sponsor: The Commonwealth Agricultural Bureaux (CAB) in the United Kingdom, the Gesellschaft für Information und Dokumentation in the Federal Republic of Germany, the Institute of Food Technologists (IFT) in the United States, and the Centrum voor Landbouwpublikaties en Landbouwdocumentatie (PUDOC) in the Netherlands.

IFIS's major service to the food science and technology community is the production of *Food Science and Technology Abstracts*. New indexing/abstracting services have been produced or are planned in areas where there has been an ongoing need, for instance in the field of packaging, viticulture and enology, and cereal science.

Other IFIS services are the publication of bibliographies, a document delivery service supplying most items abstracted in *Food Science and Technology Abstracts*, computer literature search services direct to users and through major database vendors, and a current awareness service in the form of SDI searches of items newly added to the FS&TA database.

Included in this section are indexing/abstracting services and online databases providing access to the food science and technology literature in general. A person looking for published research on a subject in the area of food science and technology will in all probability search *Food Science and Technology Abstracts* first. However, for any given area within this broad field, indexing/abstracting services mentioned in other parts of this book may be equally suitable or even more appropriate.

Indexing/Abstracting Services

624. **Food Science and Technology Abstracts**. Vol. 1- . Shinfield, England: International Food Information Service, 1969- . monthly. ISSN 0015-6574.

This monthly abstracting service provides international coverage of over 1,800 journals, patents, standards, conference proceedings, books, and miscellaneous publications in food science and technology. (See figure 8.)

Online Equivalent: Food Science and Technology Abstracts.

Arrangement: Approximately 1,400 abstracts are contained in each monthly issue. These are numerically arranged within the following broad subject categories: "Basic Food Science," "Food Microbiology," "General Food Economics and Statistics," "Food Engineering," "Commodity Technologies," "Alcoholic and Nonalcoholic Beverages," "Fruits, Vegetables and Nuts," "Cocoa and Chocolate Products," "Sugars, Syrups, Starches and Candy," "Cereals and Bakery Products," "Fats, Oils and Margarine," "Milk and Dairy Products," "Fish and Marine Products," "Meat, Poultry and Game," "Food Additives," "Spices and Condiments," and "Standards, Laws and Regulations."

Indexes: Subject and author indexes appear in each issue and are cumulated annually.

List of Periodicals Indexed: A list of periodicals indexed appears in the January issue of each year.

IFIS Thesaurus: This lists the official vocabulary used in indexing.

Comments: Though most nutrition literature is out of the scope for *FS&TA*, this is a good source for chemical composition, nutrient composition, and processing as it affects nutrients.

625. **Packaging Science and Technology Abstracts—Referatedienst Verpackung**. Vol. 1- . Frankfurt am Main, W. Germany: International Food Information Service, in cooperation with Frauenhofer-Institut für Lebensmitteltechnologie und Verpackung, 1982- . monthly. ISSN 0722-3218.

Identical in format to *Food Science and Technology Abstracts*, *PS&TA* covers literature on all aspects of packaging from about 200 periodicals. Books, pamphlets, standards and specifications, legislation, conference papers, and other types of materials are also included.

Arrangement: The abstracts are in English and in German and are arranged in 25 sections covering such subjects as economic aspects, environmental aspects, standardization, design, preserving materials, types of goods to be packaged, packaging machines, operations such as weighing, filling, filling and sealing, testing, interactions between packages and contents, transportation, etc.

Indexes: Author and subject indexes are included. There are actually two distinct subject indexes, one in English and one in German.

FOOD SCIENCE AND TECHNOLOGY ABSTRACTS

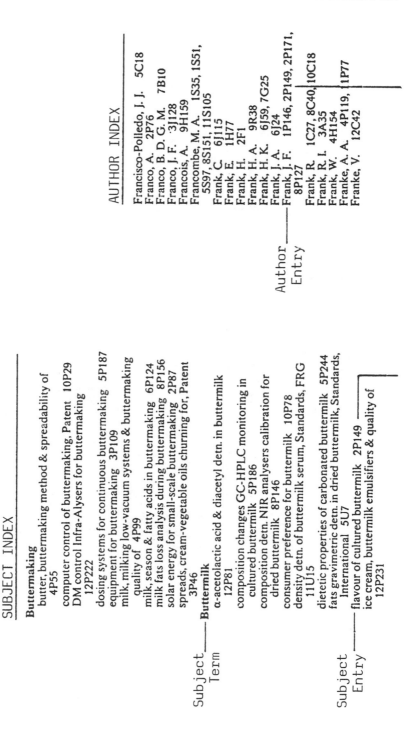

SUBJECT INDEX

Buttermaking
butter, buttermaking method & spreadability of 4P55
computer control of buttermaking, Patent 10P29
DM control Infra-Alysers for buttermaking 12P222
dosing systems for continuous buttermaking 5P187
equipment for buttermaking 3P109
milk, milking low-vacuum systems & buttermaking quality of 4P99
milk, season & fatty acids in buttermaking 6P124
milk fats loss analysis during buttermaking 8P156
solar energy for small-scale buttermaking 2P87
spreads, cream-vegetable oils churning for, Patent 3P46

Buttermilk
α-acetolactic acid & diacetyl detn. in buttermilk 12P81
composition changes GC-HPLC monitoring in cultured buttermilk 5P186
composition detn. NIR analysers calibration for dried buttermilk 8P146
consumer preference for buttermilk 10P78
density detn. of buttermilk serum, Standards, FRG 11U15
dietetic properties of carbonated buttermilk 5P244
fats gravimetric detn. in dried buttermilk, Standards, International 5U7
flavour of cultured buttermilk 2P149
ice cream, buttermilk emulsifiers & quality of 12P231

Subject Term

Subject Entry

AUTHOR INDEX

Francisco-Polledo, J. J.   5C18
Franco, A.   2P76
Franco, B. D. G. M.   7B10
Franco, J. F.   3J128
Francois, A.   9H159
Francombe, M. A.   1S35, 1S51, 5S97, 8S151, 11S105
Frank, C   6J115
Frank, E.   1H77
Frank, H.   2F1
Frank, H. A.   9R38
Frank, H. K.   6J59, 7G25
Frank, J. A.   6J24
Frank, J. F.   1P146, 2P149, 2P171, 8P127
Frank, R.   1C27, 8C40, 10C18
Frank, R. I.   3A35
Frank, W.   4H154
Franke, A. A.   4P119, 11P77
Franke, V.   12C42

Author Entry

(Fig. 8 continues on page 228.)

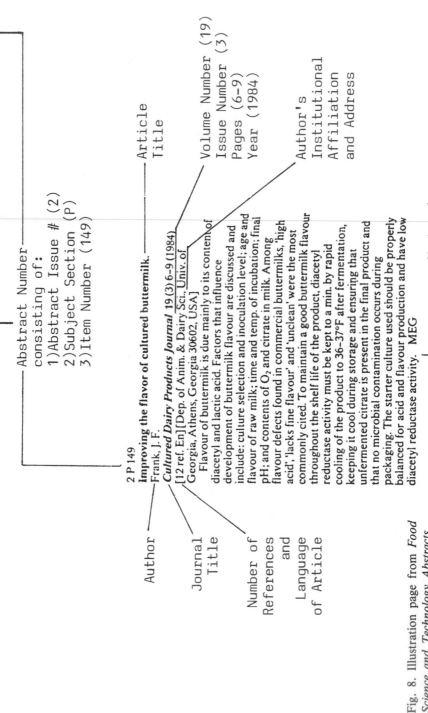

Abstract Number
consisting of:
1) Abstract Issue # (2)
2) Subject Section (P)
3) Item Number (149)

Article Title

Volume Number (19)
Issue Number (3)
Pages (6-9)
Year (1984)

Author's Institutional Affiliation and Address

Author

Journal Title

Number of References and Language of Article

2 P 149
Improving the flavor of cultured buttermilk.
Frank, J.F.
Cultured Dairy Products Journal 19 (3) 6–9 (1984)
[12 ref. En] [Dep. of Anim. & Dairy Sci., Univ. of Georgia, Athens, Georgia 30602, USA]

Flavour of buttermilk is due mainly to its content of diacetyl and lactic acid. Factors that influence development of buttermilk flavour are discussed and include: culture selection and inoculation level; age and flavour of raw milk; time and temp. of incubation; final pH; and contents of O_2 and citrate in milk. Among flavour defects found in commercial buttermilks, 'high acid', 'lacks fine flavour' and 'unclean' were the most commonly cited. To maintain a good buttermilk flavour throughout the shelf life of the product, diacetyl reductase activity must be kept to a min. by rapid cooling of the product to 36–37°F after fermentation, keeping it cool during storage and ensuring that unfermented citrate is present in the final product and that no microbial contamination occurs during packaging. The starter culture used should be properly balanced for acid and flavour production and have low diacetyl reductase activity.   MEG

Abstract

Fig. 8. Illustration page from *Food Science and Technology Abstracts.*
Reprinted by permission of International Food Information Service.

Online Databases

626. Food Science and Technology Abstracts (FS&TA)
This database corresponds to the printed abstracting service of the same name and covers all aspects of the food science and technology literature from 1969 on. Topics included parallel those in the printed product, including basic food science, food microbiology, food hygiene and toxicology, packaging, individual foods or food groups, and food additives. FS&TA covers 1,800 journals from 75 countries as well as standards, patents, and legislation on a more limited basis. Books are also included. In addition to the indexes in the printed version, the database can be searched by corporate name, publication type, and language.

627. Foods Adlibra
This is a database of literature related to the food industry, produced by General Mills and dating from 1974. It contains citations on all aspects of the food industry and trade including new products, marketing, agribusiness, retailing, packaging and importing, as well as major scientific and technological advances. It covers over 250 periodicals. An additional 500 research journals are scanned for relevant materials. It also provides indexing of food-related patents from the *Official Gazette* of the United States Patent Office.

BIBLIOGRAPHIES AND GUIDES

There are numerous one-time, specialized bibliographies available in the field. The National Agricultural Library has issued a large number of brief bibliographics on special topics in its Quick Bibliography Series. Many are on food science subjects of current interest, including food irradiation, sugar substitutes, and alternative sweeteners. The International Food Information Service has compiled more than 50 specialized bibliographies based on searches of the FS&TA database. These are issued under the collective title: *Food Annotated Bibliographies*. Topics range from acidulants to microwaves in food processing.

628. Green, Syd. Keyguide to Information Sources in Food Science and Technology. London, New York: Mansell, 1985. 231p. ISBN 0720117488.
This excellent, extensive, and very useful guide to information sources in the field covers all types of literature including theses and dissertations, technical reports, patents, journal literature, conferences, indexing/abstracting services, bibliographies, directories, encyclopedias, tables, handbooks, methods of analysis, government publications, and translations. It is particularly strong in food industry sources relating to specific commodities. One would have expected a British emphasis, but the coverage is international for English-language materials. There is an index.

629. Lehman, Clifford. GRAS (Generally Recognized As Safe) Food Ingredients: A Bibliography with Abstracts. updated ed. Springfield, Va.: National Technical Information Service, 1979. 2v. NTIS/PS-79/0650.

Based on a search of the NTIS database, this bibliography with abstracts describes about 650 reports relating to food additives on the GRAS list. An update has been issued for July 1979-June 1985 (PB 861631/LAK).

630.   Lilley, G. P., ed. **Information Sources in Agriculture and Food Science**. London: Butterworths, 1981. 603p. (Butterworths Guides to Food Information Sources). ISBN 0408106123.

Written in narrative form, this guide is devoted to agricultural reference sources. The food science chapter is brief.

631.   Nakazawa, Ryeoji. **Bibliography of Fermentation Organisms**. Tokyo: Keigaku Publishing Co., 1970-1973. 3v.

This English-language bibliography covers the period 1941 to 1965.

632.   Niskern, Nancy. **Food Additives**. Washington, D.C.: Library of Congress, 1982. 9p. (LC Tracer Bullet TB 82-1). LC33.10:82-1.

This is a brief guide to selected books, reviews, government publications, major indexing/abstracting services, journal titles, and selected articles on the subject of food additives.

633.   United Nations Industrial Development Organization. **Information Sources on the Canning Industry**. New York: United Nations, 1975. 83p. (UNIDO Guides to Information Sources, No. 19).

International and national information sources of practical value relating to the canning industry are presented. The guide covers UN, national, international, and regional organizations; directories; sources of statistics; basic reference materials; monograph series; current periodicals; indexing and abstracting services; selected films and film catalogs; and miscellaneous sources of information. Selected items are annotated.

634.   United Nations Industrial Development Organization. **Information Sources on the Packaging Industry**. New York: United Nations, 1977. 110p. (UNIDO Guides to Information Sources, No. 27).

Practical international and national information sources relating to the packaging industry are included here. Covered are UN, national, international, and regional organizations; directories; sources of statistics; basic reference materials; monograph series; current periodicals; indexing and abstracting services; selected films and film catalogs; and miscellaneous sources of information. Selected items are annotated.

635.   Wallace, Richard E. **Food Science and Technology: A Bibliography of Recommended Materials**. Beltsville, Md.: National Agricultural Library, 1978. 231p. A106.110:F73.

Originally compiled for a Food and Nutrition Division Seminar at the annual SLA meeting, June 1976 and updated through 1977 by NAL, this bibliography covers primarily books on basic food science and technology, microbiology, toxicology, economics and statistics, nutrition, marketing, advertising, packaging, alcoholic and nonalcoholic beverages, fruits, vegetables, nuts, starch, sweeteners, cereals and bakery products, fats and oils, milk and dairy products, egg and egg products, spices, herbs, flavor materials, food additives, fish, meat, and poultry.

636. Wylie-Rosett, Judith, et al. **Aspartame, a Summary and Annotated Bibliography.** Chicago: Diabetes Care and Education Practice Group, American Dietetic Association, 1982. 16p.

This highly selective bibliography contains lengthy annotations.

DICTIONARIES

Bibliographies and Guides to Dictionaries

637. Lück, Erich. **Bibliography of Dictionaries and Vocabularies on Food, Nutrition, and Cookery.** Frankfurt, W. Germany: International Food Information Service, 1985. 139p. (FSTA Reference Series, No. 4). ISBN 3922961046 (pbk).

This bibliography lists 436 monolingual, bilingual, or multilingual dictionaries, thesauri, encyclopedias, and vocabularies. The arrangement is by a subject classification system similar to that used in *Food Science and Technology Abstracts*. Entries are annotated with the number of terms included and other descriptive phrases used to show that they include tables, illustrations, bibliographies, etc. The material listed is predominantly in food science and technology. Author and subject indexes are included.

Food Science and Technology Dictionaries

638. Igoe, Robert S. **Dictionary of Food Ingredients.** New York: Van Nostrand Reinhold, 1983. 173p. ISBN 0442240023.

Over 1,000 definitions stress functional categories and uses are given. These functional categories are defined and described in a second, smaller section following the definitions. A bibliography is included.

639. Lück, Erich. **The Compact Dictionary of Food Technology: English-German.** 1985 ed. Hamburg, W. Germany: Behr's Verlag, 1985. 443p. ISBN 392252883X.

The German title is *Kompaktwörterbuch der Lebensmitteltechnologie.*

640. Morton, Ian Douglas. **Elsevier's Dictionary of Food Science and Technology: In Four Languages, English, French, Spanish, German.** Amsterdam, Netherlands: Elsevier Scientific Publishing Co., 1977. 207p. ISBN 0444415599.

Morton's dictionary lists 2,087 English-language terms with French, Spanish, and German equivalents. There are indexes in each of these languages as well as one giving Latin names of plants and animals.

641. Winter, Ruth. **A Consumer's Dictionary of Food Additives.** New York: Crown Publishing, 1984. 260p. ISBN 0517552876.

Intended for the nonspecialist, this dictionary provides approximately 1,800 definitions of varying length. A brief introductory section sets the stage and discusses basic categories of additives.

ENCYCLOPEDIAS

642. Hall, Carl S., ed. **Encyclopedia of Food Engineering**. 2nd ed. Westport, Conn.: AVI, 1986. 882p. ISBN 0870554514.

Devoted to engineering aspects of food processing operations, this alphabetically arranged encyclopedia has entries on equipment, facilities, machinery, processes, relevant engineering concepts, and physical properties of selected foods. Entries vary in length from several paragraphs to several pages. Most have bibliographies. There is no index.

643. Johnson, Arnold Harvey, and Martin S. Peterson, eds. **Encyclopedia of Food Technology**. Westport, Conn.: AVI, 1974. 993p. (Encyclopedia of Food Technology and Food Science Series, Vol. 2). ISBN 0870551574.

This encyclopedia contains roughly 275 entries, dealing with all aspects of food technology, including biographical information for important individuals in the history of the field. There are entries under individual foods, processes, food components, and flavorings. Even major awards and their recipients are listed under "Awards." Articles are accompanied by bibliographies. An index is included.

644. Leung, Albert Y. **Encyclopedia of Common Natural Ingredients Used in Food, Drugs, and Cosmetics**. New York: Wiley, 1979. 409p. ISBN 0471049549.

This encyclopedia covers about 300 natural ingredients currently used in food, cosmetics, and drugs. Each entry gives genus and species, synonyms, general description, chemical composition, pharmacologic or biological activity, uses, commercial preparation, regulatory status, and references. The arrangement is alphabetical. It has a general index and a chemical index.

645. Peterson, Martin S., and Arnold H. Johnson. **Encyclopedia of Food Science**. Westport, Conn.: AVI, 1978. 1005p. (Encyclopedia of Food Technology and Food Science Series, Vol. 3). ISBN 0870552279.

This volume consists of short, individually authored articles in an alphabetical arrangement, each with a brief bibliography. A section entitled "Food Science around the World" includes information on food science and the food industry in various countries. A brief glossary of food science terms and temperature conversion charts are appended. There is an index.

HANDBOOKS, MANUALS, AND OTHER DATA COMPILATIONS

646. American Frozen Food Institute. **Frozen Food Pack Statistics**. Washington, D.C.: American Frozen Food Institute, 1946- . annual. ISSN 0469-7405.

Calendar year production statistics of frozen foods are listed by individual commodity.

647. American Institute of Baking. **Basic Food Plant Sanitation Manual**. 3rd rev. ed. Manhattan, Kans.: American Institute of Baking, 1979. 255p.

This concise manual on topics fundamental to food plant sanitation includes material on regulatory aspects, inspections, liability, good manufacturing practice in processing, packaging and holding food, sanitation programs, and insect and rodent infestation.

648. Bryan, Frank L. **Diseases Transmitted by Foods: (A Classification and a Summary).** 2nd ed. Atlanta, Ga.: Department of Health and Human Services, Public Health Service, Centers for Disease Control, Center for Professional Development and Training, 1982. 101p. (HHS Publication, No. (CDC) 83-8237). HE20.7002:F73/982.

"This reference summarizes the following data: etiologic agents and their nature, sources and important reservoirs, epidemiology, foods frequently involved in outbreaks, specimens and samples to take in outbreak investigations, laboratory approaches and general control measures." Included are a bibliography and an index of diseases.

649. Buell, Norman S., et al. **Safety and Health Reference Handbook for the Food and Beverage Industry.** Indianapolis, Ind.: Bosley Studios, 1979. 700p.

This extensive treatment of all aspects of safety and accident prevention in food and beverage plants emphasizes hazard control and worker education. An extensive appendix, a bibliography, a glossary, and an index are included.

650. Chadwick, Ann Collins. **A Manual for Successful Resolution of Consumer Complaints in the Food Industry.** Washington, D.C.: Food Processing Institute, 1983. 32p.

"This manual is addressed primarily to those persons responsible for the complaint response function. In addition, it can serve as a guide to management in reviewing and establishing complaint handling policies and procedures."

651. Chan, Harvey T., ed. **Handbook of Tropical Foods.** New York: Marcel Dekker, 1983. 639p. ISBN 0824718801.

This handbook deals with 15 major commodities or groups of commodities from the tropics, such as amaranth, cassava, palm oil, papaya, macadamia nuts, etc. While the emphasis is on horticultural aspects, articles contain information on nutrient composition, products, and uses. There is an author and subject index.

652. Charalambous, George, ed. **Handbook of Food and Beverage Stability: Chemical, Biochemical, Microbiological, and Nutritional Aspects.** Orlando, Fla.: Academic Press, 1986. 840p. ISBN 0121690709.

This handbook contains 17 individually authored chapters with detailed information on storage characteristics and chemical and microbiological changes of specific foods, such as bread, cheeses, fruits, meat, fish, coffee, chocolate, wine, and other alcoholic beverages. Numerous tables appear throughout. The chapter on fish and shellfish alone includes tables over 200 pages long. The index in the back of the book excludes material in the fish and shellfish chapter, which has its own index.

653. **A Complete Course in Canning: A Technical Reference Book and Text-book for Students of Food Technology, Food Plant Managers, Product Research and Development Specialists, Food Brokers, Technical Salesmen, Food Equipment Manufacturers and Salesmen, and Food Industry Suppliers.** 11th ed. Baltimore, Md.: The Canning Trade, 1981. 2v.

The first volume contains general material on canning, including information on plant location, steam requirements, equipment, sanitation, waste disposal, food laws, regulations and standards, microbiology, containers, quality control, canning operations, sterilization, retort pouch packaging, warehousing, spoilage, and ingredients. Also included is an appendix with temperature conversion tables, weights and measures, normal pH ranges of canned goods, a glossary of terms, and a subject index.

The second volume deals with specific canned products. Covered are over 40 vegetables, about 25 fruits, juices and soft drinks, fish and seafood, over 50 meats and meat products, soups, and miscellaneous types of products. The tables and glossary from the first volume are repeated here. There is a subject index.

654. Fazzalari, F. A., ed. **Compilation of Odor and Taste Threshold Data**. Philadelphia, Pa.: American Society for Testing and Materials, 1978. 497p. (ASTM Data Series, No. 48A). ISBN 0504801036.

This compilation presents data on odor and taste thresholds, with bibliographic citations. Includes separate listings by chemical (with data and bibliography), by item or code number, molecular formula, Wiswesser Line Notation, and journal codes.

655. Fenaroli, Giovanni. **Handbook of Flavor Ingredients: Adapted from the Italian Language Works of Giovanni Fenaroli**. 2nd ed. Edited, translated, and revised by Thomas E. Furia and Nicolo Bellanca. Cleveland, Ohio: CRC Press, Inc., 1975. 2v. ISBN 0878195335.

This set covers natural as well as synthetic flavoring agents with FDA regulatory status and Flavor and Extract Manufacturers Association proposals. It contains an extensive bibliography on natural flavorings and extensive references in the table of synthetic flavors. An index appears in each volume.

656. **Flavor and Fragrance Materials — 1985: Worldwide Reference List of Materials Used in Compounding Flavors and Fragrances**. 4th ed. Wheaton, Ill.: Allured Publishing, 1985. 303p. ISBN 0931710073.

This compilation is based on the computer files of the Flavor and Extract Manufacturer's Association (FEMA).

657. **Food Products Formulary**. Vol. 1-3. Westport, Conn.: AVI, 1974-1982. ISBN 0870551523 (vol. 1); 0870551701 (vol. 2); 0870552033 (vol. 3).

Volume 1 is entitled *Meats, Poultry, Fish, Shellfish*, volume 2 is *Cereals, Baked Goods, Dairy and Egg Products*, and volume 3 is *Fruit, Vegetable and Nut Products*. The set includes recipes for a great variety of commercial food products such as sausages, smoked and cured meats, fish and seafood products, cereal and baked goods of all types, cheeses and ice creams, frozen fruits and vegetables, jams, jellies, sauces, fruit confections, vegetable juices and purées, dried and dehydrated vegetables, pickled vegetables, vegetable soups, as well as peanut and other nut products.

658. **Food Products Formulary**. Vol. 1- . 2nd ed. Westport, Conn.: AVI, 1982- . ISBN 0870553925 (vol. 1); 0870554042 (vol. 4).

This new edition has a more extensive section of new recipes using plant protein extenders in meat products and meat dishes. Individual volumes are not being issued in sequence.

659. Freydberg, Nicholas. **The Food Additives Book**. Toronto: Bantam Books, 1982. 717p. ISBN 0553013769 (pbk).

Intended for the consumer, this compendium of additives in name brand foods also provides information on the additives themselves and their relative safety.

660. Furia, Thomas E., ed. **CRC Handbook of Food Additives**. 2nd ed. Cleveland, Ohio: CRC Press, Inc., 1972-1980. 2v. ISBN 084930542X (vol. 1); 0849305438 (vol. 2).

In volume 1 additives are discussed by broad categories (e.g., enzymes, antioxidants, colors, acidulants, etc.). A lengthy table identifies the regulatory status of food additives, giving pertinent FEMA numbers and FDA regulation numbers. Bibliographies appear at the ends of sections. There is an index. Volume 2 updates volume 1.

661. Glaubitz, Max, and Richard Koch. **Atlas der Gärungsorganismen: Leitfaden für Mikrobiologische Übungen an Fach- und Hochschulen und für die Betriebskontrolle in der Gärungs- und Lebensmitteltechnik**. 4. aufl. Berlin: Parey, 1983. 90p. ISBN 3489616146.

This atlas of fermenting organisms contains illustrations of nearly 100 yeasts, fungi, and bacteria used in the food and beverage industry. The accompanying descriptive text is in German only.

662. Heath, Henry B. **Source Book of Flavors**. Westport, Conn.: AVI, 1981. 863p. (AVI Sourcebook and Handbook Series, Vol. 2). ISBN 0870553704.

This is an extensive compilation of information on flavor chemistry and the flavor industry, natural flavoring ingredients, including fruit flavors, herbs and spices, plant materials, essential oils, chemical flavorings, food colorants, manufacturing methods, regulations in foreign countries, and toxicology and consumer safety. It contains an extensive bibliography and a section devoted to flavoring formulations. There is a subject index.

663. Jacobson, Michael F. **The Complete Eater's Digest and Nutrition Scoreboard**. Garden City, N.Y.: Anchor Press/Doubleday, 1986. 392p. ISBN 0385182457.

Intended for a lay audience, this book is actually a complete revision of two of Jacobson's previous works: *Eater's Digest*, a book about food additives, and *Nutrition Scoreboard*, a general book on nutrition outlining a method for scoring the nutritional quality of foods, giving "credit" for nutrients and deducting for undesirable qualities such as sodium and high fat content.

The Complete Eater's Digest is a useful source of information about commonly used food additives with emphasis on their safety. It contains background information about why additives are used, how they are tested, and what agencies are responsible for protecting consumers against harmful substances in food. The major part of the book is an alphabetical list of specific food additives with information on how they are used and their relative safety. References to the literature are included. Also included are a glossary of terms, a bibliography, and an index.

664. Marmion, Daniel M. **Handbook of U.S. Colorants for Foods, Drugs, and Cosmetics**. 2nd ed. New York: Wiley, 1984. 466p. ISBN 0471093122.

This attempt to gather together information on coloring agents widely distributed in the literature provides general background information as well as data on individual colorants and analytical techniques.

665. National Research Council. Committee on GRAS List Survey, Phase III. **The 1977 Survey of Industry on the Use of Food Additives**. Springfield, Va.: National Technical Information Service, 1980. 3v. PB80-113418.

"Detailed information with regard to the data collected in the 1977 Survey of the Industry on the Use of Food Additives ... under sponsorship of the Food and Drug Administration.... Volume 1 presents an overview of the entire survey.... Volume 2 contains aggregated food additive data from the survey including annual poundage, reported technical effects, and use levels in greater than 200 food subcategories. Volume 3 contains estimates of the daily intake of substances reported in the survey."

666. Ockerman, Herbert W. **Source Book for Food Scientists**. Westport, Conn.: AVI, 1978. 926p. (AVI Sourcebook and Handbook Series, Vol. 1). ISBN 0870552287.

Part 1, about 300 pages long, consists of a dictionary of terms and relevant data on properties, formulas, uses, etc.

Part 2 provides data on the properties and composition of various types of foods or food ingredients (e.g., acidulants, honey, cheese), and miscellaneous information such as cooking times and yield of dry beans, beef cuts, roasting times and temperatures, and fish and shellfish composition. Although this section is arranged in alphabetical order, it is not easy to locate information without an index.

667. Paine, Frank A., and Heather Y. Payne. **A Handbook of Food Packaging**. Glasgow, Scotland: Leonard Hill, 1983. 394p. ISBN 0249441640.

This volume is divided into three parts: "Materials and Machinery"; "Packaging Needs of Foods"; and "Development, Evaluation, and Control." There is an index.

668. Prescott, Samuel Cate. **Prescott and Dunn's Industrial Microbiology**. 4th ed. Edited by Gerald Reed. Westport, Conn.: AVI, 1982. 883p. ISBN 0870553747.

The revised edition of this standard work covers chiefly those fermentation processes involved in food production—the making of cheese and other fermented dairy products, lactic acid fermentations (sauerkraut, pickles and olives), fermented sausage, yeast-raised baked goods, wine and brandy, beer, alcohol as a beverage and as a fuel, oriental fermented foods (soy sauce, tempeh, and natto), vinegar, baker's yeast, amino acids, microbial biomass, single cell protein, and other products. There is an index.

669. Rechcigl, Miroslav, ed. **CRC Handbook of Foodborne Diseases of Biological Origin**. Boca Raton, Fla.: CRC Press, Inc., 1983. 518p. (CRC Series in Nutrition and Food). ISBN 0849339642.

"An overview of different biological agents and important toxins that may cause diseases on ingestion with food or water." Covered are bacterial toxins;

mycotoxins; algal toxins; protozoal, helminth, and shellfish toxins; aflatoxins; brucellosis, etc. Extensive bibliographies are included.

670. Schwimmer, Sigmund. **Source Book of Food Enzymology.** Westport, Conn.: AVI, 1981. 967p. (AVI Sourcebook and Handbook Series). ISBN 0870553690.

This extensive compendium of information on the role of enzymes in food production covers basics of enzymology; enzyme production; control of enzyme action; enzyme action on food color, flavor, and texture; enzyme action in food transformations; the role of enzymes in protein modification; health and safety aspects; and the use of enzymes in assay, testing, and analysis. It contains an extensive bibliography of nearly 150 pages, an enzyme index, and a general subject index.

671. Steinkraus, Keith, et al., eds. **Handbook of Indigenous Fermented Foods.** New York: Marcel Dekker, 1983. 671p. (Microbiology Series, Vol. 9). ISBN 0824718488.

Indigenous fermented foods such as tempeh, kimchi, kefir, and soy sauce are not only important dietary staples in the developing world, but are becoming increasingly common in Western countries. This extensive treatment of these foods covers Indonesian tempeh and related fermentations, foods involving lactic acid fermentations, such as kimchi, foods in which alcohol is the major product, soy sauces, fish sauces and pastes, and mushrooms and single-cell microbial protein. There are a section of general papers on fermented foods and an index.

672. Stumbo, C. R., et al. **CRC Handbook of Lethality Guides for Low-acid Canned Foods.** Boca Raton, Fla.: CRC Press, Inc., 1983. 2v. ISBN 0849329612 (vol. 1); 0849329620 (vol. 2).

"These two books present lethality guides for low-acid canned foods by conduction (Vol. I) and convection (Vol. II).

In Vol. I detailed tables are presented, giving processing times required for production of a 'safe' product.... The second volume deals with process time evaluation in convection packs, for producing 'safe' and 'commercially sterile' products" (*Journal of Food Technology* 19 [1984]: 276-77).

673. Sutherland, Jane P., A. H. Varnham, and M. G. Evans. **A Colour Atlas of Food Quality Control.** London: Wolfe, 1986. 272p. ISBN 0723408157.

Intended for professionals, students, and trainees as well as nontechnical food personnel, this atlas illustrates technical quality defects in food resulting from microbes and other organisms, poor storage conditions, infestation by rodents or insects, the presence of foreign materials, and poor processing techniques. To give the user a point of reference, there are many photographs of products illustrating acceptable as well as poor quality. The arrangement is by food groups—dairy products, fresh meat, fresh meat products, cured meat, delicatessen meat, poultry, fish, grocery products, baked goods and flours, prepared salads, produce, frozen foods, canned foods and alcoholic beverages. There are also brief chapters on food quality assurance and foreign bodies and infestations in food. There is an index.

674. Wyllie, Thomas D., and Lawrence G. Morehouse, eds. **Mycotoxic Fungi, Mycotoxins, Mycotoxicoses: An Encyclopedic Handbook**. New York: Marcel Dekker, 1977-1978. 3v. ISBN 0824765508 (vol. 1).

"A wealth of knowledge about mycotoxic fungi, their toxins, and the resulting toxicoses has been documented in scientific literature throughout the world. This encyclopedic handbook brings this large volume of knowledge together through the collective efforts of experts analyzing the documentation in every facet of the field."

Volume 1 is entitled *Mycotoxic Fungi and Chemistry of Mycotoxins*, volume 2, *Mycotoxicoses of Domestic and Laboratory Animals, Poultry and Aquatic Invertebrates and Vertebrates*, and volume 3, *Mycotoxicoses of Man and Plants: Mycotoxin Control and Regulatory Practices*. Each volume has an author and subject index. A brief glossary is included in volume 3.

DIRECTORIES

Bibliographies and Guides to Directories

675. Uhlan, Miriam, ed. **Guide to Special Issues and Indexes of Periodicals**. 3rd ed. Washington, D.C.: Special Libraries Association, 1985. 160p. ISBN 0871112639.

This volume describes 1,352 U.S. and Canadian periodicals which publish special issues such as directories, buyer's guides, and industry statistics on a continuing basis. The periodicals are listed alphabetically. Included are a subject index to special issues and a classified list of periodicals arranged by broad subjects.

Food Science and Technology Directories

676. **The Almanac of the Canning, Freezing, Preserving Industries: Annual Compilation of Basic References for the Canning, Freezing, Preserving, and Allied Industries**. 1st- . Westminster, Md.: Edward E. Judge & Sons Inc. 1958?- . annual.

This extensive reference manual and directory of the industry contains addresses, names of officers, and convention dates of industry organizations; FDA offices and field officials; extensive sections on food law and regulations, labeling and packaging, FDA standards of identity, quality and fill, and U.S. grade standards; statistics on vegetable and fruit production; U.S. pack statistics (tin, glass and frozen); industry statistics; exports, imports; canned food prices; miscellaneous data on consumption; and government food purchases and food programs. A section of yellow pages lists manufacturers of machinery and suppliers and services.

677. Araullo, E. V., comp. **Directory of Food Science and Technology in Southeast Asia**. Ottawa, Ont.: International Development Research Center, 1975. 267p. ISBN 0889360278.

Although the listing of research projects is now out-of-date, the names and addresses of food science and technology institutes in this directory are still useful.

678.   **Chilton's Food Engineering Master.** Radnor, Pa.: Chilton, 1978/79?- . annual. ISSN 0192-6098.

"The master is the only prefiled source for buyers and specifiers of equipment, supplies, and ingredients in the food and beverage industry." It is divided into two major sections: equipment, supplies, and services; and ingredients. In each there is a product index with product listings. Also included are addresses of manufacturers' home offices and sales offices.

679.   **The Directory of the Canning, Freezing and Preserving Industries.** 1st ed.- . Washington, D.C.: E. E. Judge, 1966/67- . annual. ISSN 0419-3717.

This directory lists processors of canned and frozen foods, including those packed in glass and plastic, with information on volume, personnel, association membership, brands, container sizes, and foods produced. There are also geographical and product listings of processors, a brand name list, and industry associations.

680.   Food and Agriculture Organization of the United Nations. **Worldwide List of Food Technology Institutions.** 3rd ed. Rome: Food and Agriculture Organization of the United Nations, 1971. 60p. (FAO Agricultural Services Bulletin, No. 9).

This geographic list of names and addresses of over 100 institutions includes academic, industrial, and governmental organizations. It does not include listings for the United States.

681.   **Food Engineering's Directory of International Food and Beverage Plants.** 1st- . Radnor, Pa.: Chilton, 1976?- . frequency unknown.

682.   **Food Engineering's Directory of U.S. Food and Beverage Plants.** 1st- . Radnor, Pa.: Chilton, 1976?- . frequency unknown.

"[Lists] every location with more than 20 employees, including headquarters and R&D locations. Published as a separate issue. Not included in the subscription price" (Miriam Uhlan, ed., *Guide to Special Issues and Indexes of Periodicals*, 1985).

683.   **Food Processing Guide & Directory.** Chicago, Ill.: Putman, 19?- . annual. ISSN 0015-6523.

This directory is issued as a part of *Food Processing: The Magazine of the Food Industry*. Most of it consists of sources of ingredients, equipment, and supplies. Over 900 manufacturers of ingredients and over 3,550 manufacturers of equipment and supplies are listed. Also included are a calendar of upcoming conventions, expositions, and meetings; a guide to government agencies; food industry associations; architects and engineers; food laboratories; and custom, contract, and special services. (Description based on the 1986/87 edition.)

684.   **Frozen Food Factbook and Directory.** 1st- . New York: National Frozen Food Association, 1952- . annual. ISSN 0071-9684.

This directory lists NFFA officers, regional and national organizations, members, packers, suppliers, warehouses, brokers, etc. A handy section of yellow pages provides important telephone numbers.

685. **Good Packaging Directory**. San Jose, Calif.: Good Packaging, 1977/78?- . annual.

This directory lists Western manufacturers and suppliers of packages, packaging materials, packaging machinery, etc. The arrangement is alphabetical by manufacturer and by subject with a "cross index guide" listing subject categories. (Description based on the 1985/86 edition.)

686. Hesseltine, C. William, and W. C. Haynes. **Sources and Management of Micro-organisms for the Development of a Fermentation Industry**. Washington, D.C.: Government Printing Office, 1974. 38p. (Agriculture Handbook No. 440). A1.76:440.

This is a worldwide list of major sources of microorganisms used in the food industry and in other applications, arranged by country. It also includes a list of products with information on types of microorganisms used to produce them.

687. Institute of Food Technologists. **Institute of Food Technologists World Directory and Buyers' Guide**. 1st- . Chicago: Institute of Food Technologists, 19??- . annual. ISSN 0737-4380.

This guide contains information on IFT, a buyers' guide for ingredients, laboratory and pilot plant equipment and supplies, processing and packaging equipment and supplies, a directory of IFT members, a list of members by corporate affiliation, and a classified guide to food industry services, such as analytical and testing laboratories, consulting engineers and architects, and trade and scientific associations. It is available only to members. (Description based on the 1985 edition.)

688. **International Food Directory**. 1st- . Parkside, South Australia: International Trade Directories, 1980/81- . biennial.

Sponsored by the Australian Department of Trade and Resources, this is a country-by-country listing of companies involved in exporting or importing food products, food processing equipment, or packaging machinery; it has an extensive subject index.

689. International Union of Food Science and Technology. **Directory of Courses and Professional Organizations in Food Science and Technology**. 2nd ed. North Ryde, Australia: International Union of Food Science and Technology, 1980. 56p.

This directory lists curricula and organizations by country. No addresses are provided for organizations, although membership, grades, and number of members are given.

690. **Progressive Grocer's Marketing Guidebook**. New York: Progressive Grocer Co., 1967- . annual. ISSN 0079-6921.

Names and addresses of grocery wholesalers, retailers, and convenience stores are arranged here by region and within each region by state. The volume contains demographic and marketing data for major market areas. There is an index.

691. **Quick Frozen Foods: Annual Processors' Directory and Buyer's Guide**. Cleveland, Ohio: Harcourt Brace Jovanovich, 1950?- .

This guide lists frozen food associations and industry groups, frozen food processors (alphabetically and geographically), products, manufacturers of ingredients, brand names, processing and packaging machinery, refrigerated truck lines, leading railroads, and refrigerated warehouses. The alphabetical list of processors gives company officers and managers, production statistics, and products.

692. **Thomas Grocery Register**. New York: Thomas Publishing Co., 1899?- . annual. ISSN 0082-4151.

"The official buyer's and seller's guide of the grocery and allied trades, United States and Canada." Volume 1 lists names and addresses of supermarket chains, convenience stories, and wholesalers, the institutional food market (e.g., cafeterias, fast food outlets, hospitals), brokers and manufacturers' agents, exporters, and warehouses. Volume 2 lists food products and equipment manufacturers by subject. Volume 3 contains an alphabetic list of food suppliers and equipment manufacturers and a list of trademarks, brand names, and private labels.

SELECTED REFERENCES

Frank, Robyn C. "Information Resources for Food and Human Nutrition." *Journal of the American Dietetic Association* 80 (1982): 344-49.

Mann, E. J. "IFIS—The First 10 Years." *Food Manufacture* 54 (May 1979): 53-55.

Mann, E. J. "The International Food Information Service: Past, Present and Future." *Food Technology* 30 (May 1976): 54-58.

Mayer, William J., and Joel T. Kemp. "Foods Adlibra—A Highly Current Database for the Food Industry." *Database* 2 (September 1979): 10-23.

Mermelstein, Neil H. "Retrieving Information from the Food Science Literature." *Food Technology* 31 (September 1977): 46-55.

Schützsack, Udo, and Günter Kalbskopf, eds. *Bibliography on the International Food Information Service (IFIS) and Food Science and Technology Abstracts (FSTA)*. Berlin: Satz-Rechen-Zentrum, 1983?. 29p. (FSTA Reference Series, No. 3). ISBN 3922961034.

Schützsack, Udo, and Ernest J. Mann, eds. *Proceedings of the Symposium on Food Science and Technology Abstracts (FSTA), Berlin, October 21-23, 1980*. Berlin: Satz-Rechen-Zentrum, 1981. 200p. (FSTA Reference Series, No. 2). ISBN 3922961010.

Sze, Melanie C. "Computer-Based Information Retrieval for the Food Industry." *Food Technology* 34 (June 1980): 64-70.

Sze, Melanie C. "Meeting the Information Needs of Food Scientists through Computerized Literature Searching." *Food Technology* 35 (October 1981): 92-97.

Tchobanoff, James B. "The Databases of Food — A Survey of What Works Best ... and When." *Online* 4 (January 1980): 20-35.

19
Specific Foods or Food Groups

BEVERAGES

Bibliographies and Guides

693. Gabler, James M. **Wine into Words: A History and Bibliography of Wine Books in the English Language**. Baltimore, Md.: Bacchus Press, 1985. 403p. ISBN 0961352507.

This is a bibliography of over 3,200 books and pamphlets in the English language, regardless of place of publication. The author states that it is the most comprehensive bibliography of wine titles in English. About 1,000 of the items are annotated. There are also extensive biographical and historical sketches in and between entries. Chronological and short title indexes are included.

694. Noling, A. W. **Beverage Literature: A Bibliography**. Metuchen, N.J.: Scarecrow Press, 1971. 865p. ISBN 0810803526.

This is an extensive bibliography of older, primarily English-language books and pamphlets on all types of beverages and beverage service. Most items are found in the Hurty-Peck Library of Beverage Literature. Locations are noted for items found in other libraries. Appendixes include reference works consulted; major beverage libraries; and a guide to books which include bibliographies, dictionaries, and glossaries.

695. Tudor, Dean. **Wines, Beers, and Spirits: A Consumer's Sourcebook**. Littleton, Colo.: Libraries Unlimited, 1985. 222p. ISBN 0872874559.

This annotated guide to information on wines, beers, and spirits does more than just describe traditional information sources such as books, reference materials, and magazines. It includes information on organizations and clubs, maps, posters, audiovisual materials, courses and seminars, computer programs, even libraries and museums with good collections.

696. United Nations Industrial Development Organization. **Information Sources on the Beer and Wine Industry**. New York: United Nations, 1977. 81p. (UNIDO Guides to Information Sources, No. 25).

Covered are international and national information sources of practical value on the brewing and wine industries. The guide includes organizations (professional, scientific, UN, international, national, and regional), directories, statistics sources, basic reference works, current periodicals, indexing/abstracting services, bibliographies, selected audiovisual materials, and miscellaneous sources of information. Selected items appear with annotations.

697. United Nations Industrial Development Organization. **Information Sources on the Coffee, Cocoa, Tea, and Spices Industry**. New York: United Nations, 1977. 74p. (UNIDO Guides to Information Sources, No. 28).

International and national information sources of practical value on coffee, tea, and spices are covered. Included are professional, scientific, trade, and research organizations; UN, international, national, and regional organizations; directories; statistics sources; basic reference materials; periodicals; indexing/abstracting services; selected films and film catalogs; fairs and exhibitions; meetings and conferences; and other types of information sources. Selected items are annotated.

698. United Nations Industrial Development Organization. **Information Sources on the Non-alcoholic Beverage Industry**. New York: United Nations, 1975. 72p. (UNIDO Guides to Information Sources, No. 15).

National and international sources of practical information on soft drinks and fruit juices are included in this guide. Covered are national, regional, international, as well as UN organizations, directories, statistics sources, basic reference materials, monograph series, current periodicals, indexing/abstracting services, selected films and film catalogs, and miscellaneous sources of information, including fairs and exhibitions. Many of the items are annotated.

Dictionaries

699. European Brewery Convention. **Elsevier's Dictionary of Brewing in English, French, German, and Dutch**. Amsterdam, Netherlands, New York: Elsevier Scientific Publishing Co., 1983. 264p. ISBN 0444421319.

This dictionary lists 3,757 English-language terms with French, German, and Dutch equivalents. No definitions are included. Indexes are in French, German, and Dutch.

700. Mendelsohn, Oscar A. **The Dictionary of Drinks and Drinking**. New York: Hawthorn, 1965. 382p.

This is a dictionary of terms related to wine, wine growing and production, beer, and spirits.

Directories

701. **Beverage World Databank**. 1985/86- . Dayton, Ohio: Keller International Publishing Corp., 1986- . annual.

This directory of products, equipment, and services in the beverage industry contains marketing information, environmental agencies and organizations, updates on relevant legislation, addresses of federal agencies, manufacturers' representatives, parent/franchise companies, beer importers, packagers, wineries, breweries, bottled water companies, soft drink plants, distilleries, juice plants in the United States and Canada, and industry associations.

702. **Coffee International Directory**. London: International Trade Publications, 19?- . frequency unknown.

This directory contains statistical information on production, exports, prices, as well as names and addresses of associations, principal roasters, manufacturers and packers of soluble coffee, manufacturers of decaffeinated coffee, exporters, importers, brokers, specialist services, machinery and equipment manufacturers, and brand names. (Description based on the 1982 edition.)

703. **Wines and Vines: Buyer's Guide Issue**. San Francisco, Calif.: Hiaring Co., 19?- . annual. ISSN 0043-583X.

Information on wineries and wine bottlers in the United States, Canada, and Mexico is provided. Addresses, principals, capacity, and acreage are listed. Products and brands are listed geographically, with an alphabetical index and a roster of names. Included are a buyer's guide to equipment, supplies and services, state laws and regulations, federal tariffs, and excise taxes. There is an advertisers' index.

Encyclopedias, Handbooks, Manuals, and Other Data Compilations

704. Amerine, Maynard Andrew, et al. **The Technology of Wine Making**. Westport, Conn.: AVI, 1980. 794p. ISBN 087055333X.

This useful reference text contains 20 extensive chapters on such subjects as wines and wine regions of the world, the composition of grapes, the chemistry of wine making, winery operations, production techniques for red and white wines, sherry, dessert and sparkling wines, specialty wines and brandies, and legal restrictions on wine making. There is an index.

705. Grossman, Harold J. **Grossman's Guide to Wines, Beers and Spirits**. 7th ed. New York: Scribner, 1983. 638p. ISBN 0684177722.

A standard work for information on alcoholic beverages and beverage service, this guide covers the process of fermentation and wine making, the major wine growing areas of the world and the wines produced there, specialty wines, beers, all types of distilled spirits, purchasing, bar operation, beverage service, storage, merchandising, and beverage control and regulation. Extensive appendixes include a multilingual glossary, production and consumption statistics, wineries in the United States, a quick reference guide to wines and spirits, vintage information, standards, and a lengthy bibliography. There is an index.

706. Johnson, Hugh. **The World Atlas of Wine: A Complete Guide to the Wines and Spirits of the World**. rev. and enlarged ed. New York: Simon and Schuster, 1985. 320p. ISBN 0671508938.

This newly revised edition presents a general introduction to wine, including maps of the world's vineyards with comparative statistics for world wine production and consumption. It covers history, enology, viticulture, wine buying, tasting, and storage. The bulk of the work is "a region-by-region exploration of the wine-growing areas of the world, with descriptions of the products and the styles of each" (*Bon Appetit* 31 [December 1986]: 30). A final chapter on spirits is included.

707.   Lichine, Alexis. **New Encyclopedia of Wines and Spirits**. 4th rev. ed. New York: Alfred A. Knopf, 1985. 733p. ISBN 0394546725.

Expressly written for the consumer, this revised edition of a standard work contains prefatory chapters on the history and production of wines and spirits. The main body of the encyclopedia has over 500 pages of alphabetical entries and *see* references. Extensive appendixes include lists of French wine production by region, and German wine growing areas and vineyards; containers and measures; and a comparative table of spirit strength, conversion tables, and vintage charts. The volume contains a select bibliography and an index.

CEREALS AND CEREAL PRODUCTS

Indexing/Abstracting Services

708.   **Flour Milling and Baking Research Association Abstracts**. Vol. 1- Chorleywood, Rickmansworth, England: Flour Milling and Baking Research Association, 1948- . bimonthly. ISSN 0430-7941.

Former titles: *British Baking Industries Research Association. Abstracts* and *Baking Research Association. Abstracts*. Each issue contains about 240 abstracts on all aspects of cereal milling and baking and covers nearly 300 periodicals from 20 countries, as well as patent literature. It is organized by broad subject categories: cereals and cereal products, bakery raw materials, bakery processes, laboratory techniques and equipment, nutrition and pharmacology, microbiology, hygiene and sanitation, plant, equipment, buildings, packaging and preservation, administration, and legislation.

Bibliographies and Guides

709.   United Nations Industrial Development Organization. **Information Sources on the Flour Milling and the Bakery Products Industries**. New York: United Nations, 1981. 100p. (UNIDO Guides to Information Sources, No. 39).

Similar in format to the other UNIDO guides, this title lists trade, professional, and research organizations; information services; directories; statistical sources; basic books; conference publications; reports; periodicals; indexing/abstracting publications; bibliographies; dictionaries; and encyclopedias.

Dictionaries

710.   Daniel, Albert R. **The Bakers' Dictionary**. 2nd ed. London: Elsevier, 1971. 254p.

711. Schneeweiss, R., comp. **Dictionary of Cereal Processing and Cereal Chemistry in English, German, Latin, and Russian**. Amsterdam, Netherlands, New York: Elsevier Scientific Publishing Co., 1982. 520p. ISBN 0444420495.

This multilingual dictionary lists 6,932 English-language terms with German and French equivalents, but no definitions. Indexes in German, French, and Russian refer to the numbered items in this list.

Directories

712. **Bakery Production and Marketing Buyers Guide**. Chicago: Gorman Publishing Co., 19?- . annual. ISSN 0005-4127.

Published as a number of *Bakery Production and Marketing*, this directory of products and services is divided into the following categories: ingredients, equipment, packaging, shipping and delivery, maintenance and sanitation, and supplies and services. Within each of these categories providers of products or services are listed by subject. Also given are names and addresses of associations, names and addresses of sources, an index to editorial features from the previous year's issues, and popular quantity recipes. (Description based on the 1986 edition.)

713. **Bakery Production and Marketing Red Book**. Chicago: Gorman Publishing Co., 19?- . annual. ISSN 0005-4127.

Issued as a part of *Bakery Production and Marketing*, this title contains data on the top 100 baking companies, statistics on the baking industry, directory of major bakeries, sources of ingredients, equipment, supplies and services, and bakery distributors. (Description based on the 1986 edition.)

Handbooks, Manuals, and Other Data Compilations

714. American Institute of Baking. **Quality Assurance Manual for Food Processors**. Manhattan, Kans.: American Institute of Baking, 1980. 474p.

Although this manual has the appearance of being more general, it emphasizes quality control of bakery products. It covers pertinent federal regulations, labeling, standards, storage and handling of food ingredients, product recalls, handling consumer complaints, sanitation, analytical procedures, etc.

715. D'Appolonia, B. L., and W. H. Kunerth, eds. **The Farinograph Handbook**. 3rd ed. St. Paul, Minn.: American Association of Cereal Chemists, 1984. 64p. ISBN 0913250376.

"A revised and expanded but still compact-sized handbook, this third edition is valuable source material for operators of the farinograph as well as for scientists in the field of rheology. Several new chapters are found in this Handbook" (*Food Technology* 39 [October 1985]: 167).

716. Hulse, Joseph H., et al. **Sorghum and the Millets: Their Composition and Nutritive Value**. London, New York: Academic Press, 1980. 997p. ISBN 0123613507.

This lengthy reference text includes information on composition, analysis, history, nutritional inhibitors, toxic factors, processing, and interrelationships with other nutrient sources. It contains a section of over 250 pages containing tables with data on composition, nutrient values, production statistics, etc., and a separate bibliography (over 100 pages). A detailed subject index is included.

717.   Juliano, Bienvenido O., ed. **Rice: Chemistry and Technology**. 2nd ed. St. Paul, Minn.: American Association of Cereal Chemists, 1985. 16, 774p. ISBN 0913250414.

The second edition of this reference text has been greatly expanded and emphasizes developments in the 1970s and 1980s. It includes 19 individually authored chapters, several by the editor. Topics covered are production and utilization, gross composition, polysaccharides, proteins and lipids, biochemical properties, physical and mechanical properties, drying and storage, parboiling, milling, enrichment and fortification, quality criteria, tests for quality, rice in infant foods, rice flours, canned rice foods, miscellaneous rice foods, rice in brewing, rice bran, and rice hulls. There are numerous tables throughout. Each chapter has extensive bibliographies. There is an index.

718.   Luh, Bor S., ed. **Rice: Production and Utilization**. Westport, Conn.: AVI, 1980. 925p. ISBN 0870553321.

An extensive reference text with 24 individually authored chapters on all aspects of rice production and use, the emphasis of this work is on the composition, processing, and technology of producing a large variety of rice products. The appendix includes U.S. standards for rice. An index is included.

719.   Pomeranz, Y., ed. **Wheat Chemistry and Technology**. 2nd ed., rev. St. Paul, Minn.: American Association of Cereal Chemists, 1971. 821p. (American Association of Cereal Chemists Monograph, No. 3).

This lengthy reference text discusses production and utilization of wheat, wheat quality, milled products, principal components of wheat and flour, dough, wheat products such as bread and other baked goods, and durum wheat and paste products. There are numerous tables throughout. There are bibliographies and an index.

DAIRY PRODUCTS

Indexing/Abstracting Services

720.   **Dairy Science Abstracts**. Vol. 1- . Shinfield, England: Commonwealth Bureau of Dairy Science and Technology, 1939- . monthly. ISSN 0011-5681.

One of a series of specialized agricultural indexing and abstracting services published by CAB International, this covers all aspects of dairy science and technology including milk, cream, butter, cheese, ice cream, dried and concentrated products, whey, milk proteins, processing equipment, nutrition, legislation, economics, public health, and the chemistry and physics of dairy products.

Online Equivalent: CAB Abstracts.

Arrangement: Abstracts in monthly issues are arranged in a continuous numerical sequence, according to subject categories.

Indexes: Subject and author indexes in each issue are cumulated annually.
CAB Thesaurus: DSA has used index terms in the *CAB Thesaurus* since 1984.

Bibliographies and Guides

721. United Nations Industrial Development Organization. **Information Sources on the Dairy Product Manufacturing Industry**. New York: United Nations, 1976. 88p. (UNIDO Guides to Information Sources, No. 23).

Following the format of the other guides in the series, this volume provides practical sources of information on dairy product manufacture. It lists names and addresses of national and international trade, professional, and scientific organizations; UN agencies; and regional organizations. It lists directories and basic reference materials, sources of statistics and economic data, current periodicals, indexing/abstracting services, bibliographies, conference publications, selected films and film catalogs, and other potential information sources such as fairs and exhibitions.

Dictionaries

722. International Dairy Federation. **Dictionary of Dairy Terminology: In English, French, German, and Spanish**. Amsterdam, Netherlands, New York: Elsevier Scientific Publishing Co., 1983. 328p. ISBN 0444421017.

This dictionary contains 3,909 English-language terms with equivalents in French, German, and Spanish, but no definitions. Separate indexes in these languages refer the reader to the English-language listing.

Encyclopedias, Handbooks, Manuals, and Other Data Compilations

723. Androuet, Pierre. **The Complete Encyclopedia of Cheese**. 1st ed. New York: Harper's Magazine Press, 1973. 545p. ISBN 0061202290.

This is a translation of *Guide du Fromage*. General tips on selecting cheeses, selection by flavor and season, and information on month-by-month availability precede an extensive dictionary of French cheeses describing sources, best seasons, fat content, type of milk used, appearance, accompaniments, and other gastronomic considerations. Appended are a small chapter on special and non-French cheeses and a glossary of terms.

724. Battistotti, Bruno, et al. **Cheese: A Guide to the World of Cheese and Cheesemaking**. New York: Facts on File, 1984. 168p. ISBN 0871969815.

This is a translation of *Formaggi del Mundo*. It contains general information on the history of cheese and cheesemaking and a dictionary of world cheeses. It is well illustrated with color plates. There is an index.

725. Eekhof-Stork, Nancy. **The World Atlas of Cheese**. New York: Paddington Press, 1976. 240p. ISBN 0846701332.

This English-language translation is edited by Adrian Bailey. Included in this country-by-country guide to the cheeses of the world is information about the history, production, and consumption of cheese in each country. Detailed cheese maps are included only for major cheese-producing countries. Special features include 45 cheese recipes; an index of cheese names; a glossary of cheese terms; and a general introduction to the origin, history, and manufacture of cheese.

726. United States. Agricultural Research Service. Dairy Laboratory. **Cheese Varieties and Descriptions**. Washington, D.C.: Government Printing Office, 1978. 151p. (Agriculture Handbook No. 54). A1.76:54.

This book describes more than 400 varieties of cheese in a dictionary format. Entries range from a line or two to more than a page and emphasize raw materials and methods of production.

HERBS AND SPICES

Bibliographies and Guides

727. Simon, James F., Alena F. Chadwick, and Lyle E. Craker. **Herbs: An Annotated Bibliography, 1971-1980: The Scientific Literature on Selected Herbs, and Aromatic and Medicinal Plants of the Temperate Zone**. Hamden, Conn.: Archon Books, 1984. 770p. ISBN 0208019901.

More than 7,000 references to the literature on 64 herbs from scientific journals, books, and general and trade magazines are included. The entries for the individual herbs in part 1 contain general information, data on plant chemistry, botany, horticulture, pharmacology, and use. They lead to bibliographic references on chemistry, botany, horticulture, production ecology, culinary studies, pharmacology, and other topics found in part 2, the subject classification. Part 3 contains the author and subject indexes.

Dictionaries

728. American Spice Trade Association. **A Glossary of Spices**. New York: American Spice Trade Association, 1966. 20p.

Handbooks, Manuals, and Other Data Compilations

729. Farrell, Kenneth T. **Spices, Condiments, and Seasonings**. Westport, Conn.: AVI, 1985. 415p. ISBN 0870554646.

Written both as a work of reference and as a text, this volume contains brief chapters on the history and the nature of spices and descriptive information on individual spices, herbs, and condiments. Also included is information on sauces and other seasonings and seasoning mixes for commercial use with recipes for large quantities. Individual descriptions include historical information, origin and sources, extractives, physical description, available forms, federal specifications, composition, as well as household and commercial uses. There is an index.

730.   Purseglove, J. W., et al. **Spices**. London: Longman, 1981. 813p. 2v. ISBN 0582468116 (vol. 1); 0582463424 (vol. 2).

This two-volume compendium has individual chapters on pepper, cinnamon and cassia, nutmeg and mace, cloves, pimento, chilies, ginger, turmeric, cardamom, and vanilla. The treatment of each individual spice is extensive (sometimes 80-90 pages). Included is information on history, botany, ecology, cultivation, products and end uses, processes and manufacture, chemistry, standard specifications, production, trade and markets. Each chapter has an extensive bibliography. A glossary and an index are found in volume 2.

731.   Rosengarten, Frederic. **The Book of Spices**. Wynnewood, Pa.: Livingston Publishing Co., 1969. 489p. SBN 870980319.

This is essentially a dictionary of herbs and spices with detailed information on the history, lore, and cultivation. Included are equivalent names in 12 languages, a few recipes featuring each herb or spice, a glossary of terms, a detailed bibliography, a recipe index, and a general index. It is well illustrated throughout, with black-and-white and color plates.

732.   Stobart, Tom. **Herbs, Spices and Flavorings**. Woodstock, N.Y.: Overlook Press, 1982. 320p. ISBN 0879511486.

This encyclopedic dictionary has entries ranging from ten lines to two or more pages in length and covers botany; history; and uses of herbs, spices, and flavorings such as olives and mushrooms. It gives genus and species, plant families, and equivalent names in French, German, Italian, and Spanish. There is an index.

MEAT

Bibliographies and Guides

733.   Holmes, Zoe Ann. **Bibliography of Selected References on Beef**. Chicago: American Dietetic Association, 1978. 148p.

Over 1,300 references on nutritional aspects, quality, effects of processing, and cooking are provided, arranged in two separate sequences: annotated and unannotated. A keyword index is included.

734.   United Nations Industrial Development Organization. **Information Sources on the Meat-Processing Industry**. rev. ed. New York: United Nations, 1976. 88p. (UNIDO Guides to Information Sources, No. 1).

This guide to national and international sources of practical information on the meat industry lists professional, trade, and scientific organizations; UN agencies and regional organizations; directories; sources of statistics and economic data; basic reference materials; current periodicals; indexing/abstracting services; special documents; conference publications; and other potential sources of information. Many items are annotated.

Handbooks, Manuals, and Other
Data Compilations

735.   Levie, Albert. **Meat Handbook**. 4th ed. Westport, Conn.: AVI, 1979. 338p. ISBN 0870553151.

Basic information is provided on livestock; slaughter and inspection; grading; distribution; purchasing; specifications; merchandising; quarters and cuts of beef, lamb, veal, and pork; and packaged and processed, smoked, and variety meats. The book also contains information on cooking methods and palatability. Numerous black-and-white photographs illustrate cutting techniques and cuts. There is an index.

NUTS, OILS, AND FATS

Bibliographies and Guides

736.   United Nations Industrial Development Organization. **Information Sources on the Vegetable Oil Processing Industry**. rev. ed. New York: United Nations, 1977. 101p. (UNIDO Guides to Information Sources, No. 7).

Practical sources of national and international information on all types of vegetable oils and vegetable oil production are presented. Following the format of the other books in the series, this volume lists national and international professional and scientific organizations, as well as UN agencies and regional organizations, directories, sources of statistics and economic data, basic reference materials, monograph series, current periodicals, indexing/abstracting services, conference publications, and other sources of information. Many of the citations are annotated.

Handbooks, Manuals, and Other
Data Compilations

737.   Bailey, Alton Edward. **Bailey's Industrial Oil and Fat Products**. 4th ed. New York: Wiley, 1979-1982. 2v. ISBN 0471839574 (vol. 1); 0471839582 (vol. 2).

The chemistry and technology of fats and oils and their products are covered, including edible oils and fats and industrial products such as paints, varnishes, and soaps. Included is information on composition, methods of analysis and extraction, hydrogenation, refining and bleaching, and the preparation of secondary products. Each volume has a separate index. Bibliographies appear throughout.

738.   Menninger, Edwin Arnold. **Edible Nuts of the World**. Stuart, Fla.: Horticultural Books, 1977. 175p. ISBN 0960004645.

Information on over 30 familiar and exotic nuts is well illustrated with black-and-white photographs. This book provides basic information on horticulture, varieties, growing areas, economics, history, and uses. A bibliography and an index are included.

739. Rosengarten, Frederic. **The Book of Edible Nuts**. New York: Walker, 1984. 384p. ISBN 0802707696.

This book provides extensive information on 42 edible nuts. Covered are natural history, cultivation, lore, and use. Nutritional information is generally omitted, although recipes are included. A bibliography and an index are included.

SEAFOOD

740. Dore, Ian. **Frozen Seafood, the Buyer's Handbook: A Guide to Profitable Buying for Commercial Users**. Huntington, N.Y.: Osprey Books, 1982. 310p. ISBN 0943738008.

Provided are general hints on purchasing, with an alphabetically arranged guide to individual seafoods and associated geographic locations and concepts. Entries include descriptions of the animal varieties or types, seasonal availability, and geographic source. There is an index.

741. Seafood Business Report. **The Seafood Handbook**. Camden, Maine: Seafood Business Report, 1984. 72p.

This is a brief but excellent source of basic information on seafood and freshwater fish. Numerous color photographs help identify finfish, shellfish, and crustaceans. A useful chart provides information on seasonal availability. Included are tips for purchasing, successful retailing, restaurant use, resources for promotion, and step-by-step illustrations for cutting and cleaning. There is an index.

SUGAR

Indexing/Abstracting Services

742. **Sugar Industry Abstracts**. Vol. 1- . Keston, England: Tate & Lyle Refineries, Inc., 1938- . bimonthly. ISSN 0250-2887.

This bimonthly indexing/abstracting service covers all aspects of sugar cane and beet sugar manufacture internationally. It contains about 3,400 abstracts per year, primarily from journal literature, but also monographic materials and patents. Topics covered include health and nutritional aspects and uses for by-products such as bagasse. There are annual author, subject, and patent indexes. A for-fee translation service is available for foreign articles. A document delivery system exists for articles and patents.

Bibliographies and Guides

743. Schalit, Michael. **Guide to the Literature of the Sugar Industry: An Annotated Bibliographical Guide to the Literature on Sugar and Its Manufacture from Beet and Cane**. Amsterdam, Netherlands, New York: Elsevier Scientific Publishing Co., 1970. 184p. SBN 444408398.

This is an excellent and still useful guide to the literature relating to sugar cane or beet growing and processing. Reference sources are arranged chiefly according to form: bibliographies, abstracts and reviews, indexes and patents, government publications, dictionaries, directories and yearbooks, periodicals, etc. There are separate subject sections on sugar economics, agriculture, and sugar technology and chemistry. There is a name and title index.

Dictionaries

744. Chaballe, L. Y., comp. **Elsevier's Sugar Dictionary in Six Languages: English/American, French, Spanish, Dutch, German, and Latin**. Amsterdam, Netherlands, New York: Elsevier Scientific Publishing Co., 1984. 321p. ISBN 0444423761.

This dictionary contains 2,569 English-language terms with equivalents in French, German, Spanish, and Dutch. Latin equivalents are provided for names of weeds and pests. Indexes are in French, German, Spanish, and Dutch.

745. Müller, Conrad A., comp. **Glossary of Sugar Technology: In Eight Languages: English, French, Spanish, Swedish, Dutch, German, Italian, Danish**. Amsterdam, Netherlands, New York: Elsevier Scientific Publishing Co., 1970. 234p. SBN 444408118.

This contains 8,571 numbered English-language terms with foreign equivalents and an index in each of these languages.

Directories

746. **Sugar y Azucar: Yearbook**. Vol. 36- . New York: Palmer, 1968- . annual. ISSN 0081-9212.

This yearbook includes current production and consumption data by country and worldwide directories of cane sugar mills and cane sugar refineries. The nondirectory portion of the text appears in English and in Spanish.

Handbooks, Manuals, and Other Data Compilations

747. Chen, James C. P. **Meade-Chen Cane Sugar Handbook: A Manual for Cane Sugar Manufacturers and Their Chemists**. 11th ed. New York: Wiley, 1985. 1134p. ISBN 0471866504.

The standard reference on cane sugar manufacture and refining, this also includes analytical procedures, information on chemical process controls, and a section of reference tables nearly 160 pages long that includes data on the solubility of sucrose in water and alcohol, viscosity, refractive index, brix, apparent density, and apparent specific gravity of sucrose solutions. There is a detailed subject index.

748. Hugot, Emile. **Handbook of Cane Sugar Engineering**. 3rd rev. ed. Amsterdam, Netherlands, New York: Elsevier Scientific Publishing Co., 1986. 1166p. (Sugar Series, Vol. 7). ISBN 0444424385.

This is a detailed treatment of engineering operations in sugar production from the time of delivery and unloading of the cane at the factory to storage and drying. It contains numerous charts, drawings, and formulas. There are author and subject indexes.

749. Pancoast, Harry M. **Handbook of Sugars**. 2nd ed. Westport, Conn.: AVI, 1980. 598p. ISBN 0870553488.

This revision is almost double the size of the original edition published in 1973. It covers sucrose, corn syrups and sugars, blends, lactose and fructose, and applications of these products, and includes information on new commercially used sweeteners, such as high fructose corn syrups. There are extensive tables with added metric values. A lengthy appendix includes analytical methods. An index is included.

750. Smith, Dudley. **Cane Sugar World**. New York: Palmer, 1978. 240p. ISBN 0960206019.

This country-by-country survey of the cane sugar industry has separate chapters devoted to the 40 top production areas. It includes historical background, agriculture, factories, refining, by-products, labor, and research.

751. **Sugar Year Book**. London: International Sugar Organization, 1965?- . annual.

From 1965 to 1968 this annual was issued by the International Sugar Council. It is devoted to country-by-country statistics on production, imports and exports, and consumption of member countries. Import statistics are provided by country of origin. Also included are general tables on world production, world exports, imports, consumption, and wholesale and retail prices.

VEGETABLES, VEGETABLE PRODUCTS, AND FRUITS

Bibliographies and Guides

752. Carter, Constance. **Edible Wild Plants**. Washington, D.C.: Science Reference Section, Science and Technology Division, Library of Congress, 1984. 9p. (LC Tracer Bullet TB 84-2).

This pamphlet lists books, handbooks, dictionaries, bibliographies, government publications, indexing/abstracting services, and highly selected journal articles.

753. Kader, Adel A., and Christi M. Heintz. **Gamma Irradiation of Fresh Fruits and Vegetables: An Indexed Reference List (1965-1982)**. Davis, Calif.: Department of Pomology, University of California, 1983. 55p.

This includes 648 items from 1965-1982, with subject and author indexes but no annotations or abstracts.

754. Schwartz, Diane. **Edible Wild Plants: An Annotated List of References**. Bronx, N.Y.: Council on Botanical and Horticultural Libraries, 1978. 11p. (Plant Bibliography, No. 3).

Described are some 60 books.

Dictionaries

755.   Jardin, Claude. **Kulu, Kuru, Uru: Lexicon of Food Plants in the South Pacific = Lexique des Noms de Plantes Alimentaires dans le Pacifique du Sud**. Noumea, New Caledonia: South Pacific Commission, 1974. 231p. (South Pacific Commission. Information Document = Cahier d'Information, No. 35).

Food plants are listed alphabetically by their vernacular names, "which vary from one archipelago to another, and even from one valley to another." Place names, equivalent scientific names, and French and English names are given. There are an alphabetical index of scientific names and a bibliography.

Directories

756.   Shurtleff, William, and Akiko Aoyagi. **The Soyfoods Industry and Market, Directory and Databook**. Lafayette, Calif.: Soyfoods Center, 1983- . annual.

This continues *Soyfoods Industry Directory and Databook*. It lists soyfoods manufacturers and the soyfoods support industry by product, subarranged by state. The soyfoods section includes equipment and supplies, industry services, associations, distributors, soyfoods centers, importers, researchers, and book publishers. Also included are data on the soyfoods industry and market generally, and data for specific products, such as tofu, tempeh, soymilk, soy sauce, miso, soy oil, and soy protein. Additional features include soyfood terminology, a multilingual glossary, standards, soybean production statistics, and a worldwide directory of institutions working with soyfoods. (Description based on the 1983 edition.)

757.   **Soya Bluebook**. St. Louis, Mo.: American Soybean Association, 1980?- . annual. ISSN 0275-4509.

This lists domestic, foreign, and international organizations; U.S. and state government agencies and universities; domestic and foreign oil extraction plants and refineries; U.S. and foreign producers of soy products; equipment and supplies; marketing and related services; soybean suppliers; breeders; seed suppliers; and exporters and importers. It also includes extensive statistics on the industry, a glossary, and standards. There is an index.

Handbooks, Manuals, and Other Data Compilations

758.   Bianchini, Francesco, and Francesco Corbetta. **The Complete Book of Fruits and Vegetables**. New York: Crown Publishers, 1976. 303p. ISBN 0517520338.

Originally published in Italy as *I Frutti della Terra*, this book is lavishly illustrated with 110 color paintings by Marilena Pistoia. It describes over 400 food plants grouped into categories according to use: cereals, vegetables, fungi, herbs and spices, stimulants, and starch- and oil-yielding plants. A brief glossary of botanical terminology precedes the main part of the text. Entries in the main part provide information on botany, origin, history, geographic distribution, and uses. The appendix is a special section keyed to the main text, with more detailed botanical descriptions of plants and a complete key to the illustrations. A bibliography, an index of Latin names, and an index of common names complete the text.

759.   Yamaguchi, Mas. **World Vegetables: Principles, Production and Nutritive Values**. Westport, Conn.: AVI, 1983. 415p. ISBN 0870554336.

This is a useful guide to over 100 common and exotic vegetables. Although the emphasis is on agriculture, it does contain information on origin, botany, toxicants, antivitamins, harvesting, storage, nutritional value (not extensive), and food uses. Bibliographies appear at the end of each plant family group. A detailed index is appended.

20
Methods of Analysis and Examination

This chapter is devoted to the most frequently used or established sources containing methods for the chemical analysis or examination of foods. These are often the standard or "official" methods of the major societies, such as the Association of Official Analytical Chemists. Included are methods for the analysis of nutrients, pesticides, additives, determination of bacteria, viruses, insects, fungi, etc.

New methods are frequently published in the journal literature, particularly in chemistry and food science and technology journals and microbiology journals. Therefore, it may occasionally be necessary to use an indexing/abstracting service to search through the journal literature if a desired method is not contained in any of the sources listed below. Usually a search of *Analytical Abstracts* is the best choice, if the method is a chemical one. When *Analytical Abstracts* is not available, *Chemical Abstracts* is a useful source.

INDEXING/ABSTRACTING SERVICES

760. **Analytical Abstracts**. Vol. 1- . London: Royal Society of Chemistry, January 1954- . monthly. ISSN 0003-2689.

"A monthly journal with world-wide coverage of the literature on all branches of analytical chemistry." It covers general literature relating to analytical chemistry and relevant literature in inorganic and organic chemistry, biochemistry, pharmaceutical chemistry, food, agricultural and environmental chemistry, as well as apparatus and techniques.

Arrangement: Continuously numbered abstracts are arranged according to broad subject categories.

Indexes: Each issue has a subject index. The annual index cumulates the monthly subject indexes and also includes an author index. Multiyear indexes are available for the earlier years.

Comments: Analytical Abstracts is the best indexing/abstracting service for analytical methods literature. *Chemical Abstracts* also provides coverage of this field; however, this subject tends to get lost in the entire body of the world's chemical literature. The indexing is superb. It is usually possible to locate material under the name of the substance analyzed for, as well as the food or material analyzed. For instance, articles on the determination of theobromine in cocoa are indexed under theobromine, but also under cocoa. Frequently the method or instrumentation is identified.

METHODS OF ANALYSIS AND EXAMINATION

761. American Association of Cereal Chemists. **Approved Methods of the American Cereal Chemists**. 8th ed. St. Paul, Minn.: American Association of Cereal Chemists, 1983. 2v. (looseleaf). ISBN 0913250317.

The first comprehensive revision since 1962, this edition eliminates 24 methods and adds 3 new ones. These methods cover chemical analysis of cereals and cereal products and other methods of examination. Included are test methods for baking quality of different types of flours; experimental milling procedures; methods for identifying extraneous matter; sampling procedures for micro-organisms, mycotoxins; and moisture, vitamins, minerals, fats, protein, and fiber. There is an index.

762. American Oil Chemists Society. **Official and Tentative Methods of the American Oil Chemists' Society**. 3rd ed. Chicago: American Oil Chemists Society, 1971- . 2v. (looseleaf).

Covered are sampling and analysis of vegetable oil source materials, oilseed by-products, soap and soap products, glycerin, sulfonated and sulfated oils, lecithin, industrial oils, and derivatives, etc. An alphabetical analytical methods index follows the detailed table of contents.

763. American Society of Brewing Chemists. **Methods of Analysis of the American Society of Brewing Chemists**. 7th rev. ed. St. Paul, Minn.: American Society of Brewing Chemists, 1976- . (looseleaf).

Analytical methods related to barley, malt, hops, wort, adjunct materials, brewer's grains, and beer are covered. This volume also contains microbiological methods (e.g., for yeast cell concentration), tests to determine gas retention of packaging materials, testing of filter aids, etc. The appendix contains *Tables for Extract Determination in Malt and Cereals*, third edition (1940) and *Tables Related to Determination of Wort, Beer and Brewing Sugars and Syrups* (1940).

764. American Spice Trade Association. **Official Methods of the American Spice Trade Association**. 2nd ed. Englewood Cliffs, N.J.: American Spice Trade Association, 1968. 53p.

765. American Spice Trade Association. **Official Microbiological Methods of the American Spice Trade Association**. 1st ed. Englewood Cliffs, N.J.: American Spice Trade Association, 1976. 1v. (looseleaf).

766. **Analytical Methods for Pesticides and Plant Growth Regulators**. Vol. 6- . New York: Academic Press, 1972- . irregular.

The former title of this series, *Analytical Methods for Pesticides, Plant Growth Regulators and Food Additives*, reflects its previous scope. The emphasis has always been on the full spectrum of methods to detect individual pesticides, herbicides, fungicides, and plant growth regulators. Currently no methods for food additives are included.

767. Association of Official Analytical Chemists. **FDA Training Manual for Analytical Entomology in the Food Industry**. Arlington, Va.: Association of Official Analytical Chemists, 1978. 174p.

This is also issued as FDA Technical Bulletin, No. 3. "Although the manual was designed as a training aid for government regulatory personnel, ... it may be useful also, in whole or in part to quality control personnel in industry and to teachers of entomology and food science courses in colleges and universities."

767a. Association of Official Analytical Chemists. **Official Methods of Analysis of the Association of Official Analytical Chemists**. 11th ed.- . Washington, D.C.: Association of Official Analytical Chemists, 1970- . quinquennial. ISSN 0066-961X.

Published approximately every five years and updated by annual supplements, this title contains analytical procedures for a whole range of agricultural materials (fertilizers, foods, feeds) and drugs and cosmetics. Many tests for specific substances in foods (e.g., nutrients, pesticide residues, mycotoxins, extraneous materials) are included. The index is superb—aflatoxins in peanuts can be found both under "aflatoxins" and "peanuts and peanut butter." (Description is based on the 14th edition 1984, the "centennial edition.")

768. Augustin, Jorg, et al., eds. **Methods of Vitamin Assay**. 4th ed. New York: Wiley, 1985. 590p. ISBN 0471869570.

"The fourth edition constitutes an update to the state-of-the-art in the field of vitamin analysis. Not only are the methods outlined in the chapters covering individual vitamins updated, but just as importantly, the new edition contains four additional chapters. Of these, three cover novel analytical systems, that is, chromatographic assays, radioimmunoassays, and automated assays." There is an index.

769. **Developments in Food Analysis Techniques**. London: Applied Science Publishers, 1978- . irregular. ISBN 0853347557 (vol. 1).

This series surveys recent developments in analytical techniques used to determine composition of foods, residues of toxic substances, food coloring agents, etc. Three volumes had appeared by mid 1986.

770. Dusold, Laurence R., et al. **Mycotoxins Mass Spectral Data Bank**. Washington, D.C.: Association of Official Analytical Chemists, 1978- . 1v. (looseleaf).

771. Egan, Harold, Ronald G. Kirk, and Ronald Sawyer. **Pearson's Chemical Analysis of Foods**. 8th ed. Edinburgh, Scotland: Churchill Livingstone, 1981. 591p. ISBN 044302149X.

This is a revised edition of *The Chemical Analysis of Foods*, seventh edition (1976), by David Pearson.

772. FAO/IAEA Panel on Microbiological Standards and Testing Methods for Irradiated Foods. **Microbiological Specifications and Testing Methods for Irradiated Food**. Vienna: International Atomic Energy Agency, 1970. 121p. (Technical Report Series, No. 104).

773. Gorham, John Richard, ed. **Principles of Food Analysis for Filth, Decomposition, and Foreign Matter**. 2nd ed. Washington, D.C.: Department of Health and Human Services, Public Health Service, Food and Drug Administration, 1981. 286p. (FDA Technical Bulletin, No. 1; HHS Publication No. (FDA) 80-2128). HE20.4040:1.

This contains chapters on sanitation; contaminants in foods such as fungi, protozoa, helminths, mites, insects, and hairs; and analytical techniques and tools for detection.

774. Hall, L. P. **Manual of Methods for the Bacteriological Examination of Frozen Foods**. 3rd ed. Chipping Camden, England: Camden Food Preservation Research Association, 1982. 101p.

This is a concise manual covering methods of sampling and specimen preparation, media, solutions and stains required for analysis, as well as significance of results. A brief bibliography is appended.

775. Harrigan, W. F., and Margaret E. McCance. **Laboratory Methods in Food and Dairy Microbiology**. rev. ed. London: Academic Press, 1976. 452p. ISBN 012326040X.

"The primary object of the manual is to provide a laboratory handbook for use by students following food science, dairying, agriculture, and allied courses...." It discusses sampling techniques, preparation of diluents, the detection and enumeration of indicator and pathogenic bacteria, and the microbiological examination of specific foods. Appendixes contain recipes for stains, reagents, and media; probability tables for estimating the number of microbes by the multiple tube technique; manufacturers and suppliers; and selected references.

776. Hawaiian Sugar Technologists. **Sugar Cane Factory Analytical Control: The Official Methods of the Hawaiian Sugar Technologists**. Amsterdam, Netherlands, New York: Elsevier, 1968. 190p.

This contains extensive tables preceded by a table index and a general index.

777. International Commission for Uniform Methods of Sugar Analysis. **Sugar Analysis: Official and Tentative Methods Recommended by the International Commission for Uniform Methods of Sugar Analysis**. Peterborough, England: International Commission for Uniform Methods of Sugar Analysis, 1979. 265p. ISBN 0905003012.

778. International Commission on Microbiological Specifications for Foods. **Microorganisms in Foods 1: Their Significance and Methods of Enumeration**. 2nd ed. Toronto: University of Toronto Press, 1978. 434p. ISBN 0802022936.

Part I discusses the significance of microorganisms and their toxins in foods. Part II presents recommended methods for microbiological examination of foods. Part III provides specifications for ingredients, media, and reagents. Appendixes, extensive references, and an index are included.

779.   International Commission on Microbiological Specifications for Foods. **Microorganisms in Foods 2: Sampling for Microbiological Analysis: Principles and Specific Application**. Toronto: University of Toronto Press, 1974. 213p. ISBN 0802021433.

Part I covers principles of sampling. Part II covers specific proposals for sampling, methods of sampling, sampling plans for different classes of foods (e.g., fish products, vegetables, frozen foods, milk and milk products, etc.). It contains appendixes, a brief glossary, references, and an index.

780.   International Union of Pure and Applied Chemistry. Commission on Oils, Fats and Derivatives. **Standard Methods for the Analysis of Oils, Fats, and Derivatives**. 6th ed. Oxford: Pergamon, 1979- . ISBN 0080223796.

Part I contains analytical procedures for oleaginous seeds and fruits, and oils and fats. Covered are sample preparation, determination of physical and chemical characteristics, constituents, quality and stability, and foreign substances and additives.

781.   Koniecko, Edward S. **Handbook of Meat Analysis**. 2nd ed. Wayne, N.Y.: Avery Publishing Group, 1985. 289p. ISBN 0895292548.

This revised edition of *Handbook for Meat Chemists* covers methods for conducting proximate analysis, as well as analysis for curing ingredients. It also includes microbiological tests performed in meat plants, a discussion of laboratory safety, and interpretation of laboratory results.

782.   Lange, Hans-Joachim. **Methods of Analysis for the Canning Industry**. Orpington, England: Food Trade Press, 1983. 328p. ISBN 0900379308.

This is a translation of *Untersuchungsmethoden in der Konservenindustrie*. It presents methods of analysis for canned food products, defined in the broad sense as packaged in tin, glass, plastic, laminates, or any combination of these. Included are chemical, microbiological, and other tests.

783.   Ma, Tsu Sheng. **Organic Analysis Using Ion-Selective Electrodes**. London: Academic Press, 1982. 2v. ISBN 0124629016 (vol. 1); 0124629024 (vol. 2).

"Volume 1 presents the background of ion-selective electrodes. Volume 2 which comprises Parts Two and Three of the book concentrates on the analysis of organic materials. Part Two involves an extensive survey of the literature.... The methods and procedures for determination of elements, various functional groups, biochemical substances, natural products, and pharmaceuticals are critically reviewed.... Part Three presents 38 experiments as typical examples to cover the different areas of organic analysis...."

784.   Marcus, John R., and Joseph Sherman, eds. **Animal Drug Analytical Manual**. Arlington, Va.: Association of Official Analytical Chemists, 1985. 1v. (various paging). ISBN 0935584307.

This was prepared jointly by the FDA and the association.

785.   Osborne, D. R., and P. Vogt. **The Analysis of Nutrients in Foods**. London: Academic Press, 1978. 251p. ISBN 0125291507.

Part I is on the chemistry, biological role, and analysis of nutrients in food. Part II covers methods for the analysis of nutrients in food. The volume includes material on sample preparation; methods for determining moisture; total solids;

protein and other nitrogenous compounds; carbohydrates, lipids, ash, elements and inorganic constituents, fat-soluble vitamins, and water-soluble vitamins; and the calculation of caloric values. An index is included.

786.   Richardson, Gary H., ed. **Standard Methods for the Examination of Dairy Products**. 15th ed. Washington, D.C.: American Public Health Association, 1985. 412p. ISBN 0875531180.

"A compilation of microbiological, chemical, and physical methods for analyzing dairy foods and dairy substitutes that aid quality assurance programs. Qualities of dairy products that are discernible by the consumer will generally not be considered. Tests for specific nutrient constituents are not included." There is a chapter describing the function of the standard methods, as well as 17 others dealing with such subjects as pathogens in milk and milk products, sampling, media, tests for various types of microorganisms, and antibiotic residues and sediment. There is an index.

787.   Sikyta, B. **Methods in Industrial Microbiology**. New York: Halsted Press, 1983. 349p. ISBN 0470274433.

Methods used in fermentation technology in food and food production, alcoholic beverages, and in medicine and other applications are presented.

788.   Speck, Marvin L., ed. **Compendium of Methods for the Microbiological Examination of Foods**. 2nd ed. Compiled by the APHA Technical Committee on Microbiological Methods for Foods. Washington, D.C.: American Public Health Association, 1984. 914p. ISBN 0875531172.

This new edition has been greatly revised and expanded and is the result of the collective effort of 120 authors and contributors. Eight chapters are devoted to laboratory techniques and procedures; 16 deal with the types of microorganisms involved in food spoilage; 13 deal with indicator microorganisms and pathogens; 5 with food-borne illnesses; 16 with microorganisms in specific types of foods; and 1 with the preparation of microbiological materials. The volume contains extensive references throughout and a detailed index.

789.   United States. Food and Drug Administration. **Pesticide Analytical Manual**. Vol. 1- . Washington, D.C.: U.S. Department of Health, Education and Welfare, Public Health Service, Food and Drug Administration, 1977- . (looseleaf). HE20.4008:P43.

This is a manual of analytical procedures used by the Food and Drug Administration for the analysis of pesticide residues in food and feeds. Volume 1 contains methods for the detection of multipesticide residue methods. Volume 2 has methods for individual pesticides.

790.   United States. Food and Drug Administration. Center for Food Safety and Applied Nutrition. **Bacteriological Analytical Manual of the Division of Microbiology**. 6th ed. Arlington, Va.: Association of Official Analytical Chemists, 1984. 1v. (looseleaf). ISBN 0935584293.

"The purpose ... is to provide the Food and Drug Field Laboratories with a series of methods that have been found to be effective for the detection of microorganisms in foods.... Contains methods for virus isolation, for the detection of parasites, and for the examination of cosmetics." (Description based on the 5th edition published in 1978.)

791.   Warner, C., et al. **Food Additives Analytical Manual: A Collection of Analytical Methods for Select Food Additives**. rev. ed. Arlington, Va.: Association of Official Analytical Chemists, 1983- . ISBN 0935584226 (vol. 1).

This is a joint effort of the Association of Official Analytical Chemists and the Food and Drug Administration.

21
Food Standards, Regulations, and Inspection

UNITED STATES

The U.S. food industry is one of the most regulated industries in the country. The major federal agencies involved in assuring the integrity and quality of our food supply are the Department of Agriculture, the Food and Drug Administration, the National Marine Fisheries Service, and the U.S. Public Health Service.

Among the many types of regulations issued by these agencies are standards relating to food. These food standards are of four types:

1. *Grade Standards*, which classify farm and fishery products into various levels of quality for marketing purposes (e.g., U.S. No. 1 peas or Grade A eggs).

2. *Standards of Identity*, which define what a given food product is supposed to be or how it is to be constituted. Their major purpose is to prevent deception. For instance, to be called mayonnaise, a product must contain eggs.

3. *Standards of Quality*, which set a minimum standard of quality for a specific food product.

4. *Standards of Fill of Container*, which specify how full a container must be to prevent deception.

The U.S. Department of Agriculture's Food Safety and Inspection Service (formerly Food Safety and Quality Service) is responsible for the inspection of all meat and poultry sold in the United States. In addition to inspecting meat for wholesomeness, the USDA issues standards of identity and minimum quality for meat and meat products.

The USDA's Federal Grain Inspection service is responsible for the inspection of whole dry peas, split peas, lentils, and beans, and grains such as wheat, corn, barley, oats, rye, sorghum, flax seed, and mixed grains. The USDA has also been charged with developing grade standards for agricultural products to facilitate trade. These are entirely voluntary, but they are widely used in wholesale and retail purchasing of food. Grade standards have been established for over 300 agricultural commodities including meat and poultry, dairy products, fresh fruits and vegetables, grains, and nuts.

The Food and Drug Administration is responsible for the safety and quality of our entire food supply. This includes inspecting plants; regulating food additives, animal food, and feed additives; overseeing labeling; and issuing standards of identity for many foods. These standards assure that the jar of mayonnaise purchased in Hawaii will not differ substantially from the same product bought in New York. They specify allowable ingredients, the percentage of fat or moisture the product may contain, or the type of processing a product must undergo.

The FDA also has issued many minimum standards of quality. In contrast to USDA grade standards, both standards of identity and of minimum quality are mandatory. A product not meeting a minimum standard of quality may still be sold, but it must bear labeling indicating that it is below standard in quality or not high grade. Additionally, the FDA is responsible for standards of fill of container. These essentially tell a food packer how full "full" is so that the consumer gets the quantity paid for.

The Environmental Protection Agency is responsible for monitoring pesticide residues in foods, and for establishing tolerances, generally in parts per million, for specific substances (e.g., captan or paraquat) to be permitted in the food supply.

The U.S. Public Health Service is charged with surveillance of food-borne diseases and with developing model ordinances for states and local communities relating primarily to food sanitation. The *Grade A Pasteurized Milk Ordinance* is an example of this type of activity.

Searching for Information on U.S. Food Regulations

The laws passed by Congress — including those dealing with agriculture, food, and cosmetics — are codified and printed in the *United States Code*. The *United States Code* contains the laws investing agencies in the executive branch with the authority and responsibility to carry out the intent of Congress, frequently specifying how this will be done.

The myriad of current federal regulations relating to foods, drugs, and agriculture, issued by federal agencies, are first announced in the *Federal Register* and are then codified (arranged according to subject) in the *Code of Federal Regulations* (*CFR*). These are the executive orders or regulations actually carrying out the law set forth in the *United States Code*.

For instance, Title 21, Section 341 of the *U.S. Code* gives the Secretary of Health and Human Services the authority to develop definitions and standards for food, whereas Title 21 of the 1985 *Code of Federal Regulations Part 135 Frozen Desserts* actually contains the standards for frozen desserts such as ice cream, goat's milk ice cream, ice milk, goat's milk ice milk, sherbet, and water ices.

As a general rule, the nutritionist, dietitian, or food scientist will have occasion to use the *Code of Federal Regulations* rather than the *U.S. Code*. It should be emphasized that these regulations are constantly in a state of flux and that currency of information is crucial. When searching for information on the current regulatory status of a food additive, for instance, begin by using an index to the *CFR*. Except for the most cursory and casual searches, it is essential to update information in the *CFR* by searching the *Federal Register*, its indexes, and its *List of CFR Sections Affected* (*LSA*), or by using a tool such as *The Chemical News Guide*.

The following section describes the major sources or search tools required for locating information relating to food laws, regulations, and standards. Under the heading "Bibliographies and Guides" are special materials that guide the user through the maze of regulatory information and discuss how to do searches relating to these subjects.

BIBLIOGRAPHIES AND GUIDES

792.   Hallstrom, Curtis H., Harvey G. Johnson, and William J. Moyer. "A Food Scientist's Guide to Food Regulatory Information." **Food Technology** 32 (October 1978): 72-77.

793.   Hui, Yiu H. **United States Food Laws, Regulations, and Standards**. New York: Wiley, 1979. 616p. ISBN 0471031828.
    This useful book provides basic information to help the user understand the complexity of our food laws, the function of our federal regulatory agencies, and the regulations and standards which they issue. The book is divided into seven chapters, each discussing the regulatory activities of a particular agency. There is an index. A new edition in two volumes has been announced for 1986.

794.   Schultz, H. W. **Food Law Handbook**. Westport, Conn.: AVI, 1981. 662p. (AVI Sourcebook and Handbook Series). ISBN 0870553720.
    An extremely useful book providing descriptive information on food laws and regulations in the United States, this volume includes a background chapter on the history of food law, a chapter on the U.S. legal system, and one on the publications which contain federal food laws and regulations and how to use them. There is a separate chapter on the *CFR* and the *Federal Register*. The book also gathers together the texts of widely scattered U.S. food laws. There are appendixes and indexes to laws cited and to subjects.

795.   United States. Department of Agriculture. Food Safety and Quality Service. **USDA Grade Standards for Food and Farm Products**. Washington, D.C.: Government Printing Office, 1979. 19p. (Agriculture Handbook No. 553). A1.76:533.
    Revised periodically, this publication lists grade standards developed by the USDA Food Safety and Quality Service, the Agricultural Marketing Service, and the Federal Grain Inspection Service. It provides references to the *Code of Federal Regulations* which contains all of these standards.

796.   United States. National Archives and Records Administration. Office of the Federal Register. **The Federal Register: What It Is and How to Use It: A Guide for the User of the Federal Register, Code of Federal Regulations System**. Washington, D.C.: Office of the Federal Register, National Archives and Records Administration, 1985. 113p. AE2.108:F31.

This useful guide to the entire Federal Register System (*FR*, *CFR*, and *LSA*) was developed for educational workshops conducted by the Office of the Federal Register.

U.S. CODE

797.   United States. **United States Code**. Prepared and published under the authority of Title 2, U.S. Code, Section 285b, by the Law Revision Counsel of the House of Representatives. Washington, D.C.: Government Printing Office, 1940- . Y1.2/5: .

Issued every six years with annual cumulative supplements, the *U.S. Code* contains all laws passed by Congress currently in effect. Title 21 contains food and drug legislation. Title 7 contains agricultural laws. The multivolume *General Index* to the set is a detailed subject index. (Description based on the 1982 edition.)

CODE OF FEDERAL REGULATIONS AND ITS INDEXES

798.   United States. National Archives and Records Administration. Office of the Federal Register. **Code of Federal Regulations**. 1st- . Washington, D.C.: Government Printing Office, 1938- . annual. AE2.106/3.

The *CFR* contains current regulations of the federal agencies. It is divided into 50 broad subjects called titles. Each title is divided into subtitles, chapters, parts, and subparts. The parts are continuously numbered from chapter to chapter. Therefore, the title and the part numbers are the most important elements in citations to the *CFR*.

The *CFR* has a subject index (see pp. 272-73) which unfortunately is not very detailed, frequently making it useless for searching specific food products and chemicals entered under a larger category. When possible, it is wise to use the commercially published *Index to the Code of Federal Regulations* (Washington, D.C., Congressional Information Service). If this is not available, try the *CFR* subject index under a more general subject or examine the tables of contents of individual *CFR* titles likely to contain the information needed.

The titles most relevant to food science and nutrition are: *Title 7, Agriculture*; *Title 9, Meat and Poultry Inspection*; and *Title 21, Food and Drugs*. Outlined below are the most pertinent parts of these titles:

Title 7, Agriculture, Part:

51.   "Inspection, Certification, and Grade Standards for Fresh Fruits, Vegetables, Nuts and Miscellaneous Products."

52.   "Grade Standards for Processed Fruits and Vegetables."

53.   "Livestock Grading, Certification, and Standards."

54. "Inspection, Certification, and Grade Standards for Meats, Prepared Meats, and Meat Products."

55. "Voluntary Inspection and Grading of Egg Products."

56. "Grading and Grade Standards for Shell Eggs."

58. "Inspection and Grade Standards for Processed Dairy Products."

59. "Inspection of Eggs and Egg Products."

68. "Inspection and Grade Standards for Grains, Dry Beans, Peas and Lentils."

70. "Voluntary Grading of Poultry and Rabbit Products as Well as Classes, Standards, and Grades."

Title 9, Part:

301-85. "Meat and Poultry Inspection."

Title 21, Food and Drug, Part:

100. "General."

101. "Food Labeling."

102. "Common or Usual Name for Nonstandardized Foods."

103. "Quality Standards for Foods with No Identity Standards."

104. "Nutritional Quality Guidelines for Foods."

105. "Foods for Special Dietary Use."

106. "Infant Formula Quality Control Procedures."

107. "Infant Formula."

108. "Emergency Permit Control."

109. "Unavoidable Contaminants in Food for Human Consumption and Food-Packaging Material."

110. "Current Food Manufacturing Practice in Manufacturing, Processing, Packing, or Holding Human Food."

113. "Thermally Processed Low-Acid Foods Packaged in Hermetically Sealed Containers."

114. "Acidified Foods."

118. "Cacao Products and Confectionery."

123. "Frozen Raw Breaded Shrimp."

129. "Processing and Bottling of Bottled Water."

130. "Food Standards: General."

131. "Milk and Cream."

133. "Cheeses and Related Cheese Products."

135. "Frozen Desserts."

136. "Bakery Products."

137. "Cereal Flours and Related Products."

139. "Macaroni and Noodle Products."

145. "Canned Fruits."

146. "Canned Fruit Juices."

150. "Fruit Butters, Jellies, Preserves, and Related Products."

152. "Fruit Pies."

155. "Canned Vegetables."

156. "Vegetable Juices."

158. "Frozen Vegetables."

160. "Eggs and Egg Products."

161. "Fish and Shellfish."

163. "Cacao Products."

164. "Tree Nut and Peanut Products."

165. "Non-Alcoholic Beverages."

166. "Margarine."

168. "Sweeteners and Table Syrups."

169. "Food Dressings and Flavorings."

170-89. "Food Additives, Food Irradiation, Substances Generally Recognized as Safe (GRAS List), Substances Prohibited in Human Food."

193. "Tolerances for Pesticides in Food."

197. "Seafood Inspection."

261. "Grade Standards for Whole or Dressed Fish."

262. "Grade Standards for Fish Steaks."

263. "Grade Standards for Fish Fillets."

264. "Grade Standards for Frozen Fish Blocks and Products Made Therefrom."

265. "Grade Standards for Crustacean Shellfish Products."

266. "Grade Standards for Molluscan Shellfish."

500. "Animal Food Labeling, Animal Drugs, Food Additives in Animal Foods, Substances Not Permitted in Animal Foods or Feeds."

1220. "Tea."

799. **Index to the Code of Federal Regulations**. Bethesda, Md.: Congressional Information Service, 1978- . annual. ISSN 0198-9014.

This is the preferred index to the *CFR*. There are five distinct sections: *Subject Index, Geographic Index, Geographic Proper Name Index, List of Descriptive Headings*, and *List of Reserved Headings*. References are to title, subtitle, chapter, subchapter, part, subpart, and page. The extensive and detailed subject index has numerous cross-references. The *List of Descriptive Headings* lists all of the headings that have been assigned by federal agencies to each title, subtitle, chapter or subchapter, part or subpart.

800. United States. National Archives and Records Administration. Office of the Federal Register. **Code of Federal Regulations. LSA List of CFR Sections Affected**. Washington, D.C.: Government Printing Office, 1977- . monthly. AE2.106/2.

Issued monthly with March, June, September, and December issues being cumulative from January, this periodical is "designed to lead users of the *Code of Federal Regulations (CFR)* to recent amendatory actions published in the *Federal Register (FR)*.

FEDERAL REGISTER AND ITS INDEXES

801. United States. National Archives and Records Administration. Office of the Federal Register. **Federal Register**. Vol. 1- . Washington, D.C.: Government Printing Office, 1936- . daily. AE2.106: .

Issued daily, the *Federal Register* is the chief medium for announcing the countless new regulations emanating from the executive agencies to the public. It is organized by agency and each issue has a list of *CFR* parts affected. The Office of the Federal Register issues an index, the *Federal Register Index*, in cumulative form each month. However, *FR* users are urged to use the commercially published *CIS Federal Register Index* if that is available.

802. United States. National Archives and Records Administration. Office of the Federal Register. **Federal Register Index**. Vol. 1- . Washington, D.C.: Government Printing Office, 19?- . monthly. AE2.106: .

Each issue is cumulative, with the December issue being the annual index. This is a difficult-to-use index because it is organized by issuing agency rather than by keywords or true subjects. It is preferable to use the commercially produced *CIS Federal Register Index*.

803. **CIS Federal Register Index**. Vol. 1- . Bethesda, Md.: Congressional Information Service, 1984- . weekly. ISSN 0741-2878.

This weekly index is the preferred tool for locating material in the *Federal Register*. It covers all rules, proposed rules, notices, and presidential documents contained in that publication. Cumulations are issued every five weeks and every fifteen weeks. These are then replaced by permanent semi-annual cumulations. The major part of the publication is the *Index by Subjects and Names*. Material is indexed by specific subjects, general policy area, responsible federal agency, authorizing legislation, affected industries, organizations, corporations, individuals or geographic areas. (See figure 10, pages 274-75.) Other parts are the *Index*

(Text continues on page 276.)

CODE OF FEDERAL REGULATIONS

CFR Index

Floods

Federal Highway Administration, Federal aid highways
Location and hydraulic design of encroachments on flood plains, 23 CFR 650
Mitigation of environmental impacts to privately owned wetlands, 23 CFR 777

Justice Department, floodplain management and wetland protection procedures, 28 CFR 63

National Aeronautics and Space Administration, flood plain and wetlands management, 14 CFR 1216

Postal Service, floodplain management and protection of wetlands procedures, 39 CFR 776

Small Business Administration, policies of general application, 13 CFR 116

Soil Conservation Service, flood plains management and wetlands protection, 7 CFR 650

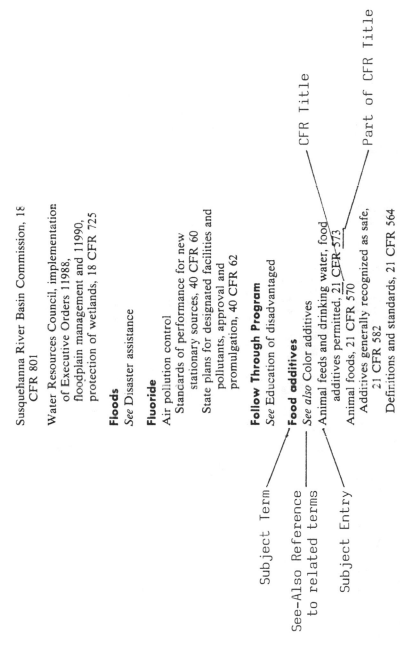

Susquehanna River Basin Commission, 18 CFR 801

Water Resources Council, implementation of Executive Orders 11988, floodplain management and 11990, protection of wetlands, 18 CFR 725

Floods
See Disaster assistance

Fluoride
Air pollution control
Standards of performance for new stationary sources, 40 CFR 60
State plans for designated facilities and pollutants, approval and promulgation, 40 CFR 62

Follow Through Program
See Education of disadvantaged

Food additives
See also Color additives
Animal feeds and drinking water, food additives permitted, 21 CFR 573
Animal foods, 21 CFR 570
Additives generally recognized as safe, 21 CFR 582
Definitions and standards, 21 CFR 564

Subject Term

See-Also Reference to related terms

Subject Entry

CFR Title

Part of CFR Title

Fig. 9. Illustration page from *Code of Federal Regulations, CFR Index.*

CIS FEDERAL REGISTER INDEX

Index by Subjects and Names

Subject Term

Descriptive Annotation

Name of Legislation

Issuing Agency (Bureau of Alcohol, Tobacco & Firearms)

Page in Federal Register

Date (2/4)
Document Type (Rule)
Correction (ex)

Sabotage
Intl Organizations Employees Loyalty Bd, evaluation stds revision: OPM *(3/11/PR)* 8329
James River VA security zone and anchorage, estab re Newport News Shipbuilding and Drydock Co naval vessels protection: USCG *(2/27/PR)* 6921

Saccharin
Alcoholic beverage labeling rqmts, saccharin warning statement estab: ATF *(2/4/R-cx)* 4338

Saccharin Study and Labeling Act
Alcoholic beverage labeling rqmts, saccharin warning statement estab: ATF *(2/4/R-cx)* 4338

Sack, Stephen H.
DOE Office of Hearings and Appeals case filing: OHA *(2/10/N)* 4978

Saco River
Hydroelectric license appls and actions, descriptive listing: FERC *(2/3/N)* 4219

Page

4338   Federal Register / Vol. 51, No. 23 / Tuesday, February 4, 1986 / Rules and Regulations

Title and Parts
of CFR affected ———

Bureau of Alcohol, Tobacco and Firearms

——— **27 CFR Parts 4, 5, and 7**

[T.D. ATF–210; Correction]

Disclosure of Saccharin in the Labeling of Wine, Distilled Spirits, and Malt Beverages

AGENCY: Bureau of Alcohol, Tobacco and Firearms (ATF), Treasury.

ACTION: Treasury decision, final rule; correction.

SUMMARY: This document corrects errors made in FR Doc 85–29707, published in the Federal Register on December 20, 1985, at 50 FR 51851.

FOR FURTHER INFORMATION CONTACT: James P. Ficaretta, FAA, Wine and Beer Branch, Bureau of Alcohol, Tobacco and Firearms, 1200 Pennsylvania Avenue, NW., Washington, DC 20226. (202) 566–7626.

SUPPLEMENTARY INFORMATION:
Paragraph 1. The Treasury decision number should read "T.D. ATF–220."

Para. 2. In the left column under "Summary" in the fifth line the word "continuing" should read "containing." Para. 3. In the right column in the second and third lines remove the words", or on the basis of petitions."

Para. 4. On page 51852 in the right column the name "David D. Green" should read "David D. Queen."

Signed: January 27, 1986.
Stephen E. Higgins,
Director.

[FR Doc. 86–2416 Filed 2–3–86; 8:45 am]

BILLING CODE 4810-31-M

Fig. 10. Illustration page from *CIS Federal Register Index.* © 1986 by Congressional Information Service, Inc. (Bethesda, MD). Reprinted with permission. All rights reserved.

to CFR Section Numbers, Index to Federal Agency Docket Numbers, and *Calendar of Effective Dates and Comment Deadlines.*

SPECIALIZED INDEXES

804. **The Food Chemical News Guide**. Washington, D.C.: Food Chemical News, 196?- . weekly (looseleaf).

This looseleaf service with weekly updates covering the regulatory status of food chemicals includes information on direct and indirect additives; GRAS substances; prior sanctioned substances; additives proposed for clearance; ingredients listed for use in meat and poultry products by the USDA; additives for alcoholic beverages; pesticide tolerances for processed foods and feeds; substances banned by the FDA; color additives for foods, drugs, and cosmetics; and inert ingredients in pesticide formulations. It is indexed by chemical names and titles of food and color additive orders.

HANDBOOKS, MANUALS, AND OTHER DATA COMPILATIONS

805. Monlux, William S., and Andrew W. Monlux. **Atlas of Meat Inspection Pathology**. Washington, D.C.: Government Printing Office, 1972. 178p. (Agriculture Handbook No. 367). A1.76:367.

This atlas includes color photographs illustrating lesions found in meat animals at the time of slaughter. "Functions as a ready reference guide for meat inspectors who are searching for current terminology and for assistance in interpreting lesions and in making diagnoses."

806. National Research Council. Food and Nutrition Board. Committee on Codex Specifications. **Food Chemicals Codex**. 3rd ed. Washington, D.C.: National Academy Press, 1981- . 1v. plus supplements. ISBN 0309030900.

Revised and updated information on standards of purity and quality for nearly 800 food chemicals is presented. Included in the entries are description, requirements for identification, assays and tests, molecular formula, molecular weight, directions for packaging and storage, and identification of functional use in food. Many of the entries also have chemical structures. Also included are specifications for flavor, aromatic chemicals and isolates, general tests and apparatus, and infrared spectra for over 400 compounds, primarily the essential oils and the flavor aromatic chemicals and isolates. There is an index. Supplements were issued in 1983 and 1986.

807. United States. Department of Agriculture. Agricultural Marketing Service. **Poultry Grading Manual**. Washington, D.C.: Government Printing Office, 1977. 30p. (Agriculture Handbook No. 31). A1.76:31.

"This manual is a guide to the uniform application of the United States Classes, Standards, and Grades of Poultry. Although designed primarily to aid poultry graders, it should prove useful to those teaching poultry marketing and to the poultry industry."

808.   United States. Department of Agriculture. Federal Grain Inspection Service. **Grain Inspection Handbook**. Washington, D.C.: U.S. Department of Agriculture, Federal Grain Inspection Service, 1979- . A104.8:G76/2/trans.

This looseleaf handbook will replace the *Grain Inspection Manual* when it is completed.

809.   United States. Department of Agriculture. Federal Grain Inspection Service. **Grain Inspection Manual: Covering the Sampling, Inspection, Grading, and Certification of Grain under the United States Grain Standards Act as Amended**; Washington, D.C.: U.S. Department of Agriculture, Federal Grain Inspection Service, 1977. 487p. A104.8:G76.

"A guide to the proper sampling, inspection, grading, and certification of the various grains under the provisions of the United States Grain Standards Act." It covers wheat, corn, barley, oats, rye, sorghum, soybeans, flaxseed, and mixed grain.

810.   United States. Department of Agriculture. Federal Grain Inspection Service. **Rice Inspection Handbook**. Washington, D.C.: U.S. Department of Agriculture, Federal Grain Inspection Service, 1982- . (looseleaf). A104.8:R36.

"This Handbook [sic] provides guidelines for the proper sampling, inspection, grading and certification of rough rice, brown rice, for processing and milled rice under the provisions of the agricultural Marketing Act of 1946 ... for use by official inspection personnel."

811.   United States. Department of Agriculture. Food Safety and Quality Service. **Chemistry Laboratory Guidebook**. rev. basic ed. Washington, D.C.: U.S. Department of Agriculture, Food Safety and Quality Service, 1986- . (looseleaf). A110.8/3 March 1986.

"The purpose of this publication is to provide a readily available reference book of methods suitable for the analysis of the natural constituents, additives, and biological and environmental residues that may occur in meat and poultry products. In addition, the book covers policy ... on the use of additives, both direct and indirect, that is applicable to meat and poultry products."

812.   United States. Department of Agriculture. Food Safety and Quality Service. **Egg Grading Manual**. (Slightly revised May 1978). Washington, D.C.: Government Printing Office, 1978. (Agriculture Handbook No. 75). A1.76:75/978.

"This manual was prepared as an aid in teaching both beginning and experienced egg graders the correct interpretation and application of the U.S. standards, grades and weight classes for shell eggs."

813.   United States. Department of Agriculture. Food Safety Inspection Service. **List of Proprietary Substances and Nonfood Compounds Authorized for Use under USDA Inspection and Grading Programs**. Washington, D.C.: Government Printing Office, 1982- . annual. (Miscellaneous Publication No. 1419). A1.38:1419.

This publication, distributed to depository libraries on microfiche, supersedes *List of Chemical Compounds Authorized for Use under USDA Inspection and Grading Programs*. It "lists proprietary substances used in the preparation of product and nonfood compounds used in the plant environment which are authorized by the Food Ingredient Assessment Division (FIAD), Science, Food Safety and Inspection Service (FSIS), for use in slaughtering and processing plants operating under the USDA poultry, meat, rabbit, shell egg grading and egg products inspection programs."

814.   United States. Department of Agriculture. Meat and Poultry Inspection Program. **Meat and Poultry Inspection Manual**. Washington, D.C.: Government Printing Office, 1973- . (looseleaf). A110.8/2.

"An official publication of procedural guidelines and instructions to aid all MPI employees in enforcing laws and regulations related to federal meat and poultry inspection. It also contains information on MPI's organization and relevant material directly affecting meat and poultry activities issued by other federal agencies."

DIRECTORIES

815.   United States. Department of Agriculture. Meat and Poultry Inspection Program. **Meat and Poultry Inspection Directory**. Washington, D.C.: U.S. Department of Agriculture, Food Safety and Inspection Service, July/December 1977- . semi-annual. A103.9: .

This publication contains names and addresses of Food and Safety Inspection Service personnel, personnel in regional offices, Compliance Division field locations and personnel, international programs, scientific personnel, accredited laboratories, veterinary services, FDA field offices, state officials, meat and poultry establishments under USDA inspection by number, USDA certified export establishments, USDA import inspection, inedible fat shippers, and USDA establishments by state and city. There is a name index to USDA meat and poultry inspection establishments. Foreign meat and poultry establishments are listed by country. (Description based on the 1983 edition.)

816.   United States. Food and Drug Administration. **Directory of State Officials: 85-1**. Rockville, Md.: Department of Health and Human Services, Food and Drug Administration, 1985. unpaged. HE20.4037/2:985.

Names and addresses of officials from state departments of health, agriculture, and other regulatory bodies are listed.

INTERNATIONAL AND FOREIGN

Internationally, food standards are issued by the Joint FAO/WHO Codex Alimentarius Commission (sometimes known simply as the Codex Alimentarius Commission), the Joint FAO/WHO Expert Committee on Food Additives, the International Organization for Standardization, and specialized organizations such as the International Dairy Federation.

The Codex Alimentarius Commission was established in 1963 by the Food and Agriculture organization of the United Nations and the World Health Organization for the purpose of issuing international food standards to protect consumers and to facilitate trade. Most of these standards are combined standards of identity and minimum quality. They define quality, composition, additives and contaminants, labeling, etc. A few are standards for sanitation and methods of analysis. Some set limits for pesticide residues. The goal is eventually to arrive at international standards for all major foods.

The first set of Codex standards was issued in several series beginning with 1969. A new revised Codex began publication in 1979, and as before it is being issued in series.

Member countries may accept Codex standards in full, indicate that they are accepting by a certain date (target acceptance), or accept a standard with certain specified deviations.

The Joint FAO/WHO Expert Committee on Food Additives exists to advise its parent organization on food additives. It is concerned with formulating general principles on the use of food additives and has issued a number of specifications for identity and purity of additives.

Joint FAO/WHO Codex Alimentarius Commission

817. Joint FAO/WHO Codex Alimentarius Commission. **Codex Alimentarius.** Rome: Food and Agriculture Organization of the United Nations and World Health Organization, 1981- . (looseleaf).

The *Codex* is intended to replace the Commission's recommended international standards and methods of analysis and sampling, previously issued in the *CAC/RS* series and the *CAC/RM* series as appropriate.

There are now over 200 international commodity standards available for all principal foods, whether processed, semiprocessed or raw. Their purpose is to protect the health of consumers and to ensure fair trade practices.

Volume 1 is *Explanatory Notes on the Joint FAO/WHO Foods Standards Programme and on the Codex Alimentarius Commission*; volume 2, *Codex Standards for Processed Fruits and Vegetables and Edible Fungi*; volume 3, *Codex Standards for Sugars (including Honey)*; volume 4, *Codex Standards for Processed Meat and Poultry Products and Soups and Broths*; volume 5, *Codex Standards for Fish and Fishery Products*; volume 6, *Codex Standards and Guidelines for the Labelling of Foods and Food Additives*. Volume 7 is *Codex Standards for Cocoa Products and Chocolate*; volume 8, *Codex Standards for Quick-Frozen Fruits and Vegetables*; volume 9, *Codex Standards for Foods for Special Dietary Uses including Foods for Infants and Children and Related Code of Hygienic Practice*; volume 10, *Codex Standards for Fruit Juices, Concentrated Fruit Juices, Fruit Nectars*. Volume 11 is *Codex Standards for Edible Fats and Oils*; volume 12, *Codex Standards for Natural Mineral Waters and Edible Ices and Ice Mixes*; volume 13, *Codex Maximum Limits for Pesticide Residues*; volume 14, *Food Additives*; volume 15, *Codex General Standard for Irradiated Foods and Recommended International Code of Practice for the Operation of Radiation Facilities Used for the Treatment of Foods*; volume 16, *Code of Principles Concerning Milk and Milk Products and International Individual Standards for Cheeses*; and volume 17, *Contaminants*.

818. Joint FAO/WHO Codex Alimentarius Commission. **Codex Alimentarius: CAC/RCP.** No. 1- . Rome: Food and Agriculture Organization of the United Nations and World Health Organization, 1979- . irregular.

This series of the *Codex Alimentarius* contains the "Recommended International Code of Practice," individual standards dealing with hygienic practice in the processing of various foods. Standards are also designated alphabetically as volumes (e.g., *Codex Alimentarius*, Volume B, CAC/RCP10-76).

819. Joint FAO/WHO Codex Alimentarius Commission. **Guide to Codex Recommendations Concerning Pesticide Residues: CAC/PR**. No. 1- . Rome: Food and Agriculture Organization of the United Nations and World Health Organization, 1984- . (looseleaf). irregular.

This set of standards updates the *Guide to Codex Maximum Limits for Pesticide Residues* (CAC/PR1-1978).

820. Joint FAO/WHO Codex Alimentarius Commission. **Procedural Manual**. 5th ed. Rome: Food and Agriculture Organization of the United Nations and World Health Organization, 1981. 120p.

The *Procedural Manual* describes the rules and procedures of the Codex Alimentarius Commission; the purposes, scope, and value of the codex; procedures for arriving at and revising Codex standards; format of the standards; subsidiary bodies; members; committee guidelines; and definitions of methods of analysis.

821. Joint FAO/WHO Codex Alimentarius Commission. **Summary of Acceptances of Recommended Worldwide and Regional Codex Standards and Recommended Codex Maximum Limits for Pesticide Residues: As of October, 1978**. Rome: Food and Agriculture Organization of the United Nations and World Health Organization, 1978. 1 portfolio (about 336 leaves).

This work summarizes degree of acceptance by various countries of individual Codex Alimentarius standards.

Joint FAO/WHO Expert Committee on Food Additives

GENERAL

822. Joint FAO/WHO Expert Committee on Food Additives. **FAO/WHO Food Additives Data System**. Rome: Food and Agriculture Organization of the United Nations, 1984. 233p. (FAO Food and Nutrition Paper, No. 30). ISBN 925101471X.

This is an index to toxicological evaluations of food additives performed since 1956 by the Joint Committee and the Codex Committee on Food Additives of the WHO and FAO. Information contained in each entry includes chemical names and synonyms, functional classes, permitted uses, latest evaluation status with references, and previous evaluation status, with information on acceptable daily intake.

823. Joint FAO/WHO Expert Committee on Food Additives. **Guide to Specifications for General Notices, General Methods, Identification Tests, Test Solutions, and Other Reference Materials**. Rome: Food and Agriculture Organization of the United Nations, 1983. 304p. (FAO Food and Nutrition Paper, No. 5, rev. 1). (looseleaf). ISBN 925101406X.

"These General Notices provide in summary form a commentary on how specifications of the Joint FAO/WHO Expert Committee on Food Additives are to be interpreted." Covered are general methods, methods for enzyme preparations, fats and related substances, flavoring substances, phosphates, identification tests, standard buffer solutions, test solutions, and volumetric solutions. The apendix includes a Bertrand table and a bibliography of reports and other documents resulting from previous sessions of the Committee.

824. Food and Agriculture Organization of the United Nations. **Manual of Food Quality Control**. Rome: Food and Agriculture Organization of the United Nations, 1979- . (FAO Food and Nutrition Paper, No. 14).
"This manual has been prepared to provide a single source book on methods and useful information in the microbiological examination, quality control and monitoring of food in developing countries."

> No. 14/1. *Food Control Laboratory*. By P. G. Martin. ISBN 9251008396.
>
> No. 14/2. *Additives, Contaminants, Techniques*. ISBN 9251008671.
>
> No. 14/3. *Commodities*. By P. G. Martin. ISBN 9251008442.
>
> No. 14/4. *Microbiological Analysis*. By M. K. Refai. ISBN 9251008361.
>
> No. 14/5. *Food Inspection*. ISBN 9251014051.
>
> No. 14/6. *Food for Export*. By O. P. Dhamija. ISBN 9251008493.

SPECIFICATIONS FOR IDENTITY
AND PURITY

The Joint FAO/WHO Expert Committee on Food Additives has published many standards for identity and purity of food additives. These are being issued as *FAO Food and Nutrition Papers*. To date they have dealt with topics such as food colors, carrier solvents, flavoring agents, emulsifiers, stabilizers, sweetening agents, enzyme preparations, buffering agents, and antioxidants.

International Organization for Standardization

825. International Organization for Standardization. **International Standards**. Geneva: International Organization for Standardization, 1972- .
The International Organization for Standardization is a federation of national standards organizations in 90 countries. It issues standards in all fields except electrical and electronic engineering. Prior to 1972 these were published as *ISO Recommendations*. They are entirely voluntary and generally serve as models in the development of national standards. Food standards are developed by Technical Committee 34 (Agricultural Food Products) and now number approximately 340. Some are issued in revised editions.

826.   International Organization for Standardization. **ISO Catalogue**. Geneva: International Organization for Standardization, 19?- . ISSN 0303-3309.
This annual catalog serves as a subject and numeric index to ISO standards.

Other

827.   British Food Manufacturing Industries Research Association. **Overseas Food Legislation**. 2nd ed. Leatherhead, England: British Food Manufacturing Association, 1984. 2v. (looseleaf).

828.   Flowerdew, Dorothy W. **A Guide to the Food Regulations in the United Kingdom**. 2nd ed. Leatherhead, England: British Food Manufacturing Industries Association, 1981. 1v. (looseleaf).
The second edition incorporates the first supplement to this guide.

829.   International Dairy Federation. **International Standard FIL-IDF: Norme Internationale FIL-IDF**. Brussels: International Dairy Federation, General Secretariat, 1955- . ISSN 0538-7094.
The text is in English and French. Some standards are issued in revised editions.

830.   Japan. Kōseishō. **The Japanese Standards of Food Additives**. 4th ed. Tokyo: Ministry of Health and Welfare, 1979. 678p.
Similar to our *Food Chemicals Codex*, this is a translation of *Shokuhin Tenkabutsu Kōteisho*, the standards for food additives in Japan.

831.   Université Libre de Bruxelles. Food Law Research Centre. **Food Additives Tables**. Amsterdam, Netherlands: Elsevier Scientific Publishing Co., 1980-1984. 3v. ISBN 0444419381.
Data on the regulatory status of food additives used in specific foods in 19 countries are included. The arrangement is by classes of foods.

SELECTED REFERENCES

Allen, R. J. "Nutrition and the Work of the Codex Alimentarius Commission." *Food and Nutrition* 7 (1981): 22-27.

"Codex Alimentarius Commission." *Food and Nutrition* 9 (1983): 50-51.

Grange, George R. "USDA Grade Standards for Foods." In *Encyclopedia of Food Technology*, A. H. Johnson and M. H. Peterson, eds., 917-22. Westport, Conn.: AVI, 1974.

Hutt, P. B. "Government Regulation of the Integrity of the Food Supply." *Annual Review of Nutrition* 4 (1984): 1-20.

Janssen, Wallace F. *The U.S. Food and Drug Law: How It Came, How It Works.* Washington, D.C.: U.S. Department of Health, Education and Welfare, Food and Drug Administration, 1979. 7p. (HEW Publication No. (FDA) 79-1054). HE20.4002.F73/21.

National Research Council. Food and Nutrition Board. Committee on the Scientific Basis of the Nation's Meat and Poultry Inspection Program. *Meat and Poultry Inspection: The Scientific Basis of the Nation's Program.* Washington, D.C.: National Academy of Science, 1985. 209p. ISBN 0309035821.

Stine, Bryan J. "Codex Alimentarius." In *Encyclopedia of Food Technology*, A. H. Johnson and M. H. Peterson, eds., 234-39. Westport, Conn.: AVI, 1974.

United States. Department of Agriculture. *USDA Standards for Food: How They Are Developed and Used.* Washington, D.C.: U.S. Department of Agriculture, 1977. 19p. (Program Aid, No. 1027). A1.58:1027/3.

United States. Department of Agriculture. Agricultural Marketing Service. *Codex Alimentarius Commission: The United States Role in International Standards for Food Products.* Washington, D.C.: U.S. Department of Agriculture, Agricultural Marketing Service, 1976. 6p. (AMS 568). A88.40:568.

United States. Department of Agriculture. Federal Grain Inspection Service. *Federal Grain Inspection Service: Standardization Division.* Kansas City, Mo.: U.S. Department of Agriculture, 1980. 6p. A104.2:G76/2.

United States. Department of Agriculture. Food Safety and Quality Service. *Federal Food Standards.* Washington, D.C.: U.S. Department of Agriculture, Food Safety and Quality Service, 1981. 4p. (FSQS No. 19). A103.14:19.

United States. Department of Agriculture. Food Safety and Quality Service. *Meat and Poultry Inspection: A Program That Protects.* Washington, D.C.: U.S. Department of Agriculture, Food Safety and Quality Service, 1981. 4p. (on one sheet). (FSQS No. 50). A103.14:50.

United States. Food and Drug Administration. *We Want You to Know about Today's FDA.* Washington, D.C.: U.S. Department of Health, Education and Welfare, Public Health Service, Food and Drug Administration, 1979. 6p. (HEW Publication, No. (FDA) 79-1021). HE20.4002:F73/8 1979.

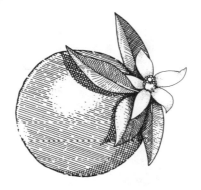

Part VI

RELATED
AREAS

22
Food Service
and Food Preparation

Literature of interest to the food service professional is scattered through-out periodicals relating to the restaurant and hotel industry, institutional food service, cooking, dietetics, hospitals, and management and business. There is no indexing/abstracting service in the field. The most useful continuing bibliography is the *Bibliography of Hotel and Restaurant Administration*. The *Food and Nutrition Quarterly Index* and its predecessor, *Food and Nutrition Bibliography*, also cover some of the food service literature. For business- and management-related literature, it is useful to consult the *Business Periodicals Index*.

BIBLIOGRAPHIES AND GUIDES

832. **Bibliography of Hotel and Restaurant Administration**. No. 39- . Ithaca, N.Y.: School of Hotel Administration, Cornell University, 1980- . annual. ISSN 8756-9388.

Formerly published in the *Cornell Hotel and Restaurant Administration Quarterly*, this bibliography is the major access tool for food service literature appearing in periodicals. Recently, books have also been covered in some of the issues. A list of indexing terms and a list of periodical publishers' addresses are included.

833. Coyle, Patrick L. **Cook's Books: An Affectionate Guide to the Literature of Food and Cooking**. New York: Facts on File, 1985. 239p. ISBN 0971966832.

This bibliographic survey is organized as follows: history of cookbooks; classic books by great chefs; famous cookbooks by food and cookery experts; general cookbooks; cuisine cookbooks; cookbooks by type of food or special ingredients; cookbooks by course, process, or technique; shopping for food and equipment; and food appreciation. Coyle is to be commended for a rare bibliography indeed—one that is readable from cover to cover. However, some important authors and books have escaped his attention. The vegetarian section is brief and excludes Mollie Katzen's *Moosewood Cookbook*, one of the all-time bestsellers of this genre. The section on Chinese cooking omits Irene Kuo's *Key to Chinese Cooking*, a book widely recognized as a classic, and the section on the books of great chefs excludes Fernand Point.

834.   Feret, Barbara L. **Gastronomical and Culinary Literature: A Survey of Historically Oriented Collections in the U.S.A.** Metuchen, N.J.: Scarecrow Press, 1979. 124p. ISBN 0810812045.

Part ·1 discusses major works in the history of gastronomy by country and time period. Part 2 describes major library and private collections on the history of cookery. Appendices list culinary bibliographies and secondary historical texts. There is an index.

835.   Lowenstein, Eleanor. **Bibliography of American Cookery Books, 1742-1860.** 3rd ed. Worcester, Mass.: American Antiquarian Society, 1972. 132p.

This is a revised edition of Lowenstein's earlier work, *American Cookery Books, 1742-1860* (1954), which in turn was a revision of Waldo Lincoln's *American Cookery Books* (1929). This checklist of 835 items has an author and a title index.

836.   Pickworth, Barbara A. **An Annotated Bibliography of Food Service Articles in the Journal of the American Dietetics Association from 1965 to 1982.** Toronto: Ryerson Polytechnical Institute Library, 1983. 1v. (various paging).

Organized by broad but useful subject categories, this bibliography has no index.

837.   Tudor, Nancy, and Dean Tudor. **Cooking for Entertaining.** New York: R. R. Bowker, 1976. 256p. ISBN 0835208850.

This annotated guide to culinary reference materials and cookbooks arranged by concepts, foods, and geographic areas also lists societies, periodicals, book clubs, and cooking classes. There is a title and author index.

838.   Wixon, Emily, and John Norback. **Foodservice Bibliography, 1979-82.** Chicago: Institute of Food Technologists, 1983. 1v. (various paging).

"Compiled from literature searches conducted in four bibliographic databases: *Agricola ... Food Science and Technology Abstracts ... Foods Adlibra ...* and *Management Contents.*" Citations are arranged in broad subject categories within three chronological sequences.

RECIPE INDEXES

839.   Forsman, John. **Recipe Index, 1971: The Eater's Guide to Periodical Literature.** Detroit: Gale Research, 1973. 764p.

"A key to over 6600 recipes published in popular magazines, arranged according to recipe name, principal ingredient, nationality, and type of dish." Included are recipes from *Gourmet.*

840. Torgeson, Kathryn W., and Sylvia J. Weinstein. **The Garland Recipe Index**. New York: Garland, 1984. 314p. (Garland Reference Library of the Humanities, Vol. 414). ISBN 0824091248.

Indexed are recipes appearing in approximately 50 cookbooks published in the last 10 years. The following food categories are included: basic, foreign and ethnic, U.S. regional, and specialty. Recipes are indexed according to name, major food ingredients, and cooking style. A bibliography is included.

DICTIONARIES

841. Dahl, Crete M., and Julie Wilkinson, eds. **Food and Menu Dictionary**. Boston: Cahners Books, 1972. 135p. ISBN 0843605561.

Brief definitions of more than 2,000 terms, with pronunciation of foreign terms, are given. Entries range from one word to one-half page.

842. De Sola, Ralph, and Dorothy De Sola, comps. **A Dictionary of Cooking: Approximately Eight Thousand Definitions of Culinary Ingredients, Methods, Terms, and Utensils**. New York: Meredith Press, 1969. 246p. SBN 696580128.

The number of definitions in this dictionary is large, but many are extremely brief and in some cases inadequate. This dictionary is now in need of updating.

843. **Funk and Wagnalls Cook's and Diner's Dictionary: A Lexicon of Food, Wine, and Culinary Terms**. New York: Funk and Wagnalls, 1969. 274p.

Covered are terms related to cooking methods, prepared dishes, individual foods, drinks, and food ingredients. Foreign terms are accompanied by pronunciations. The length of entries ranges from one sentence to one page.

844. Hering, Richard. **Hering's Dictionary of Classical and Modern Cookery and Practical Reference Manual for the Hotel, Restaurant, and Catering Trade**. 7th ed. Revised and translated by Walter Bickel. London: Virtue, 1981. 852p. ISBN 3805702442.

This book is essentially an English translation of *Lexikon der Küche*, a series of separately paged dictionaries defining food terms or prepared dishes. The arrangement is by subject categories (e.g., hors d'oeuvres, sauces and gravies, soups, garnishes, egg dishes). A multilingual vocabulary with index appears at the end. The volume is thumb-indexed for convenience. This can be an excellent source of reference for someone who already knows what category to consult.

845. Mariani, John E. **The Dictionary of American Food and Drink**. New York: Ticknor & Fields, 1983. 477p. ISBN 0899191991.

A dictionary of American gastronomy not unlike the well-known *Larousse Gastronomique*, this work has been highly praised by reviewers. There are roughly 1,700 major entries for foods, dishes, drinks, restaurant terms, etc., from all regions of the country. Definitions tell what ingredients a dish is made from, relate anecdotes and lore, provide historical information about its introduction, and tell where it is commonly eaten. Some entries have extremely detailed information, with many subentries. For example, the entry for candy bar has 23 subentries for individual candy bars. Recipes are tucked into 500 of the definitions. Selected by *Library Journal* as one of the best reference books of

1983, this is a particularly good source of information on regional food. It contains a bibliography and a detailed subject index.

846. Martin, Ruth Marion Somers. **International Dictionary of Food and Cooking**. New York: Hastings House, 1974. 311p. ISBN 0803833881.

This dictionary has very brief definitions, but covers a large number of terms, many of which are foreign. It is intended for the housewife or new student of cooking.

847. Root, Waverly. **Food; An Authoritative, Visual History and Dictionary of the Foods of the World**. New York: Simon and Schuster, 1980. 602p. ISBN 0671627953 (pbk).

Attractively illustrated with photographs and reproductions of paintings, this dictionary emphasizes the historical origins and proliferation of basic ingredient foods. The 200 finely crafted essays, occasionally several pages long, are a delight to read. In addition to origins, they discuss geography, growing conditions, and lore. A bibliography of source materials is included.

848. Sharman, Fay. **The Taste of France: A Dictionary of French Food and Wine**. London: Macmillan Reference Books, 1982. 320p. ISBN 0333320069.

"A dictionary of French words and French terms connected with food. It has been designed to cover anything you might encounter on a menu in a French restaurant." Included are terms relating to wines and spirits; pronunciations are omitted.

849. Simon, André Louis. **A Dictionary of Gastronomy**. New York: McGraw-Hill, 1970. 400p.

This dictionary of culinary terms, with many extensive but some brief definitions, covers ingredient foods, names of dishes (some with recipes in the body of the definition), wine terms, utensils, cooking methods, names of famous chefs, herbs, spices, and even exotic fruits and vegetables. It is illustrated with color plates and line drawings. This is an updated version of an earlier work by Simon.

850. Waldo, Myra. **Dictionary of International Food and Cooking Terms**. New York: Macmillan, 1967. 648p.

One of the most complete dictionaries of food and cooking terms available, this volume includes entries of varying length. Definitions are clear and to the point. This excellent source of reference could, however, use updating.

DIRECTORIES

851. **Restaurants and Institutions**. Vol. 88- , No. 1- . Chicago: Cahners Publishing Co., 1981- . semi-monthly. ISSN 0273-5520.

The annual "400" issue of this periodical, published in July, lists the 400 largest food service companies in rank order, and provides information on sales volume and recent developments in the company. It also provides information on market trends.

852.   Sheridan, John F., and Leo A. Rouf. **Food Service Equipment Directory for Health Care Facilities**. Columbus, Ohio: Ross Planning Associates, Ross Laboratories, 1982. 68p.

Listed is food service equipment for hospitals and nursing homes made by nearly 800 companies. A subject guide to equipment with addresses of manufacturers is appended. Also included are hints on purchasing and estimated useful life of various items. There is an index.

853.   **Who's Who in the Foodservice Industry: Membership Directory of the National Restaurant Association**. Washington, D.C.: National Restaurant Association, 1984- . frequency unknown.

ENCYCLOPEDIAS

854.   Claiborne, Craig. **Craig Claiborne's The New York Times Food Encyclopedia**. Compiled by Joan Whitman. New York: Times Books, 1985. ISBN 0812912713.

While useful, this encyclopedia is not as extensive as one would have wished. Entries range from six or seven lines to over a page and generally deal with food ingredients, prepared dishes, styles of cooking, or cuisines. Very exotic ingredients are absent. The text is enjoyable to read and draws heavily upon the author's vast experience in the culinary arts. There is a bibliography, but no index.

855.   FitzGibbon, Theodora. **The Food of the Western World: An Encyclopedia of Food from North America and Europe**. New York: Quadrangle/New York Times Book Co., 1976. 529p. ISBN 0812904273.

Containing information about the history of food and the cuisines of 34 countries, this volume has some 2,500 recipes, arranged alphabetically. There are comparative tables for American, English, and French cuts of meat, as well as a bibliography.

856.   Montagné, Prosper. **The New Larousse Gastronomique: The Encyclopedia of Food, Wine and Cookery**. New York: Crown Publishers, 1977. 1064p. ISBN 0517531372.

A major source of reference for the culinary arts, this extensive encyclopedia defines terms, describes ingredients and dishes, and provides many recipes. It is beautifully illustrated with many color plates. There is an index.

857.   Snider, Nancy. **Frozen Food Encyclopedia for Foodservice**. Hershey, Pa.: National Frozen Food Association, 1985. 133p.

Intended for institutional food purchasers and sales representatives, this book gathers information on different types of frozen foods available by category: beverages, breads, cakes, pies and desserts, prepared entrees, fish and seafood, fruits, meats, poultry and game, vegetables, and other foods. It describes items, and gives available sizes or weights, grades, preparation hints, selling points, cost comparisons, merchandising hints, and hints for specifying desirable quality. Each section contains numerous charts and tables. There is an index.

858. Stobart, Tom. **The Cook's Encyclopedia: Ingredients and Processes**. New York: Harper & Row, 1981. 547p. ISBN 0060141271.

A useful encyclopedic dictionary of ingredient foods (e.g., cardamom, almond or papaya), and cooking processes (e.g., freezing, thickening, marinating), this work contains alphabetically arranged entries ranging in length from a few lines to more than a page. There are numerous cross-references. Genera and species are provided for plants and animals.

859. Woodman, Julie G. **The IFMA Encyclopedia of the Foodservice Industry**. 5th ed. Chicago: International Foodservice Manufacturers Association, 1985. 275p.

This revised edition reflects new developments in the market place, such as consumer concern about nutrition. The entire volume emphasizes information on marketing. There are data on industry trends; menu changes to reflect consumer concerns; market surveys, size, and segments; marketing and distribution to the food service industry; the market for food, equipment, and supplies; food service chains; regional, state, and metropolitan area markets; and the impact of the federal government on markets. There is also a list of industry publications, associations, trade shows, conferences, and award programs. A detailed subject index appears at the front of the volume.

HANDBOOKS, MANUALS, AND OTHER DATA COMPILATIONS

860. American Home Economics Association. **Handbook of Food Preparation**. 1st- . Washington, D.C.: American Home Economics Association, 1946- . ISSN 0278-906X.

This handbook contains general information on recipe development and recipe writing; tables with basic proportions of common recipes; baking temperatures and times; information on thickening and gelling agents; and information on preparation of food at high altitudes, in microwave ovens, and in slow cookers. There are glossaries of terms and extensive sections on using specific types of foods, dealing with purchasing, storage, and cooking of dairy products, meat, poultry, eggs, fruits, vegetables, grains, and grain products. There are also sections dealing with leavening agents, sweeteners, and fats and oils. Other useful material provided is food buying guides converting purchased weight to number of servings, pieces or cups and approximate weight per cup as cooked, time tables for canning, freezing temperatures, and tests for syrups and candies. Included are sources of information and an index. (Description based on the 1980 edition.)

861. Avery, Arthur C. **A Modern Guide to Foodservice Equipment**. rev. ed. New York: CBI Books, 1985. 358p. ISBN 0442208375.

This survey of characteristics of available equipment covers ranges, ovens, fryers, frypans, griddles, broilers, steam jacketed kettles, steam and pressure cookers, refrigerators and freezers, dishwashers, coffee makers, mixers, serving equipment, waste disposals and trash compactors, and miscellaneous small equipment. It includes a glossary, information on kitchen layout and ergonomic design, and an index.

862. Bailey, Adrian, et al. **The Book of Ingredients.** London: Michael Joseph Ltd., 1980. 296p. ISBN 0718119150.

Although well illustrated, this book does not provide extensive information on food ingredients. The superb photographs in themselves, however, are invaluable in enabling cooks to identify ingredients such as different types of fish and seafood. A good complement to other less well illustrated books of this type.

863. Batcher, Olive. **Food Purchasing for Group Feeding.** (Revised June 1983). Washington, D.C.: Government Printing Office, 1983. 148p. (Agriculture Handbook No. 284). A1.76:284/2.

"Information helpful to food managers in estimating quantities of foods to be prepared for group feeding in small and large institutions." Tables list about 770 food items in customary market units, weight per unit, percent yield as served, description of prepared food, and purchase units for 100 portions.

864. Beard, James, et al., eds. **The Cook's Catalogue: A Critical Selection of the Best, the Necessary, and the Special in Kitchen Equipment and Utensils, Over 4000 Items Including 200 Extraordinary Recipes Plus Cooking Folklore.** New York: Harper & Row, 1975. 565p. ISBN 0060115637.

This beautifully produced catalog is adorned with old fashioned drawings and contemporary photographs of featured equipment and utensils, selected and evaluated by a team of chefs. It covers every conceivable type of equipment useful to the home cook, and to a lesser extent to the professional, from measuring cups, knives, pots and pans, to electric mixers and ice cream makers. Included are recipes using particular items, a bibliography of cookbooks, a recipe index, and a general index.

865. Birchfield, John. **Foodservice Operations Manual: A Guide for Hotels, Restaurants, and Institutions.** Boston: CBI Publishing Co., 1979. ca.500p. (various paging). ISBN 0843621451.

This manual contains basic information on the major operations in the "food management sequence" and is intended in part as a guide for food service managers to use in developing manuals for specific food service operations. Eight thumb-indexed sections cover menu planning, purchasing guidelines and storage, food production and food handling methods, sanitation standards and inspection, cost control, personnel policies and procedures, efficiency, and administrative policies. The appendix includes a menu costing chart and various types of forms. A supplement contains information on energy management. There is no index.

866. Cox, Beverly. **Cooking Techniques: How to Do Anything a Recipe Tells You to Do.** Boston: Little, Brown, 1981. 567p. ISBN 0316937525.

A compendium of photographs with text illustrating preparation and cooking techniques, this volume is arranged according to food groups. There is no index.

867. Cox, Pat M. **Deep Freezing: A Comprehensive Guide to Its Theory and Practice.** London: Faber, 1979. 482p. ISBN 0571649540.

Intended for the home economist and the housewife, this book presents theoretical and technical information on freezing food and detailed instructions for freezing specific foods. Included are recipes and an index.

868. Eckstein, Eleanor F. **Menu Planning**. 3rd ed. Westport, Conn.: AVI, 1983. 463p. ISBN 0870554395.

A standard reference work on menu planning for institutional food services, this work gives special consideration to diverse consumer groups in a variety of institutions and to foodways of American ethnic groups. It includes information on computer applications to menu planning, bibliographies, and an index.

869. Fulton, Lois. **Average Weight of a Measured Cup of Various Foods**. Washington, D.C.: Government Printing Office, 1977. 26p. (Home Economics Report, No. 41). A1.87:41.

This table provides information on the average weight in one cup of fresh and prepared foods. It is useful in dietary analysis as well as food preparation.

870. Fulton, Lois. **Buying Food: A Guide for Calculating Amounts to Buy and Comparing Costs**. Washington, D.C.: Government Printing Office, 1977. 71p. (Home Economics Report, No. 42). A1.87:42.

This guide compares foods as purchased, in terms of yield in number of servings. For instance, this table provides information on the amount of chuck steak needed per 3 oz. serving if bought with or without bone.

871. Hullah, Evelyn. **Cardinal's Handbook of Recipe Development**. Don Mills, Ont.: Cardinal Kitchens, 1984. 159p. ISBN 0920451004.

Hullah's excellent guide to planning procedures, terminology, measurement, testing, and writing principles used to develop standardized recipes is of value to home economists, dietitians, and others involved in recipe development. It contains information on recipe adaptation for microwave cooking and high altitude cooking. There are numerous charts and tables covering garnishes, spices, and herbs and their uses; smoke points of fats and oils; traditional ingredient proportions in basic recipes; thickening and gelling agents; oven temperatures; approximate baking times; roasting temperatures and times; a vegetable cookery chart; seasonal availability of fresh foods and vegetables (in Canada); a glossary of food and cooking terms; substitutions for common foods; approximate food equivalents after preparation; and volume and weight equivalents for common foods. A bibliography and an index are included. The book is very Canadian and metric, but very, very useful.

872. Mahaffey, Mary J., Mary E. Mennes, and Bonnie B. Miller. **Food Service Manual for Health Care Institutions**. Chicago: American Hospital Association, 1982. 381p. ISBN 0872583309.

A compendium of useful information for the hospital food service administrator, this book contains information on organization and management, food production and service systems, personnel, food protection practices, financial management, nutrition, menu planning, food purchasing, and equipment.

873. Matthews, Ruth H., and Young J. Garrison. **Food Yields Summarized by Different Stages of Preparation**. Washington, D.C.: Government Printing Office, 1975. 136p. (Agriculture Handbook No. 102). A1.76:102.

Food Yields is a useful publication for food service professionals who need to know yields of given quantities of raw food, in other words, how many pounds of potatoes with skin are needed to equal a given number of pounds of peeled potatoes for a mashed potato dish. A table provides description of food before preparation, yield after preparation, and average loss or gain in preparation. The appendix has sample calculations.

874.   McGee, Harold. **On Food and Cooking: The Science and Lore of the Kitchen**. New York: Scribner, 1984. 684p. ISBN 0684181320.

This extensive compendium of information on the science, history, and lore of cooking is organized by groups of foods, with additional chapters on nutrition and general principles of cooking. This excellent book provides information on topics 'as diverse as sugar refining, the making of chocolate, bread making principles, the development of the breakfast cereal industry, and why eggs whip. An extensive bibliography and index are included.

875.   Peddersen, Raymond B. **SPECS: The Comprehensive Foodservice Purchasing and Specification Manual**. Boston: Cahners Books, 1977. 1185p. ISBN 0843620846.

This comprehensive compendium includes information on varieties, marketing, season, grades, and quality standards of all foods likely to be purchased by institutions or restaurants. Included in the section on quality control are references to the *Code of Federal Regulations*, federal specifications, and military standards. There are major sections on meat, poultry, eggs, dairy, fish, convenience foods, kosher foods, fruits and vegetables, juices, jams, jellies, etc. There is an index.

876.   Roehl, Evelyn. **Food Facts: A Compendium of Information for a Whole Foods Cuisine**. Winona, Minn.: Food Learning Center, 1984. 212p. ISBN 0931149002.

Information on frequently used natural foods is grouped by categories — nuts and seeds, grains, legumes, etc. Individual entries describe food and how it is marketed, how it is grown or made, where it originated, how to use and store it, as well as major nutrients. Appended are a food composition table in the form of USDA Home and Garden Bulletin, No. 72 (1981), a brief table of vitamin E values, a bibliography, and an index.

877.   Rose, James C., ed. **Handbook for Health Care Food Service Management**. Rockville, Md.: Aspen Systems Corp., 1984. 369p. ISBN 0894438999.

Individually authored chapters on all aspects of the organization and management of food service operations in health care institutions cover topics as diverse as personnel management, training, equipment, purchasing, forecasting demand, computers in hospital food services, productivity, diet order transmittal systems, etc. There is an index.

878.   Schneider, Elizabeth. **Uncommon Fruits and Vegetables: A Commonsense Guide**. 1st ed. New York: Harper & Row, 1986. 546p. ISBN 0060154209.

Arranged alphabetically, this extensive guide provides information on a wide range of unusual fruits and vegetables used in a variety of ethnic foods. Included are entries for such diverse foods as taro, feijoa, cape gooseberry, and prickly pear. Individual entries provide alternative names; genera and species; description; recipes; and information on selection, storage, use, and preparation. Nutritional information is very sketchy. The volume contains a bibliography and a detailed index.

879.   Scriven, Carl. **Food Equipment Facts: A Handbook for the Food Service Industry**. New York: Wiley, 1982. 429p. ISBN 0471868191.

Covered are characteristics, planning, space, and organizational aspects of all types of food service equipment.

880.   Sunset Magazine. **Good Cook's Handbook**. Menlo Park, Calif.: Lane Publishing Co., 1986. 112p. ISBN 0376022027.

This is a handy collection of useful information aimed chiefly at the home cook. The first section, entitled "Kitchen Basics," defines terms, describes and illustrates kitchen equipment and herbs and spices, lists staple foods for a well-stocked kitchen, provides equivalents and substitutions, and includes a wine selection guide and an abbreviated food composition table based on USDA Home and Garden Bulletin, No. 72. Five additional sections are devoted to meat and poultry, fish and shellfish, eggs and cheese, pasta and grains, and fruits and vegetables. These provide information on purchasing, cooking techniques, storage, and cooking temperatures and times. Microwave cooking directions appear throughout. Other useful features included are adjustments for high altitude baking and directions for preparing vegetables in the food processor. Not included are standard recipe proportions for common baked goods and sauces, information on thickeners, and cooking with a slow cooker. The book is well illustrated with color drawings, and has an index.

881.   Terrell, Margaret E. **Professional Food Preparation**. 2nd ed. New York: Wiley, 1979. 741p. ISBN 0471852023.

An extensive reference text on the organization of quantity food preparation operations, Terrell's book includes material on cooking; baking; preparation of vegetables, fruits, soups, and sauces; etc. Appendixes include a table of equivalent measures of food; a glossary; a table of food quantities for 100 portions; required utensils for each type of activity; and suggestions for toppings, garnishes, and accompaniments. There is an index.

882.   Thorner, Marvin Edward. **Convenience and Fast Food Handbook**. Westport, Conn.: AVI, 1973. 358p. ISBN 0870551345.

This manual for the preparation of convenience foods in food service operations covers food preparation areas, equipment, quality control, and specific convenience foods. There is an index.

883.   United States. Department of Agriculture. Food and Nutrition Service. **Menu Planning Guide for School Food Service**. rev. ed. Washington, D.C.: Government Printing Office, 1983. 1v. (Program Aid, No. 1260). A1.68:1260/2.

This is a guide for planning nutritious school lunch menus which reduce plate waste and comply with federal requirements, recommendations, and policies. There is an index.

884.   United States. Department of Health, Education and Welfare. Food and Drug Administration. Division of Retail Food Protection. **Food Service Sanitation Manual: Including a Model Food Service Sanitation Ordinance**. Washington, D.C.: Government Printing Office, 1978. 96p. (DHEW Pub. No. (FDA) 78-2081). HE20.4008:F73/3.

This manual includes information on the need for and conducting of an effective food sanitation program. Section VI contains the Food and Drug Administration's Food Service Sanitation Ordinance (1976 recommendations).

885. Von Welanetz, Diana, and Paul Von Welanetz. **The Von Welanetz Guide to Ethnic Ingredients: With More Than 150 Recipes and Information on Buying, Storage, Preparation, and Use.** Los Angeles, Calif.: J. P. Tarcher, 1982. 731p. ISBN 0874772257.

This extensive guide to ethnic ingredient foods and seasonings from all parts of the world is arranged by region—Africa, Asia, Europe, Latin America, Middle East—and regional American foods. It includes recipes; shopping sources; equivalents for food names in French, German, Italian, and Spanish; and genera and species where applicable. There is an index.

886. Wenzel, G. L. **Wenzel's Menu Maker.** Boston: CBI Publishing Co., 1979. 1167p. ISBN 0843621354.

Sometimes referred to as "the bible" of the food service industry, this voluminous compendium of practical information is virtually indispensable to the food service professional. It is divided into 17 major sections: management, purchasing, soups, salads, pantry, beef, veal, pork, lamb, poultry, seafood, international dishes, meatless dishes, sauces, bakery products, dessert service, and breakfast. Each has purchasing information where relevant and basic recipes. The extensive section on management provides information on staff and kitchen organization, setting up menus, inventory control, etc. The general purchasing section has descriptions and U.S. grades of fresh fruits and vegetables and miscellaneous items. Purchasing information on meats and fish is found in sections dealing with those subjects. The appendix contains a glossary, weights and measures, and a metric conversion chart. It is thumb-indexed only.

887. West, Bessie Brooks, Grace Severance Shugart, and Fay Maxine Wilson. **Food for Fifty.** 6th ed. New York: Wiley, 1979. 676p. ISBN 0471026883.

A classic work on quantity cookery, this book contains a full spectrum of recipes from appetizers to desserts. It also contains information on menu planning and charts showing the amounts of food as purchased to serve 50, food weights and approximate equivalents, adjusting yield, a guide for rounding off weights and measures, approximate equivalent substitutions, baking temperatures, a glossary of terms, etc. There is an index.

888. Zaccarelli, Herman E. **Cost Effective Contract Food Service: An Institutional Guide.** Rockville, Md.: Aspen Systems Corp., 1982. 289p. ISBN 0894433997.

In addition to general material on contracted food services, this guide to the economics of contract health care food service management includes chapters on legal aspects, costs of facility-operated services versus contracted services, writing requests for proposal, administration, personnel, and other topics. A bibliography and an index are included.

STANDARDS

889. Eckel, Peter J. **College & University Food Service Management Standards**. Westport, Conn.: AVI, 1985. 175p. (L. J. Minor Foodservice Standards Series, No. 6). ISBN 0870554808.

"This book considers those standards of good management that are necessary for survival in the increasingly competitive business of college foodservice." Included are chapters dealing with public relations, menus, purchasing, budgeting, food conservation, sanitation, vending, and other topics. Included are a bibliography of food service trade publications and associations and an index.

890. Kotschevar, Lendal Henry. **Standards, Principles, and Techniques in Quantity Food Production**. 3rd ed. Boston: Cahners Books, 1974. 661p. ISBN 0843605839.

"Emphasizes the basic production of food from the standpoint of techniques, standards and principles." There are three major sections, each with five to seven chapters on management in quantity food production, kitchen production, and bakeshop production. The appendix contains a glossary, tables of substitutions and equivalents, standard portions, etc. An index is included.

891. Lawson, Harry W. **Standards for Fats & Oils**. Westport, Conn.: AVI, 1985. 235p. (L. J. Minor Foodservice Standards Series, No. 5). ISBN 0870554670.

Written as a reference text on the use of oils and fats in the foodservice industry, this volume is divided into three parts. Part I discusses the chemical structure of fats and oils; physical properties; sources; processing technology; and analytical tests to determine rancidity, degree of saturation, etc. Part II describes good practice in deep frying, pan frying, preparation of salad dressings, and the use of oils in baking. Part III deals with the nutritional aspects of fats and oils and new product development. The book is indexed.

892. McIntosh, Robert Woodrow. **Employee Management Standards**. Westport, Conn.: AVI, 1984. 194p. (L. J. Minor Foodservice Standards Series, No. 4). ISBN 087055459X.

McIntosh discusses good practice in employee management. Topics covered include the development of leadership; human relations and communication skills; selecting, training, supervising, and motivating staff; and avoiding legal problems. Appendixes have selected job descriptions and lists of selected trade journals and book publishers. There is an index.

893. Minor, Lewis J. **Nutritional Standards**. Westport, Conn.: AVI, 1983. 281p. (L. J. Minor Foodservice Standards Series, No. 1). ISBN 0870554255.

Food and nutrition-related standards relevant to food service are covered. The book treats standards for food products, food flavor, nutrition, food product development, and the laboratory evaluation of food.

894. Minor, Lewis J. **Sanitation, Safety & Environmental Standards**. Westport, Conn.: AVI, 1983. 245p. (L. J. Minor Foodservice Standards Series, No. 2). ISBN 087055428X.

This volume provides guidelines for sanitation and food handling and discusses standard practice for controlling microbial and other food hazards, occupational health and safety measures, kitchen safety, and food waste control. It has an index.

895.   National Association of College and University Food Services. **National Association of College and University Food Services Professional Standards Manual**. East Lansing, Mich.: National Association of College and University Foodservices, 1982. 1v. (various paging).

Covered are costs, controls and accountability, satisfaction of clientele, employees and community, quality assurance systems, sanitation and safety, and administration of personnel and programs. There is no index.

896.   National Sanitation Foundation. **NSF Food Service Equipment Standards**. Ann Arbor, Mich.: The Foundation, 1978. 288p.

"NSF operates its own testing laboratory.... It tests and evaluates equipment, products and services for compliance with NSF standards and criteria; and grants and controls the use of the NSF seal." NSF suggests that regulatory agencies, manufacturers, and purchasers contact the organization to determine if revisions have been made in a particular standard.

23
Social and Cultural Factors

Locating literature on the social, behavioral, economic, and cultural aspects of food and nutrition may require the use of major indexing/abstracting services and other indexing tools in the social sciences. These are described below, with the exception of education sources, which were discussed in chapter 15. In addition to these tools, this chapter includes selected nonperiodic bibliographies useful for specific purposes.

HUMAN RELATIONS AREA FILES

The Human Relations Area Files are not an indexing/abstracting service in the traditional sense of the word. They are a collection of primary source materials, chiefly in the form of excerpts from published books on selected cultures or societies representing all major areas of the world. They are available in the libraries of many academic institutions, either on paper slips or microfiche.

These materials are organized by a unique method designed for the rapid and accurate retrieval of specific data on individual cultures and topics. Retrieval involves using the accompanying *Outline of World Cultures* to locate the alpha-numeric designation for a specific culture—OB1 for Indonesia, for instance, and then using the accompanying *Outline of World Cultural Materials* to locate an appropriate subject number for the topic. For instance, category number 26 relates to food consumption, and within that broad classification number 262 relates to diet—the staple and other foods consumed, seasonal changes in diet, proportion of various foods in diet, and so on. A person then searches for the alphanumeric designation representing the culture for that category number to locate materials on the subject of diet in Indonesia. It is recommended that the following relevant books be consulted to become more familiar with the procedure:

Lagace, Robert O. **Nature and Use of the HRAF Files: A Research and Teaching Guide**. New Haven, Conn.: Human Relations Area Files, Inc., 1974. 49p.

Murdock, George Peter, et al. **Outline of Cultural Materials**. 5th rev. ed. New Haven, Conn.: Human Relations Area Files, Inc., 1982. 247p. ISBN 0875366546.

Murdock, George Peter. **Outline of World Cultures**. 6th rev. ed. New Haven, Conn.: Human Relations Area Files, Inc., 1976. 259p. ISBN 0875366643.

INDEXING/ABSTRACTING SERVICES

897. **Nutrition Planning: An International Journal of Abstracts about Nutrition Policy, Planning, and Programs**. Vol. 1- . Boston: Oelgechlager, Gunn & Hain Publishers, Inc., 1978- . quarterly. ISSN 0149-6743.
The scope of this abstracting service is difficult to define. It includes the planning process itself, consequences of malnutrition, nutritional status assessment, nutrition education and home-centered activities, public health and curative measures, food processing, distribution and feeding problems, agriculture, economics, and social and cultural aspects. It covers journal literature, national and international government publications, and reports of private agencies engaged in nutrition planning and intervention. Most of the literature abstracted is related to developing countries. Most abstracted documents are available from *Nutrition Planning*. It now includes the "Joint WHO/UNICEF Nutrition Support Programme Newsletter."
Arrangement: Extended abstracts are numerically arranged in subject categories.
Indexes: Geographic index, source index, and subject index.

898. **Psychological Abstracts: Nonevaluative Summaries of the World's Literature in Psychology and Related Disciplines**. Vol. 1- . Arlington, Va.: American Psychological Association, 1927- . monthly. ISSN 0033-2887.
The major abstracting service in psychology, *Psychological Abstracts* covers not only the psychological and psychiatric literature, but a significant share of the total behavioral sciences literature as well. Material covered consists primarily of journal articles, dissertations, conference publications, and some books. Over 1,000 sources are regularly scanned.
Online Equivalent: PsycINFO.
Arrangement: Continuously numbered abstracts are arranged by broad subject categories.
Index: An author and a brief subject index are available in each monthly issue and are keyed to abstract numbers. These indexes are cumulated every six months.
Thesaurus of Psychological Terms: Index terms are assigned to articles from the *Thesaurus of Psychological Terms*. It is advisable to use this thesaurus to locate appropriate index terms before beginning a search. Some of the terms relevant to food and nutrition are *food, food intake, diets, eating, obesity, appetite, nutrition, nutritional deficiences, beverages,* and *food additives*.
Psychological Abstracts can be a major source of references for aspects of nutrition with strong behavioral components. The list of journals indexed appears with the cumulated index.

899.   **Social Sciences Citation Index**. Vol. 1- . Philadelphia, Pa.: Institute for Scientific Information, 1969- . 3/yr. (with annual and quinquennial cumulations). ISSN 0091-3707.

An analog of the *Science Citation Index* for social sciences literature, the *Social Sciences Citation Index* is an interdisciplinary citation index covering the major social sciences journals. Citation indexing allows literature searching without subject terms because it enables the user to trace who cited a specific book or article and where it was cited, in effect establishing subject links between books or articles and the references that subsequently cite them.

Citation indexing thus exploits the natural subject relationship between an article and the references cited there to buttress its content. This is a particularly useful feature in the social sciences, where terminology tends to be less standard than in the natural sciences. Researchers instinctively understand this concept because they are already using it when they track the references in a relevant article, moving from article to article backward in time. Citation indexes work similarly, but by consulting each year subsequent to the publication of an article, a searcher moves forward in time, instead of backward.

Online Equivalent: Social SciSearch.

Arrangement: The *Social Sciences Citation Index* has four principal parts: *Citation Index*, *Source Index*, *Corporate Index*, and *Permuterm Subject Index*. The formats of each of these indexes parallel the *Science Citation Index*.

The *Citation Index* is an alphabetical listing by author of articles referred to in a given calendar year. In chronological order under an author's name are all works cited that year. Indented under each is information about who cited these references and where. The *Source Index* should then be consulted under the author of the citing article (the author using the original article as a reference) to find the full reference for this article including the title.

The *Source Index* is an author listing of all articles appearing in the source list of journals regularly indexed. It may be used simply to find out who wrote articles in the source journals in any given year. Its major use, however, is to provide complete information to citing references, that is, those articles which cite the original reference.

The *Permuterm Subject Index* is a title word index to articles in the *Source Index*. It pairs every keyword with every other keyword, with the exception of prepositions and similar "stop" words. The paired terms may or may not be adjacent to one another. This index is used to search *SSCI* by subject when there is no reference available to enter the *Citation Index*, or when it is difficult to find a subject listed in a major indexing and abstracting service with a strictly controlled list of index terms. Because the terms in the *Permuterm Index* are actual words used in titles of articles, they are more apt to reflect currently used terminology in a particular discipline.

The *Corporate Index* consists of two parts: "Geographic" and "Organization." In the "Geographic" part, all entries from the *Source Index* are arranged alphabetically by location (state or country and city). The "Organization" part provides locations for specific institutions and organizations to facilitate their retrieval in the "Geographic" section.

List of Journals Indexed: A *Guide and Lists of Source Publications*, with an abbreviations key to periodical titles, is included in each annual set and is also published separately.

900. **Sociological Abstracts**. Vol. 1- . San Diego, Calif.: Sociological Abstracts, Inc., January-October 1952/53- . monthly (with annually cumulated indexes). ISSN 0038-0202.

Sociological Abstracts is the major abstracting service for sociology and ancillary topics, such as group interaction, complex organization, social change and economic development, culture and social structure, and rural sociology and agriculture, etc. It is much less likely to be used by nutrition and food science professionals than the other indexing/abstracting services listed in this section. However, it does index literature on topics such as the social aspects of food supply, food patterns, food beliefs, diet and fertility studies, malnutrition as a social problem, and poverty.

Online Equivalent: Sociological Abstracts.

Arrangement: The abstracts in each issue appear in a continuous alphanumeric arrangement by broad subjects.

Indexes: There are subject and author indexes in each issue which are then cumulated annually. However, at this writing they are somewhat slow to be issued.

Thesaurus of Sociological Terms: This list of index terms was made available in mid-1986.

List of Journals Indexed: A source index provides a list of the 1,200 or so source journals and other publications from which citations are gleaned.

Supplements: The supplements contain abstracts from the meetings of various organizations in the field, *IRPS International Review of Publications in Sociology*, which contains book abstracts and book reviews, and the *ISA Bulletin*, a newsletter from the International Sociological Association.

Comments: A service for the delivery of source documents is available. Some issues contain the abstracts of the annual conference of the American Sociological Association.

901. **World Agricultural Economics and Rural Sociology Abstracts**. Vol. 1- Farnham Royal, England: CAB International, 1959- . monthly. ISSN 0043-8219.

One of 46 abstracting services published by CAB International, *WAERSA* covers the literature related to agricultural economics and policy. This includes literature on supply and demand, prices, marketing, distribution, international trade, finance and credit policy, economics of production, cooperatives and collectives, education, research and extension, and rural sociology.

Online Equivalent: CAB Abstracts.

Arrangement: Numbered abstracts are arranged by subject in a continuous sequence from issue to issue.

Indexes: Author and subject indexes in each issue are cumulated annually.

CAB Thesaurus: The *CAB Thesaurus* has been the authorized list of index terms since January 1984.

Comments: The subject index provides indexing by country. *WAERSA* is a good choice for such topics as food supply, foreign agricultural investments, hunger and famine, and literature on the production of specific commodities.

ONLINE DATABASES

902. CAB Abstracts
This is the online equivalent for all of the CAB abstracting services including *World Agricultural and Rural Sociology Abstracts*. It is described in chapter 10.

903. PsycINFO
This is the online version of *Psychological Abstracts* from 1967 to the present. It now includes over 520,000 individual records from 1,300 periodicals, books, conference papers, technical reports, and other sources such as dissertations. Not all dissertations included in the online version are included in the printed product. It can be accessed using the vocabulary found in the *Thesaurus of Psychological Terms* as well as title keywords, authors, journal titles, etc.

904. Social SciSearch
This database is the online equivalent of the *Social Sciences Citation Index* from 1972 to the present. It now consists of over 1.5 million records and includes material from about 1,500 major social science journals as well as selected items from 3,000 scientific and technical periodicals. In addition to title words, article author, journal title, and corporate source, it is also possible to search by cited references.

905. Sociological Abstracts
The online version of the monthly abstracting service by the same name, this database provides detailed coverage of the world's sociological literature from 1963 to the present. It now includes over 160,000 records from over 1,200 journals, conferences, and other publications. The file is searchable by subject, title and abstract words, author, journal title, etc.

BIBLIOGRAPHIES AND GUIDES

906. Ball, Nicole. **World Hunger: A Guide to the Economic and Political Dimensions**. Santa Barbara, Calif.: ABC-Clio, 1981. 386p. ISBN 087436308X.
An excellent guide to over 3,000 books and articles on all facets of the world food problem, including economic and rural development, the Green Revolution, land tenure, and agrarian reform, this volume includes citations to numerous country-specific studies arranged geographically. Individual sections are supplemented by critical introductions. Also included are sources of further information and author and subject indexes.

907. Burgess, Ann. **Evaluation of Nutrition Interventions: An Annotated Bibliography and Review of Methodologies and Results**. 2nd ed. Rome: Food and Agriculture Organization of the United Nations, 1982. 194p. (FAO Food and Nutrition Paper, No. 24). ISBN 9251012288.
More than 110 items on evaluation methodology and 300 reports describing the outcome of nutrition interventions are included.

908.   Friedman, Robert L. **Human Food Uses: A Cross-Cultural Comprehensive Annotated Bibliography.** Westport, Conn.: Greenwood Press, 1981. 552p. ISBN 0313229015.

"This bibliography has been developed for scholars and scientists requiring data on the various aspects of food in human culture." Over 9,000 numbered, annotated references are arranged alphabetically by major author. The index provides access by place, subject, name of culture or country, as well as genera and species where relevant. A "List of Serial Title Abbreviations" is included. This excellent bibliography provides access to a large and international body of literature on cultural uses of food, covering difficult-to-trace materials from widely scattered sources, and as such is a real bibliographic achievement for the field.

909.   Friedman, Robert L. **Human Food Uses: A Cross-Cultural, Comprehensive Annotated Bibliography. Supplement.** Westport, Conn.: Greenwood Press, 1983. 387p. ISBN 0313234345.

This supplement lists over 4,000 items which could not be accommodated in the main volume because of insufficient space and time. The format and arrangement are the same as in the original volume.

"The entries in both books, taken together, present much of the known literature on the general subject of nutritional anthropology" (*Food Technology* 37 [December 1983]: 113-14).

910.   Goldsmith, Robert H. **World and National Food and Nutrition Problems: A Selected Bibliography.** Monticello, Ill.: Vance Bibliographies, 1983. 151p. (Public Administration Series — Bibliography). ISBN 0880667664.

This bibliography of approximately 1,800 citations covers journals and books on the world food problem, various social and cultural factors related to nutritional status, nutritional problems in the United States and in the developing world, and food programs and legislation.

911.   Hartog, A. P. den. **Tropical Africa.** Rome: Food and Agriculture Organization of the United Nations, 1974. 88p. (FAO Library Occasional Bibliographies, No. 10).

"A selected bibliography on food habits (socio-economic aspects of food and nutrition)."

912.   Institute for Food and Development Policy. **Food First Resource Guide: Documentation of the Roots of World Hunger and Rural Poverty.** San Francisco, Calif.: Institute for Food and Development Policy, 1979. 79p.

This introduction to world hunger for the uninitiated contains extensive references to source materials.

913.   Leung, Woot-tsuen Wu, Ritva R. Butrum, and Flora Huang Chang. **A Selected Bibliography on East-Asian Foods and Nutrition Arranged According to Subject Matter and Area.** Bethesda, Md.: National Institutes of Health, 1973. 296p. (DHEW Publication No. (NIH) 73-466). HE20.3316Ea7a.

This useful bibliography of older literature was collected during the preparation of *Food Composition Table for Use in East Asia.* Geographic areas covered are East Asia generally, Burma, Cambodia, Mainland China, Republic of China, Hong Kong, Indonesia, Japan, Korea, Laos, Malaysia, Philippines, Singapore,

Thailand, and Vietnam. Within each geographic area material is organized by topics: food composition, food technology, food habits, nutrition and dietary surveys, food resources, etc.

914. MacDonald, Donna. **Resources on Food, Nutrition and Culture**. Toronto: Nutrition Information Service, Ryerson Polytechnical Institute Library, 1983. 21p. ISBN 0919351115.

MacDonald's bibliography of background materials on theories of the relationship of food, nutrition and culture, as well as the social history of food and culture and ethnic cuisine also lists basic nutrition materials for the lay public and sources of translated teaching aids. The volume was prepared to accompany *Eating Right*, a slide/tape presentation aimed at immigrant women in Canada.

915. Newman, Jacqueline M. **Melting Pot: An Annotated Bibliography and Guide to Food and Nutrition Information for Ethnic Groups in America**. New York: Garland, 1986. 194p. (Garland Reference Library of Social Science, No. 351). ISBN 082404326X.

"In chapters devoted to each ethnic group, an overview of food preferences, eating styles, and nutrition needs are given in an introductory essay. This is followed by an annotated list of the most recent and vital books, scholarly journals, and resources for recipes. Over 700 entries are listed.... A final section includes general information on all ethnic groups, cites multiethnic works and recipe sources." This is an excellent source of reference for material on cultural food patterns.

916. Rechcigl, Miloslav. **World Food Problem: A Selective Bibliography of Reviews**. Cleveland, Ohio: CRC Press, Inc., 1975. 211p. ISBN 087819066X.

Unfortunately now somewhat dated, this bibliography of approximately 5,000 literature reviews may nonetheless prove useful for access to some of the ·older literature on the subject.

917. Schofield, Sue. **Village Nutrition Studies: An Annotated Bibliography**. Brighton, England: Village Nutrition Programme, Institute of Development Studies, University of Sussex. 1975. 285 columns. ISBN 0903354152.

Schofield's bibliography of nutrition studies relating to villages in developing countries, arranged geographically, includes detailed annotations describing research methods and results with comments. A substantial amount of older literature is included. There is no index.

918. United States. Agency for International Development. Office of Nutrition. **Food Consumption and Nutrition Effects of International Development Projects and Programs: An Annotated Bibliography**. Washington, D.C.: Office of Nutrition, Bureau of Science and Technology, U.S. Agency for International Development, 1983. 100p.

"Intended for a multi-disciplinary audience, this bibliography provides 196 citations dealing with technical agriculture, economics, nutrition, anthropology, project management, etc. The material is divided into three categories: (1) malnutrition: causes and solutions; (2) the impacts of agriculture and rural development programs on nutrition; and (3) guidelines and techniques for measuring these impacts" (*LIFE* (*League for International Food Education*) 17 [February/March 1984]: 6).

919. Wilson, Christine S. "Foods—Custom and Nurture: An Annotated Bibliography on Sociocultural and Biocultural Aspects of Nutrition." **Journal of Nutrition Education. Supplement 1** 11(4) (October/December 1979): 211-64.

This annotated bibliography of over 600 books and articles on nutritional anthropology and related literature covers food symbolism, paleodietetics, cannibalism, drugs and stimulants, taboos, traditional diet, foods for infants, children and pregnant women, and indigenous foods. The references are chiefly in English. There is an author index, but no subject index.

DIRECTORIES

920. Kutzner, Patricia L., and Nickola Lagoudakis, eds. **Who's Involved with Hunger: An Organization Guide for Education and Advocacy.** 4th ed. Washington, D.C.: World Hunger Education Service, 1985. 46p.

"A guide to 400 organizations in the U.S. which do research, education, community organizing, or political advocacy on hunger, poverty, and development issues both in the U.S. and Third World. Each organizational listing includes: address, telephone number, director or contact person, program description, and publications information."

921. Miller, Duncan, and Morag Soranna. **Directory of Food Policy Institutes.** Guildford Surrey, England: Published for the Development Centre of the Organization for Economic Co-operation and Development, Paris, by Butterworths Scientific, Ltd., 1981. 100p. ISBN 0861030559.

"The Directory has two major purposes: to provide readers/users with basic information about food policy institutes in all regions of the world; and, to undertake at least some preliminary analysis of the comparative characteristics and priorities of these institutes." The text is in English and French.

922. Trzyna, Thaddeus C., et al. **World Food Crisis: An International Directory of Organizations and Information Resources.** Claremont, Calif.: Public Affairs Clearinghouse, 1977. 140p. (Who's Doing What Series, No. 4). ISBN 0912102217.

World Food Crisis is a guide to governmental agencies and national and international organizations involved in some way with the world food problem.

HANDBOOKS, MANUALS, AND OTHER DATA COMPILATIONS

923. American Dietetic Association. **Cultural Food Patterns in the U.S.A.** Chicago: American Dietetic Association, 1976. 15p.

Brief information is provided on the basic food groups as they apply to various ethnic diets, with suggestions for optimizing nutrition and economy while meeting nutritional needs. There are sections relating to Chinese, Italian, Japanese, Jewish, Polish, Puerto Rican, Spanish or Mexican American, and Southern foods.

924.   Bringas, Juliet G., and Teresa Y. Chan. **Spanish Aid in Clinical Dietetics**. Culver City, Calif.: Nutrition in the Life Cycle, Inc., 1979. 135p. ($9.00, Nutrition in the Life Cycle, Inc., P.O. Box 546, Culver City, CA 90230. Also available from EDRS on microfiche only, ED 215 825).

Written in English with some parallel text in Spanish, this book is intended to help dietitians, nutritionists, and other health professionals better serve their Hispanic clienteles. It describes the eating patterns of Mexican, Cuban, and Puerto Rican Americans, with special attention to Mexican Americans. Included are examples of dietary questionnaires, vocabulary for patient interviews, Spanish-language equivalents of frequently used terms, basic food groups in English and in Spanish, and dietary suggestions for specific problems, as well as common modified diets such as low-cholesterol, sodium restricted, and diabetic. Also included is information on the nutritive value of foods found in Hispanic markets.

925.   Crabbe, David, Simon Lawson, and Sandra Young. **The World Food Book: An A-Z, Atlas, and Statistical Source Book**. London: Kogan Page; distr., New York: Nichols Publishing Co., 1981. 240p. ISBN 0893970956.

This encyclopedia includes brief entries relating to food and the world food supply. Appended are numerous maps showing land use, arable land, production of various vegetable and animal foods, and statistical tables showing production and yield of various types of crop and animal foods.

926.   Dairy Council of California. **Asian Food Guide for Teachers**. Los Angeles, Calif.: Dairy Council of California, 1981?. 12p.

This brief but useful guide covers basic vocabulary and food practices for Korea, China, Japan, and Indochina (Vietnam, Cambodia, Laos, and Thailand).

927.   Ghosh, Pradip K., ed. **Health, Food and Nutrition in Third World Development**. Westport, Conn.: Greenwood Press, 1984. 617p. (International Development Resource Books, Vol. 6). ISBN 0313241422.

Ghosh's book provides information on current trends in the development of health, food, and nutrition policy relating to Third World countries; it also serves as a guide to information sources on this topic. Part I includes 18 chapters dealing with population growth and food supply, food and nutrition policy, and health care planning, with extensive bibliographies. Part II provides a bibliography of statistical reference sources and statistical tables, with data on global indicators of health and nutrition, calories per day, comparative economic data, health expenditures, etc. Part III is an annotated bibliography of relevant books and articles with a special subject index. Part IV lists relevant UN information sources, databases, libraries, a directory of periodicals, relevant research institutions, etc. There are an appendix and an author index.

928.   Mothershead, Alice Bonzi. **Dining Customs around the World, with Occasional Recipes**. Garret Park, Md.: Garrett Park Press, 1982. 150p.

Brief information is provided on dining and food customs in 53 countries, with roughly two to four pages of text per country. The volume includes background information on meal patterns, popular foods, and occasional recipes for typical dishes. An index to foods and beverages is included.

929. United States. Food and Nutrition Service. **Southeast Asian American Food Habits.** Washington, D.C.: U.S. Department of Agriculture, Food and Nutrition Service, 1980. 10p. (FNS 225). A98.9:225.

Discussed are diets, staple foods, and meal patterns of Southeast Asian Americans. There is a bibliography.

STATISTICS

930. Food and Agriculture Organization of the United Nations. **FAO Production Yearbook.** Vol. 30- . Rome: Food and Agriculture Organization of the United Nations, 1976- . annual. ISSN 0071-7118.

The yearbook contains country production statistics for individual agricultural commodities and per capita production of nutrients (calories, protein, fat, calcium, iron, retinol, beta carotene, thiamin, riboflavin, niacin, and ascorbic acid). There are extensive explanatory notes on the tables.

931. Food and Agriculture Organization of the United Nations. **Food Balance Sheets: 1979-81 Average.** Rome: Food and Agriculture Organization of the United Nations, 1984. 272p. ISBN 925102149X.

Data on supply and utilization of roughly 300 primary food and agricultural commodities for 146 countries and territories are included. "A food balance sheet represents a comprehensive picture of the pattern of a country's food supply during a specified reference period. The food balance sheet shows for each food item—i.e., for each primary commodity and a number of processed commodities potentially available for human consumption, the sources of supply and its utilization."

932. Food and Agriculture Organization of the United Nations. **The Fourth World Food Survey.** Rome: Food and Agriculture Organization of the United Nations, 1977. 128p. (FAO Statistics Series, No. 11; FAO Food and Nutrition Series, No. 10). ISBN 9251004293.

The three previous *World Food Surveys* were published in 1946, 1952, and 1963. This survey presents data on the growth of food and agricultural production, the food supply in relation to the population, and the prevalence of poverty and malnutrition, by countries. There are extensive tables throughout the volume as well as a lengthy appendix with tables. There is no index.

933. Food and Agriculture Organization of the United Nations. **The State of Food and Agriculture: World Review.** Rome: Food and Agriculture Organization of the United Nations, 19?- . annual. ISSN 0081-4539.

This survey of the current world agricultural outlook, long-term trends and issues, such as urbanization and its effect on food systems contains numerous tables.

934. Food and Agriculture Organization of the United Nations. **World Food Report.** Rome: Food and Agriculture Organization of the United Nations, 1983- . annual.

This is a concise survey of agricultural production, food supply, and malnutrition along with reports of FAO activities for the year and a reference section with data in the form of graphics and tables. There are extensive illustrations in color, particularly in the data section. "Intended for use by the media, non-governmental organizations and all individuals responsible for mobilizing support for agricultural and rural development. It is not a technical document; readers requiring technical data should refer to publications such as the State of Food and Agriculture and various statistical periodicals of the FAO."

935.   United States. Department of Agriculture. **Agricultural Statistics**. Washington, D.C.: Government Printing Office, 1936- . annual. ISSN 0082-9714. A1.47.

"Published each year to meet the diverse need for a reliable reference book on agricultural production, supplies, consumption, facilities, costs and returns."

Arranged by commodity groups (e.g., grains, oilseeds, fats and oils, vegetables and melons), this statistical compilation contains detailed production statistics for individual commodities in the United States, import statistics where relevant, value of products, and consumption figures of selected commodities. Included is a detailed index.

936.   United States. Department of Agriculture. Economic Research Service. **World Food Aid Needs and Availabilities**. Washington, D.C.: Government Printing Office, 1981?- . annual.

"Report prepared by an Interagency Food Analysis Working Group established to provide the U.S. Government with assessments of food needs in the developing world."

Appendix A
Purchasing Information
for Books

Books in Print. New York: R. R. Bowker, 1948- . annual. ISSN 0068-0214.

This guide to "available books, new and old, indexed by author and by title with full ordering information" covers "hardbounds, paperbacks, trade books, textbooks, adult books, juveniles." Over 700,000 books are listed in separate author and title sections. A publishers' directory identifies publishers' and distributors' abbreviations and provides addresses and telephone numbers. Though excellent for book trade publications in the United States, this source does not include many publications of societies or organizations.

British Books in Print. London: J. Whitaker; distr., New York: R. R. Bowker, 1965- . annual. ISSN 0068-1350.

Over 400,000 currently available British books are listed in one alphabetical sequence by author, title, and subject. A list of publishers with addresses is included.

Cumulative Book Index. A World List of Books in the English Language. New York: H. W. Wilson, 1898- . ISSN 0011-300X.

The *Cumulative Book Index* serves as a permanent record of books published in the English language. It is published monthly except in August and is cumulated quarterly and annually. It lists books by author, subject, and title and includes a directory of publishers.

Forthcoming Books. Vol. 1- . New York: R. R. Bowker, 1966- . bimonthly. ISSN 0015-8119.

This title lists books which have been published since the latest edition of *Books in Print* and those to be published in the following five months, by author and title. It also lists titles which have been indefinitely postponed. "Each bi-monthly issue updates and expands the previous ones and includes all categories, adult trade books, technical and scientific books, juveniles, and college texts, paperbacks, imports, and revised editions and reprints."

International Books in Print. Munich: G. K. Saur; distr., Detroit: Gale Research, 1979- . annual. ISSN 0170-3948.

Over 150,000 books are listed in this guide to English-language books published outside the United States and the United Kingdom. Books are entered under author, title, and subject. A list of publishers' addresses is included.

Paperbound Books in Print. New York: R. R. Bowker, 1978- . semi-annual. ISSN 0031-1235.

Paperbound books currently available in the United States and Canada are listed by author, title, and subject. A key to publishers' and distributors' abbreviations is included. Subject listings are done according to the subject headings of the American Booksellers Association and the National Association of College Bookstores. All books listed in *Paperbound Books in Print* are also found in *Books in Print*.

Subject Guide to Books in Print. New York: R. R. Bowker, 1957- . annual. ISSN 0000-0159.

A companion to *Books in Print*, the *Subject Guide to Books in Print* lists currently available books by subject. The indexing vocabulary is the *Library of Congress Subject Headings* (*LCSH*).

Subject Guide to Forthcoming Books. Vol. 1- . New York: R. R. Bowker, 1967- . bimonthly. ISSN 0000-0264.

This is a subject index to those books listed in *Forthcoming Books* which are scheduled to appear in the next five months. "Each bi-monthly issue overlaps, updates, and expands by two months the previous issue."

Appendix B
Subscription and Other
Information on Periodicals

Bowker International Serials Database Update. New York: R. R. Bowker, 1985- . quarterly. ISSN 0000-0892.

A supplement to *Ulrich's International Periodicals Directory* and *Irregular Serials and Annuals*, this directory updates both of these titles. Periodicals are listed in a classified arrangement with a title index and a separate list of cessations.

Broome, Charlotte, and Donna MacDonald. **Food and Nutrition: Newsletters, News Releases, and Journals: A Selected List**. Toronto: Nutrition Information Service, Ryerson Polytechnical Institute Library, 1981. 41p. ISBN 0919351042.

This bibliography lists 126 food and nutrition periodicals issued by industry, government agencies, community and consumer groups, private publishers, and professional organizations. Entries include bibliographic and purchasing information, information on indexing, and description of content. The emphasis is on Canadian materials. A title index is included.

Irregular Serials and Annuals: An International Directory. New York: R. R. Bowker, 1967- . biennial. ISSN 0000-0043.

A companion to *Ulrich's International Periodicals Directory*, this guide lists over 35,000 serials, annuals, continuations, and conference proceedings currently available. Entries are grouped according to 466 subject headings and include bibliographic and purchasing information, circulation figures, and information on indexing.

Oxbridge Directory of Newsletters. New York: Oxbridge Communications, 1979- . ISSN 0163-7010.

Former title: *Standard Directory of Newsletters.*
Over 14,000 American and Canadian newsletters are classified by subject. A title index is included.

Serials Directory: An International Reference Book. Birmingham, Ala.: EBSCO, 1986- . annual. ISSN 0866-4179.
An extensive directory of bibliographic, ordering, and other information on more than 113,000 domestic and foreign periodicals, this annual lists both regularly and irregularly published titles. The basic arrangement is by subject, with indexes by title and ISSN. The directory also includes a ceased title index. In addition to bibliographic and ordering information, the entries include telephone numbers, indexing information, circulation figures, and information on whether or not advertising is accepted and book reviews are published. A special feature is a succinct description of the content of many of the titles.

Standard Periodicals Directory. New York: Oxbridge Communications, 1964/65- . biennial. ISSN 0085-6630.
This directory provides information on over 65,000 periodicals published in the United States and Canada. It classifies periodicals by 280 subject categories and includes a title index. It has traditionally been strong in industry-based trade periodicals. Entries include information for purchasing, circulation figures, information on whether advertising or book reviews are included, telephone numbers, etc.

Ulrich's International Periodicals Directory. New York: R. R. Bowker, 1965- annual. ISSN 0000-0175.
This directory of over 68,000 currently published domestic and foreign periodicals is arranged by 534 subject categories and includes a title index. Other features are a list of ceased titles, periodicals available online, and an index to the names of international organizations. Indexing and abstracting publications are listed with other periodicals. In addition to bibliographic and purchasing information, entries include information on where titles are indexed, if advertising is accepted, and if book reviews are published.

WATCH OUT FOR THESE SOUND-ALIKES!

"Food and Nutrition" is a popular title for periodicals.

Food and Nutrition. Vol. 1- . Washington, D.C.: Food and Nutrition Service, U.S. Department of Agriculture, 1971- . quarterly. ISSN 0098-4604. (Volume 15 is 1985.)

Food and Nutrition. Vol. 1- . Rome: Food and Agriculture Organization of the United Nations, 1975- . biannual. ISSN 0304-8942. (Volume 11 is 1985.)

Food and Nutrition Bulletin. Vol. 1- . Tokyo: United Nations University, 1978- . quarterly. ISSN 0379-5721. (Volume 7 is 1985.)

Journal of Food & Nutrition. Vol. 38- . Canberra, Australia: Commonwealth Department of Health, 1981- . quarterly. ISSN 0728-4713. (Volume 41 is 1985. Previous title: *Food and Nutrition Notes and Reviews.*)

Author/Title Index

Reference is to pages and entry numbers. References to page numbers are preceded by "p." References to authors and titles within annotations are followed by "n." Page references are listed first and are separated from entry numbers by a semicolon.

Subject Index

Reference is to pages and entry numbers. References to page numbers are preceded by "p." and are separated from references to entry numbers by a semicolon.

343